Handbook of Clinical Nursing: MEDICAL– SURGICAL NURSING

Ronald L. Hickman, Jr., PhD, RN, ACNP-BC, FNAP, FAAN, is an associate professor and a board-certified acute care nurse practitioner at Frances Payne Bolton School of Nursing, Case Western Reserve University (CWRU) in Cleveland, Ohio. He earned a bachelor of arts in biology, a master of science (acute care nurse practitioner), and a doctorate in nursing from CWRU. He has received regional and national distinctions for his commitment and sustained contributions to nursing science and practice. Dr. Hickman is a nationally recognized nurse scientist and advanced practice nurse. In 2015, he was elected a fellow of the American Academy of Nursing and National Academies of Practice. With nearly two decades of clinical experience, he has provided evidence-based nursing care to patients and their families across tertiary care settings. He has authored more than 50 publications and numerous book chapters with a clinical focus, and serves as a contributing editor for the *American Journal of Critical Care*. As an associate editor of *A Guide to Mastery in Clinical Nursing*, Dr. Hickman's clinical expertise in the management of patients requiring life-sustaining care in emergency departments and intensive care units is highlighted in the book's content regarding emergency and critical care, medical–surgical, and nurse anesthesia care.

Celeste M. Alfes, DNP, MSN, RN, CNE, CHSE-A, is associate professor and director of the Center for Nursing Education, Simulation, and Innovation at the Frances Payne Bolton School of Nursing, Case Western Reserve University (CWRU) in Cleveland, Ohio. She earned a bachelor of science in nursing (University of Akron), master of science in nursing (University of Akron), and doctor of nursing practice at CWRU. With a background in critical care nursing, she has 20 years of experience teaching baccalaureate nursing students and has been instrumental in developing high-fidelity simulation programs nationally and internationally. She was instrumental in developing the Dorothy Ebersbach Academic Center for Flight Nursing, which features the nation's first high-fidelity Sikorsky S76® helicopter simulator adapted for interdisciplinary education and crew resource management. She received the National League for Nursing's Simulation Leader in Nursing Education award (2012) and the Joyce Griffin-Sobel Research award (2014). Her research incorporates interprofessional simulations to strengthen clinical reasoning and performance outcomes. Dr. Alfes currently serves as a reviewer for the National Science Foundation, is a coinvestigator on funded research projects with the Laerdal Foundation of Norway and the U.S. Air Force Research Laboratory, is on the editorial board of *Applied Nursing Research*, and is a reviewer for the journals *Nursing Education Perspectives* and *Clinical Simulation in Nursing*.

Joyce J. Fitzpatrick, PhD, MBA, RN, FAAN, FNAP, is Elizabeth Brooks Ford Professor of Nursing, Frances Payne Bolton School of Nursing, Case Western Reserve University (CWRU) in Cleveland, Ohio, where she was the dean from 1982 through 1997. She is also an adjunct professor, Department of Geriatrics, Ichan School of Medicine, Mount Sinai Hospital, New York, New York. She earned a bachelor of science in nursing (Georgetown University), an MS in psychiatric–mental health nursing (The Ohio State University), a PhD in nursing (New York University), and an MBA at CWRU. She was elected a fellow of the American Academy of Nursing (AAN; 1981) and a fellow in the National Academies of Practice (1996). She received the *American Journal of Nursing* Book of the Year award 20 times. Dr. Fitzpatrick received the American Nurses Foundation Distinguished Contribution to Nursing Science award for sustained commitment and contributions to the development of the discipline (2002). She was a Fulbright Scholar at University College Cork, Cork, Ireland (2007–2008), and was inducted into the Sigma Theta Tau International Research Hall of Fame (2014). In 2016, she was named a Living Legend of the AAN. Dr. Fitzpatrick's work is widely disseminated in nursing and health care literature; she has authored or edited more than 300 publications, including more than 80 books. She even served as a coeditor of the *Annual Review of Nursing Research* series, volumes 1 to 26, and she currently edits the journals *Applied Nursing Research, Archives of Psychiatric Nursing*, and *Nursing Education Perspectives*, the official journal of the National League for Nursing.

Handbook of Clinical Nursing: MEDICAL–SURGICAL NURSING

Ronald L. Hickman, Jr., PhD, RN, ACNP-BC, FNAP, FAAN

Celeste M. Alfes, DNP, MSN, RN, CNE, CHSE-A

Joyce J. Fitzpatrick, PhD, MBA, RN, FAAN, FNAP

EDITORS

SPRINGER PUBLISHING COMPANY

Springer Publishing Company, LLC
11 West 42nd Street
New York, NY 10036
www.springerpub.com

Acquisitions Editor: Joseph Morita
Compositor: Newgen KnowledgeWorks

ISBN: 978-0-8261-3078-5
ebook ISBN: 978-0-8261-3469-1

18 19 20 21 22 / 5 4 3 2 1

Extracted from *A Guide to Mastery in Clinical Nursing: The Comprehensive Reference*

Library of Congress Cataloging-in-Publication Data
Names: Hickman, Ronald, editor. | Alfes, Celeste M., editor. | Fitzpatrick, Joyce J., 1944- editor.
Title: Handbook of clinical nursing. Medical-surgical nursing / Ronald L. Hickman, Jr., Celeste M. Alfes, Joyce J. Fitzpatrick, editors.
Other titles: Medical-surgical nursing | Contained in (work): Guide to mastery in clinical nursing.
Description: New York, NY : Springer Publishing Company, LLC, [2018] |
    Contained in: A guide to mastery in clinical nursing : the comprehensive
    reference / Joyce J. Fitzpatrick, Celeste M. Alfes, Ronald Hickman,
    editors. 2018. | Includes bibliographical references.
Identifiers: LCCN 2017059922| ISBN 9780826130785 (pbk.) | ISBN 9780826134691 (ebook)
Subjects: | MESH: Medical-Surgical Nursing
Classification: LCC RT41 | NLM WY 150 | DDC 610.73—dc23
LC record available at https://lccn.loc.gov/2017059922

Contact us to receive discount rates on bulk purchases.
We can also customize our books to meet your needs.
For more information please contact: sales@springerpub.com

Printed in the United States of America.

Contents

Contributors

Consuela A. Albright, MSN, RN, FNP-BC, PPCNP-BC
Staff Nurse
Cleveland Clinic Children's Hospital for Rehabilitation
Cleveland, Ohio

Celeste M. Alfes, DNP, MSN, RN, CNE, CHSE-A
Associate Professor
Director, Center for Nursing Education, Simulation, and Innovation
Frances Payne Bolton School of Nursing
Case Western Reserve University
Cleveland, Ohio

Sarine Beukian, MSN, RN, AGACNP-BC
Cardiology Nurse Practitioner
Division of Cardiology
Department of Medicine
Bassett Medical Center, Affiliate of College of Physicians and Surgeons,
Columbia University
New York, New York

Susan V. Brindisi, MS Ed, MA, MSN, RN, CHES, CRRN
Clinical Nurse Leader
Mount Sinai Health System
New York, New York

Christina M. Canfield, MSN, RN, APRN, ACNS-BC, CCRN-E
eHospital Program Manager
Cleveland Clinic
Cleveland, Ohio

Deborah H. Cantero, DNP, RN, ARNP, FNP-C
Assistant Professor
FNP Program Coordinator
School of Nursing and Health Sciences
Florida Southern College
Lakeland, Florida

Peter J. Cebull, MSN, RN, CNP
Nurse Practitioner
Frances Payne Bolton School of Nursing
Case Western Reserve University
Cleveland, Ohio

Steven R. Collier, MS, RN, CNP
Nurse Practitioner
Department of Neurosurgery
Center for Spine Health
Cleveland Clinic
Cleveland, Ohio

Kate Cook, MSN, RN
DNP Student
Frances Payne Bolton School of Nursing
Case Western Reserve University
Cleveland, Ohio
Assistant Professor
Chamberlain University
Downers Grove, Illinois

Dianna Jo Copley, MSN, RN, APRN, ACCNS-AG, CCRN
Clinical Nurse Specialist
Cleveland Clinic
Cleveland, Ohio

Marisa A. Cortese, PhD, RN, FNP-BC
Research Nurse Practitioner
White Plains Hospital—Center for Cancer Care
White Plains, New York

Edwidge Cuvilly, MS, RN, ANP-BC, GNP, OCN
Nurse Practitioner
Bone Marrow Transplant
Weill Cornell Medicine
Division of Hematology & Medical Oncology
New York, New York

Catherine O'Neill D'Amico, PhD, RN, NEA-BC
Director
Programs and Operations
NICHE—Nurses Improving Care to Health System Elders
Rory Meyers College of Nursing
New York University
New York, New York

Danielle M. Diemer, MSN, RN, FNP-C
Nurse Practitioner
Department of Endocrinology
Cleveland Clinic
Cleveland, Ohio

Erin H. Discenza, MSN, RN
Instructor
Frances Payne Bolton School of Nursing
Case Western Reserve University
Cleveland, Ohio

Courtney G. Donahue, MS, RN, FNP-BC, PCCN
Family Nurse Practitioner, Stroke NP
Department of Neurosciences
New York–Presbyterian Brooklyn Methodist Hospital
Brooklyn, New York

Merlyn A. Dorsainvil, DHSc, MS, MPH, RN
Assistant Professor
Department of Nursing
College of Technology of the City University of New York
Brooklyn, New York

Mary Jo Elmo, MSN, RN, CNP
Nurse Practitioner
Department of Surgery
University Hospitals Cleveland Medical Center
Cleveland, Ohio

Lisa D. Ericson, MSN, RN, FNP-BC
Assistant Professor
School of Nursing
Bethel College
Mishawaka, Indiana

Charrita Ernewein, DNP, RN, ARNP, FNP-C
Adjunct Professor
College of Nursing
South University
Valrico, Florida

Yolanda Flenoury, MSN, RN, APRN-BC, CDE
Clinical Nurse Specialist
University Hospitals Cleveland Medical Center
Cleveland, Ohio

Crina V. Floruta, MSN, RN, ANP-BC, CWOCN
Nurse Practitioner—Colorectal Surgery
Cleveland Clinic
Cleveland, Ohio

Helen Foley, MSN, RN, AOCNS, ACHPN
Clinical Nurse Specialist Hematology/Oncology
Seidman Cancer Center
University Hospitals Cleveland Medical Center
Cleveland, Ohio

Ashley L. Foreman, DNP, RN, FNP-C
Family Nurse Practitioner
Chesapeake, Virginia

Carrie Foster, MSN, RN, PNP
Surgical Hospitalist
Seattle Children's Hospital
Seattle, Washington

Kari Gali, DNP, MSN, RN
CNP, Director of Quality and Population Health Design in Distance Health
Clinical Transformation
Cleveland Clinic
Cleveland, Ohio

Deborah R. Gillum, PhD, RN, CNE
Dean of Nursing
Bethel College
Mishawaka, Indiana

Maricar P. Gomez, MSN, RN, FNP-BC, PCCN
Nurse Practitioner
Cleveland Clinic
Cleveland, Ohio
DNP Student
Frances Payne Bolton School of Nursing
Case Western Reserve University
Cleveland, Ohio

Jennifer Gonzalez, MSN, RN, APRN, AGCNS-BC
Clinical Nurse Specialist
University Hospitals Cleveland Medical Center
Cleveland, Ohio

Mary T. Quinn Griffin, PhD, RN, FAAN, ANEF
Professor
Frances Payne Bolton School of Nursing
Case Western Reserve University
Cleveland, Ohio

Rebecca Witten Grizzle, PhD, MSN, RN, NP-C
Clinical Assistant Professor
College of Nursing
Sacred Heart University
Fairfield, Connecticut

Mary de Haan, MSN, RN, ACNS-BC
Instructor
Frances Payne Bolton School of Nursing
Case Western Reserve University
Cleveland, Ohio

Andrea Marie Herr, MS, RN, ANP-BC
New York–Presbyterian Weill Cornell Medical Center
New York, New York

Una Hopkins, DNP, RN, FNP-BC
Administrative Director
Center for Cancer Cure
White Plains Hospital
White Plains, New York

Bette K. Idemoto, PhD, RN, ACNS-BC, CCRN
Clinical Nurse Specialist
University Hospitals Cleveland Medical Center
Cleveland, Ohio

Elsie A. Jolade, DNP, EdM, RN, FNP-BC, ACNS, APRN, CCRN
Clinical Professor
Hunter College
School of Nursing
City University of New York
New York, New York

Colleen Kurzawa, MSN, MFA, RN
PhD Student
Frances Payne Bolton School of Nursing
Case Western Reserve University
Cleveland, Ohio

Leslie J. Lockett, MS, RNC, CNE, CMSRN
Director of RN-BSN Program
Instructor
College of Nursing
University of South Florida
Tampa, Florida

Rebecca M. Lutz, DNP, RN, APRN, FNP-BC, PPCNP-BC
Assistant Professor
College of Nursing
University of South Florida
Tampa, Florida

Kelly Ann Lynn, MS, MA, RN
Manager
Center for Advanced Digestive Care
New York–Presbyterian Hospital
New York, New York

Alaa Mahsoon, MSN, RN
PhD Student
Frances Payne Bolton School of Nursing
Case Western Reserve University
Cleveland, Ohio

Jane F. Marek, DNP, MSN, RN
Assistant Professor
Frances Payne Bolton School of Nursing
Case Western Reserve University
Cleveland, Ohio

Kathleen Marsala-Cervasio, PhD, EdD, RN, ACNS-BC, CCRN
Associate Professor
Harriet Rothkopf Heilbrunn School of Nursing
Long Island University
Brooklyn Campus
Brookville, New York

Visnja Maria Masina, MSN, RN, APRN, AGCNS-BC
Clinical Nurse Specialist
Cleveland Clinic
Cleveland, Ohio

Kerry Mastrangelo, DNP, RN, APRN, NP-C
Assistant Professor of Nursing
The Barbara H. Hagan School of Nursing
Molloy College
Rockville Center, New York

Kelly K. McConnell, DNP, MSN, RN, AG-ACNP-BC
Assistant Professor
Frances Payne Bolton School of Nursing
Case Western Reserve University
Cleveland, Ohio

Maria A. Mendoza, EdD, RN, ANP, GNP-BC, CDE, CNE
Assistant Clinical Professor
Director
Nursing Education Master's and Advanced Certificate
Programs
Rory Meyers College of Nursing
New York University
New York, New York

Jennifer E. Millman, BSN, RN
Clinical Practice Nurse
Advanced Endoscopy
Division of Gastroenterology
Weill Cornell Medical Center
New York, New York

Mary Beth Modic, DNP, RN, APRN-CNS, CDE
Diabetes Clinical Nurse Specialist
Department of Advanced Practice Nursing
Cleveland Clinic
Cleveland, Ohio

Scott Emory Moore, PhD, RN, APRN, AGPCNP-BC
Postdoctoral Fellow
Frances Payne Bolton School of Nursing
Case Western Reserve University
Cleveland, Ohio

Joseph D. Perazzo, PhD, RN
Assistant Professor
College of Nursing
University of Cincinnati
Cincinnati, Ohio

Gayle M. Petty, DNP, MSN, RN
Assistant Professor
Frances Payne Bolton School of Nursing
Case Western Reserve University
Cleveland, Ohio

Rhoda Redulla, DNP, RN-BC
Magnet® Program Director
Office of Nursing Excellence
New York–Presbyterian Hospital Weill Cornell
Medical Center
New York, New York

Shannon A. Rives, MSN, RN, ACNS-BC, CCRN, CMSRN
Clinical Nurse Specialist
Cleveland Clinic
Cleveland, Ohio

Jacqueline Robinson, MSN, MBA, RN, ACNS-BC, CCRN
Simulation Manager
Frances Payne Bolton School of Nursing
Case Western Reserve University
Cleveland, Ohio

Ronald Rock, MSN, RN, APRN, CNS
Nurse Manager/Clinical Nurse Specialist
Wound Ostomy Continence Nursing Department
Cleveland Clinic
Cleveland, Ohio

Maria G. Smisek, MSN, RN-BC
Doctoral Student
Frances Payne Bolton School of Nursing
Case Western Reserve University
Cleveland, Ohio

Marian Soat, MSN, RN, APRN, CCNS, CCRN
Clinical Nurse Specialist
Department of Advance Practice Nursing
Cleveland Clinic
Cleveland, Ohio

Karen L. Terry, DNP, MSN, RN, NP-C, GNP-BC
Nurse Practitioner
Mercy Health Physicians Lorain Geriatrics
Amherst, Ohio

Arlene Travis, MSN, RN, ANP-BC
Nurse Clinician
Mount Sinai Hospital
New York, New York
Adjunct Assistant Professor
Pace University Lienhard School of Nursing
New York, New York

Mary Variath, MSN, RN
Instructor
Frances Payne Bolton School of Nursing
Case Western Reserve University
Cleveland, Ohio

Sharon Stahl Wexler, PhD, RN, FNGNA
Associate Professor
Pace University
Lienhard School of Nursing
New York, New York

Heidi Youngbauer, MSN, RN
Adjunct Professor
Department of Nursing
Sacred Heart University
Onalaska, Wisconsin

Preface

In the United States and worldwide, medical–surgical nursing is the most common nursing specialty practiced by registered nurses. Medical–surgical nursing consists of the delivery of evidence-based nursing care to adult patients who are hospitalized owing to an acute condition, exacerbation of a chronic illness, or a surgical procedure. Medical–surgical nursing is a specialty area of nursing that directs nursing practice toward the prevention of disease, attenuation of disease progression, and promotion of symptom palliation and health-related quality of life across the adult life span. The practice of medical–surgical nursing requires knowledge across disciplinary domains, such as the physiological, cognitive, psychosocial, environmental, and behavioral mechanisms that influence the health and susceptibility of disease among hospitalized patients. The care of the hospitalized patients and their family systems requires medical–surgical nurses to maintain an up-to-date knowledge base that guides the formulation of a nursing diagnosis and initiation of evidence-based nursing actions to optimize the health of hospitalized patients and family systems.

The knowledge base of medical–surgical nurses is wide ranging and reflects the diversity of care needs of patients and their family systems. For medical–surgical nurses, the health care environments in which they practice are dynamic, and the complexity of care needs of patients is steadily increasing. Adding to the complexity of providing medical–surgical nursing care, registered nurses are finding it more difficult to acquire and make use of an evolving knowledge base of evidence to guide their nursing practice. Although the challenges of a dynamic health care environment, increasing complexity of patients, and an expanding evidence base for nursing care are not unique challenges restricted to medical–surgical nurses, these challenges pose a significant threat to the quality of care delivered by novice and even expert medical–surgical nurses.

The *Handbook of Clinical Nursing: Medical–Surgical Nursing* was conceptualized to assist the novice or the expert medical–surgical nurse reviewing up-to-date content on a variety of clinical topics pertinent to the care of hospitalized patients and their family systems, and is included in *A Guide to Mastery in Clinical Nursing: The Comprehensive Reference*, a comprehensive reference for individuals across the life span. This handbook includes a compendium of clinical topics with a structured format to aid the comprehension and application of the content to nursing practice. The *Handbook of Clinical Nursing: Medical–Surgical Nursing* has selected clinical topics curated by Dr. Jane Marek and contributions from expert practitioners in specialty areas of medical–surgical nursing. The objective of the *Handbook of Clinical Nursing: Medical–Surgical Nursing* is to provide detailed information on the most important topics in clinical nursing practice for both new registered nurses and those transitioning to a new clinical area.

For each clinical topic, there is an overview of the clinical problem, relevant clinical background, clinical aspects for the nurse (assessment; nursing interventions, management, and clinical implications; and outcomes), and a summary. Key references are provided for each entry, including both classic references and current citations from clinical and research literature. Although there are a number of comprehensive textbooks, this handbook provides information that is both concise and practical for the students as they enter each clinical area, and for registered nurses searching for up-to-date content that will guide their nursing practice.

In summary, the *Handbook of Clinical Nursing: Medical–Surgical Nursing* has particular relevance to several groups of nurses. Nurse faculty will find this handbook useful as it provides concise synopses of clinical topics relevant to the care of a hospitalized patient. Clinicians transitioning to new clinical areas will have a ready resource for key clinical problems they may face in their new clinical area. And, importantly, newly licensed registered nurses will find that this guide to clinical mastery will chart their way in addressing the important clinical problems that their patients experience.

Ronald L. Hickman, Jr.
Celeste M. Alfes
Joyce J. Fitzpatrick

■ ADDISON'S DISEASE

Yolanda Flenoury

Overview

The adrenal glands are an important part of the endocrine system. They secrete vital hormones (glucocorticoids, mineralcorticoids, and androgens) that play a part in response to stress, blood pressure, sodium, potassium, and water balance (Michels & Michels, 2014). Addison's disease is an illness characterized by destruction of the adrenal glands. Adrenal gland destruction may occur because of an autoimmune process, infectious or fungal disease, medications, or malignancy. The goal in caring for these patients is the ability to recognize the disease, treat the symptoms, maintain their health status, and avoid a crisis state. Nurses play a vital role in providing education so that the patients can manage and treat their disease appropriately (Bornstein et al., 2016).

Background

In 1855, Thomas Addison published a book describing his patient case studies and subsequent autopsy findings. He described a disease in his patients that had an insidious onset and was characterized by patterns of progressive, distinctive skin discoloration, nausea, weakness, delirium, and weak pulse with the ultimate demise of the patient. On autopsy, he found that all of his patients had diseased adrenal glands (Addison, 1855).

Addison's disease can manifest as the result of autoimmune processes. This form of Addison's disease accounts for 70% to 90% of cases. The second most common cause of Addison's disease is caused by tuberculosis. A less common cause of Addison's disease includes pathological disorders that include fungal infections, malignancies, and medications (National Endocrine and Metabolic Disease Information Service, 2014). A good history, including geographic location and travel, is vital when making the diagnosis. Patients who live or have been in areas with a high prevalence of tuberculosis or other infectious diseases will have a higher proportion of Addison's disease caused by these conditions (Bornstein et al., 2016). In Western countries, the prevalence of Addison's disease had been estimated at 35 to 60 million people. In the first two decades of life, Addison's disease is diagnosed more often in males, more evenly divided in the third decade and then mostly female in the subsequent decades of life. The gender differential, however, shifts to female, if patients have polyglandular autoimmune syndrome, a condition in which more than one endocrine gland is destroyed (Nieman, 2016).

The adrenal glands have two layers, the cortex and the medulla. The adrenal cortex is responsible for the synthesis of cortisol, aldosterone, and androgens. Most notable in Addison's disease, the lack of cortisol leads to diminished hepatic and muscle glycogen stores, hepatic glucose output and hypoglycemia, muscle weakness, anemia, hyponatremia, and postural hypotension (Brandão Neto & Carvalho, 2014). Cortisol is a glucocorticoid hormone that is secreted in response to pituitary secretion of ACTH. Cortisol is also secreted in response to circadian rhythms, eating, activity, and in response to stress. Cortisol is secreted rapidly after the onset of a physical stressor. This lack of response and release of cortisol results in an addisonian crisis during times of physical stress, such as illness or surgery, and is characterized by shock, hypotension, and volume depletion (Michels & Michels, 2014). In Addison's disease, the distinctive darkening of the skin that can be seen around the neck, axilla, groin, and between digits is related to the ACTH- mediation stimulation of melanocytes (Michels & Michels, 2014). Patients with Addison's disease often have decreased levels of the mineralocorticoid aldosterone due to adrenal cortex destruction. Aldosterone deficiency can lead to hyponatermia, hyperkalemia, and hypotension (Quinkler, Oelkers, Remde, & Allolio, 2014).

Clinical Aspects

It is recommended that acutely ill patients with unexplained symptoms suggestive of Addison's disease (volume depletion, hypotension, hyperkalemia, hyponatremia, fever, abdominal pain, hyperpigmentation, or hypoglycemia) are tested to exclude Addison's disease as a diagnosis (Bornstein et al., 2016). Confirmatory testing with corticotropin-stimulation testing is recommended for patients who have suggestive symptoms. Patients who have severe adrenal insufficiency or are in an adrenal crisis should be treated with intravenous (IV) hydrocortisone to prevent life-threatening consequences, even in the absence of definitive test results (Bornstein et al., 2016).

Diagnosis of Addison's disease can be made using the short synacthen test, also known as the ACTH stimulation test. Peak cortisol levels less than 500 nmol/ L indicate adrenal insufficiency. Measurement of plasma ACTH is recommended to establish diagnosis of Addison's disease (primary adrenal insufficiency) versus secondary adrenal insufficiency related to decreased ACTH levels. Plasma renin and aldosterone can also be measured to determine whether the patient has a mineralocorticoid deficiency (Bornstein et al., 2016).

Patients who have Addison's disease need to have glucocorticoid replacement therapy. Glucocorticoids can be replaced with hydrocortisone, cortisone acetate, or prednisolone. Generally, the doses of hydrocortisone and cortisone acetate are given in divided doses, with the largest in the morning to mimic the circadian cycle of cortisol release (Bornstein et al., 2016). If the patient has an aldosterone deficiency, he or she should also have mineralocorticoid replacement with fludrocortisone (Quinkler et al., 2014).

Patients who are having an adrenal crisis should be treated emergently with IV glucocorticoids and fluid resuscitation. The preferred drug is hydrocortisone, followed by prednisolone. Dexamethasone should be used if no other glucocorticoid is available (Bornstein et al., 2016).

ASSESSMENT

It is imperative that patients who have Addison's disease have a thorough medication reconciliation. The nurse needs to be aware that these patients cannot be without their glucocorticoid replacement and that the other routes of medication administration must be provided if the patient is unable to take oral doses. The nurse should collaborate with the other members of the medical team to facilitate medication adjustments in the face of worsening illness, surgical procedures, or labor to prevent an Addisonian crisis. Nursing assessment should include monitoring for worsening symptoms of adrenal insufficiency; hypotension, elevated potassium, decreased sodium, and hypoglycemia could indicate an impending crisis (Craven, 2016).

NURSING INTERVENTIONS, MANAGEMENT, AND IMPLICATIONS

Addison's disease is a chronic condition with the vast majority of the disease being managed at home by the patient. Nurses play a vital role in educating and advocating for patients with Addison's disease. Patients should be educated about the types of physical stressors (illness, surgery, severe injury, and pregnancy) that can precipitate a crisis (Bornstein et al., 2016; Craven, 2016). Education should also include symptoms, such as fever, nausea and vomiting, anorexia, weakness, lethargy, and decreased urinary output, that may indicate an impending crisis state (Craven, 2016). Patient education should include the importance of medication timing to mimic normal cortisol release, as well as emergency medication dosing if they are having crisis symptoms in a nonhospital settings (Bornstein et al., 2016; Craven, 2016).

OUTCOMES

Nursing evaluation of treatment response to glucocorticoid replacement includes assessment of weight stability, postural hypotension, reported energy levels, and signs of glucocorticoid excess (cushighoid symptoms). Treatment response to mineralocorticoid replacement should be assessed by presence of postural hypotension, peripheral edema, and reported salt craving (Bornstein et al., 2016).

Summary

Addison's disease or primary adrenal insufficiency is a disease characterized by destruction of the adrenal glands. Cortisol produced by the adrenal gland plays a vital role in the body's response to stress, and helps to maintain blood pressure, sodium, potassium, and water balance. Without lifelong cortisol replacement, patients with Addison's disease are at risk for life-threatening hypovolemia, hypoglycemia, and hypotension. The goal in caring for these patients is the ability to recognize the disease, treat the symptoms, maintain their health status, and avoid a crisis state. The nurse is responsible for providing close observation and careful nursing assessments to monitor for signs of adrenal insufficiency. As most of the management of Addison's disease is done outside of a health care setting, medication and disease management education is crucial to help people with Addison's disease maintain their health.

Addison, T. (1855). In the constitutional and local effects of disease of the supra-renal capsules. Retrieved from https://archive.org/details/b21298786

Bornstein, S. R., Allolio, B., Arlt, W., Barthel, A., Don-Wauchope, A., Hammer, G. D., . . . Torpy, D. J. (2016). Diagnosis and treatment of primary adrenal insufficiency: An Endocrine Society clinical practice guideline. *Journal of Clinical Endocrinology and Metabolism, 101*(2), 364–389. doi:10.1210/jc.2015-1710

Brandão Neto, R. A., & de Carvalho, J. F. (2014). Diagnosis and classification of Addison's disease (autoimmune adrenalitis). *Autoimmunity Reviews, 13*(4–5), 408–411. doi:10.1016/j.autrev.2014.01.025

Craven, H. (2016). Physiological alterations of the endocrine system. In H. Craven (Ed.), *Core curriculum for medical-surgical nursing.* Sewell, NJ: Academy of Medical Surgical Nursing.

Michels, A., & Michels, N. (2014). Addison disease: Early detection and treatment principles. *American Family Physician, 89*(7), 563–568.

National Endocrine and Metabolic Disease Information Service. (2014). *Adrenal insufficiency and Addison's disease.* Washington, DC: U.S. DHHS.

Quinkler, M., Oelkers, W., Remde, H., & Allolio, B. (2015). Mineralocorticoid substitution and monitoring in primary adrenal insufficiency. *Best Practice & Research. Clinical Endocrinology & Metabolism, 29*(1), 17–24. doi:10.1016/j.beem.2014.08.008

■ AMYOTROPHIC LATERAL SCLEROSIS

Mary Jo Elmo

Overview

Amyotrophic lateral sclerosis (ALS) is a progressive neurodegenerative disease affecting both upper and lower motor neurons resulting in paralysis. It was first described in 1869 and became well known in the United States when famous New York Yankee baseball player Lou Gehrig was diagnosed with ALS in 1939 (Zarei et al., 2015). There is no cure for ALS and the disease is fatal with death occurring in most patients within 2 to 5 years of diagnosis. An estimated 20,000 to 30,000 people in the United States are living with ALS with an additional 5,000 newly diagnosed cases annually. Patient presentation varies, but ultimately all patients will have respiratory insufficiency, which is the most common cause of death. Because there is no cure, a primary goal in ALS is symptom management.

Background

ALS is frequently called an insidious disease with progression leading to diffuse muscle weakness, muscle wasting, dysarthria, dysphagia, and paralysis, including paralysis of the respiratory muscles. Men have a lifetime risk of ALS of 1:350 and women 1:500 (Salameh, Brown, & Berry, 2015). Only 10% of patients live more than 10 years (Paganoni, Karam, Joyce, Bedlack, & Carter, 2015). ALS is sporadic in 90% to 95% of cases and 5% to 10% of cases have familial ALS. The superoxide dismutase-1 (SOD1) gene mutation was the first identified and is the most common. An additional 18 gene mutations that cause familial ALS (FALS) have been discovered. Whether sporadic or familial, the presentations are similar with age of onset as the distinguishing feature. In ALS, the age of onset varies from 50 to 65 years old; in familial ALS the onset is generally 10 years earlier. Although the etiology of sporadic ALS is unknown, there are several risk factors. Smoking increases the probability of ALS because of inflammation, oxidative stress, and neurotoxicity associated with cigarettes. There is an association with lead and formaldehyde exposure and ALS, but a relationship between other heavy metals and chemicals has not yet been identified (Zarei et al., 2015). There is an increase in the rate of ALS in U.S. military personnel and ALS is now considered a 100% service connected disability (Weisskopf, Cudkowicz, & Johnson, 2015).

ALS is a diagnosis of exclusion and it takes an average of 11 months to confirm the diagnosis. In many patients, symptoms need to progress before a definitive diagnosis can be made (Nzwalo, de Abreu, Swash, Pinto, & de Carvalho, 2014). Common presenting symptoms include foot drop, weak hand grasp, or slurred speech. Regardless of where the weakness first presents, with disease progression weakness ultimately spreads, finally affecting the respiratory muscles (Paganoni et al., 2015).

Individual patients vary in presentation and severity of symptoms. It was once thought patients with ALS do not experience cognitive impairment, but up to 50% of persons will develop frontotemporal dementia (FTD). Pseudobulbar palsy, characterized by uncontrollable laughing or crying, is also seen in up to 50% of patients (Pattee et al., 2014). Bulbar symptoms, such as dysphagia and dysarthria, are the presenting symptoms in 30% of patients. The presence of bulbar symptoms puts patients at risk for sialorrhea, weight loss, dehydration, aspiration pneumonia, and inability to communicate. Muscle weakness or complete paralysis can affect the neck, limbs, and trunk, which may lead to complete dependence on caregivers. Paralysis of the respiratory muscle leads to respiratory failure. Central apnea and nighttime hypoventilation can occur independently from daytime respiratory function (Ahmed et al., 2016). ALS affects bowel and bladder function and 43% of persons with ALS have urinary incontinence and 46% have problems with constipation (Nübling et al., 2014). Depression can affect the patient and family members. Although there is no cure, there are management strategies to treat symptoms.

Clinical Aspects

The only U.S. Food and Drug Administration–approved medication to treat ALS is riluzole (Rilutek, Tegultik), which decreases the neurotoxic effects of glutamate. The use of riluzole prolongs survival by approximately 3 months and may delay the need for tracheostomy or dependence on a ventilator. Caring for the patient with ALS is highly complex and requires ongoing assessments. Because of the progressive nature of the disease, an intervention employed just a week ago may be obsolete the following week. Patients with ALS who attend a multidisciplinary clinic specializing in treatment of ALS have slightly improved life expectancy. Both the American Academy of Neurology and the European Federation of Neurological Services recommend ALS patients and their caregivers be referred to a multidisciplinary clinic (Zarei et al., 2015).

Respiratory failure is the leading cause of death in persons with ALS, making assessing and monitoring patients' respiratory function a priority of care. Serial pulmonary function testing and monitoring the forced vital capacity (FVC) results are recommended; there is a strong correlation between mortality and FVC less than 50%. The nurse should carefully assess the patient for signs of declining respiratory functioning. Data should be gathered regarding the patient's quality and amount of sleep. Does the patient wake up with headaches? Is the patient fatigued during the day? Is the patient sleeping with more than two pillows? The use of noninvasive ventilation (NIV) is recommended when the FVC falls to approximately 50% or sooner if the patient is symptomatic, hypercarbic, or has apnea confirmed by a sleep study (Ahmed et al., 2016). The use of NIV can prolong survival in ALS, but approximately 25% of patients are unable to tolerate the therapy (Ahmed et al., 2016). Patients should be assessed for tolerance and compliance with therapy at each visit.

Diaphragmatic (phrenic nerve) pacing has been used as a means to prolong survival and improve sleep in persons with ALS, but the results are controversial (Robinson, 2016).

Effective airway clearance is crucial in ALS. Sialorrhea, or excessive drooling, is caused by muscle weakness leading to the inability to manage normal saliva production (Banfi et al., 2015). Anticholinergic medications, such as glycopyrrolate, scopolamine, and hyoscyamine sulfate, can decrease saliva production but can also contribute to thickening of mucus. Weakness of the muscles that control cough contributes to the inability to manage saliva production and the inability to clear secretions from airways. Methods to assist in cough and airway clearance include using a mechanical insufflator/exsufflator device, air stacking followed by cough, or a cough-aid device. To ensure patients are receiving the correct therapy, it is crucial for nurses to recognize whether the patient is having a problem with managing saliva or clearing mucus.

ASSESSMENT

Assessing the patient's nutritional status, fluid volume balance, and weight is another important nursing consideration. Malnutrition and dehydration contribute to fatigue and may compound muscle weakness (Zarei et al. 2015). Patients should undergo a formal swallow study and be frequently assessed for the ability to chew/swallow food. Patients are at risk for aspiration and may benefit from a nutritional consult to determine the type and consistency of food or need for supplements. It is not uncommon for patients with upper extremity paralysis, even in the absence of bulbar symptoms, to forgo food and fluid so as not to be "too much of a bother" to their caregivers. A percutaneous endoscopic gastrostomy is recommended when a patient loses 10% of body weight or 10 pounds in a month. In addition, fluid intake needs to be monitored, especially as it may contribute to constipation.

Many patients identify the loss of speech or ability to communicate as the worst symptom of ALS (Paganoni et al., 2015). Nurses should assess and identify strategies to allow the patient to communicate. There are a myriad of augmentative alternative speech devices (AAC) that patients can use when they lose the ability to speak. Patients should be continually assessed for referral and evaluation for an AAC device. These devices can be controlled by eye gaze or head movements. Nurses should also be aware of voice banking, in which the patient's own voice is be stored for eventual transfer to the AAC when the need arises.

Depression and pseudobulbar affect (PBA) are frequently seen in persons with ALS. Anxiety and caregiver burden are also common. Medications can be used to treat depression and PBA. Nurses should be aware that depression is different from hopelessness and a wish to die. Quality of life does not always correlate with physical function in persons with ALS. In fact, quality of life is generally maintained in people with ALS and health care professionals frequently underestimate how ALS patients perceive their quality of life.

End-of-life care issues need to be addressed while the patient is able to communicate and make decisions. Palliative care and hospice are options for the patient and family to discuss. Many multidisciplinary clinics have palliative caregivers as part of their team.

OUTCOMES

The focus of care for patients with ALS is managing dyspnea and pain. Before the disease progresses to respiratory insufficiency, the patient should be made aware of the various treatment options, including tracheostomy and invasive ventilation. In the United States, between 1.4% and 15% of patients with ALS choose to go onto invasive ventilation. The number is much higher in Japan, with as many as 45% of patients opting for mechanical ventilation. Patients who choose tracheostomy ventilation are typically younger, have young children, and are less likely to be depressed (Rabkin et al., 2006).

Summary

ALS is a progressive degenerative motor neuron disease with an average survival rate of 2 to 5 years from onset of symptoms. There is no cure but there are treatment strategies to manage symptoms and prolong life. Ensuring patients are optimizing respiratory therapies is key to prolonging survival in ALS. This includes noninvasive ventilation, airway clearance therapies, and sialorrhea management. Malnutrition and dehydration are associated with other complications. Discussions regarding end-of-life care, including palliative care, hospice, and tracheostomy, are crucial in ensuring patients are given treatment options when disease progression affects respiratory functioning.

Ahmed, R., Newcombe, R., Piper, A., Lewis, S., Yee, B., Kernan, M., & Grunstein, R. (2016). Sleep disorders and respiratory function in amyotrophic lateral sclerosis. *Sleep Medicine Reviews, 26*, 33–42. doi:10.1016/j.smrv.2015.05.007

Banfi, P., Ticozzi, N., Lax, A., Guidugli, G. A., Nicolini, A., & Silani, V. (2015). A review of options for treating sialorrhea in amyotrophic lateral sclerosis. *Respiratory Care, 60*(3), 446–454. doi:10.4187/respcare.02856

Nübling, G. S., Mie, E., Bauer, R. M., Hensler, M., Lorenzl, S., Hapfelmeier, A., . . . Winkler, A. S. (2014). Increased prevalence of bladder and intestinal dysfunction in amyotrophic lateral sclerosis. *Amyotrophic Lateral Sclerosis & Frontotemporal Degeneration, 15*(3–4), 174–179. doi:10.3109/21678421.2013.868001

Nzwalo, H., de Abreu, D., Swash, M., Pinto, S., & de Carvalho, M. (2014). Delayed diagnosis in ALS: The problem continues. *Journal of the Neurological Sciences, 343*(1–2), 173–175. doi:10.1016/j.jns.2014.06.003

Paganoni, S., Karam, C., Joyce, N., Bedlack, R., & Carter, G. T. (2015). Comprehensive rehabilitative care across the spectrum of amyotrophic lateral sclerosis. *NeuroRehabilitation, 37*(1), 53–68. doi:10.3233/NRE-151240

Pattee, G. L., Wymer, J. P., Lomen-Hoerth, C., Appel, S. H., Formella, A. E., & Pope, L. E. (2014). An open-label multicenter study to assess the safety of dextromethorphan/ quinidine in patients with pseudobulbar affect associated with a range of underlying neurological conditions. *Current Medical Research and Opinion, 30*(11), 2255–2265. doi:10.1185/03007995.2014.940040

Rabkin, J. G., Albert, S. M., Tider, T., Del Bene, M. L., O'Sullivan, I., Rowland, L. P., & Mitsumoto, H. (2006). Predictors and course of elective long-term mechanical ventilation: A prospective study of ALS patients. *Amyotrophic Lateral Sclerosis, 7*(2), 86–95. doi:10.1080/14660820500515021

Robinson, R. (2016). Diaphragm pacing for ALS at crossroads following conflicting trial results. *Neurology Today, 16*(2), 18–21. doi:10.1097/01.NT.0000480659.79684.39

Salameh, J. S., Brown, R. H., & Berry, J. D. (2015). Amyotrophic lateral sclerosis: Review. *Seminars in Neurology, 35*(4), 469–476. doi:10.1055/s-0035-1558984

Weisskopf, M. G., Cudkowicz, M. E., & Johnson, N. (2015). Military service and amyotrophic lateral sclerosis in a population-based cohort. *Epidemiology, 26*(6), 831–838. doi:10.1097/EDE.0000000000000376

Zarei, S., Carr, K., Reiley, L., Diaz, K., Guerra, O., Altamirano, P. F., . . . Chinea, A. (2015). A comprehensive review of amyotrophic lateral sclerosis. *Surgical Neurology International, 6*, 171. doi:10.4103/2152-7806.169561

■ ANEMIA IN ADULTS

Kerry Mastrangelo
Mary T. Quinn Griffin

Overview

Anemia is one of the most common hematologic problems. The term "anemia" refers to a condition in which there is a decrease in the number of circulating red blood cells (RBCs), hemoglobin concentration, or the volume of packed cells (hematocrit) as compared with normal values. The most commonly accepted definition of anemia is the World Health Organization's (WHO) definition of a hemoglobin concentration less than 13 g/dL in men and less than 12 g/dL in women (Le, 2016). Older adults with anemia have increased hospitalizations and higher mortality rates making anemia a relevant public health concern in light of the predicted increase in the population aged 65 years and older. Anemia is associated with higher utilization of health care resources and an overall increase in morbidity and mortality (Le, 2016).

Background

The prevalence of anemia in the United States is estimated at 5.6% of adults with 1.5% of anemias diagnosed as moderate to severe. The prevalence of anemia in adults has increased from 4.0% to 7.1% over the years 2003 to 2012 (Le, 2016). Anemia is a common problem and is found in 20% to 30% of all hospitalized patients, making it a significant concern for nurses. Most anemias in adults result from blood loss, inadequate RBC production, or destruction of RBCs. Anemias are generally categorized according to cause or morphology.

Clinical manifestations of anemia are dependent on the degree of anemia and whether the anemia is acute or chronic. Common manifestations, regardless of the etiology, are fatigue, dyspnea with exertion, weakness, lightheadedness, palpitations, and pallor of the skin, mucous membranes, and conjunctiva. Tachycardia and hypotension occur as anemia becomes more severe. Severe anemia leads to increased cardiac output to compensate for tissue hypoxia, resulting in a systolic ejection murmur. Sustained tachycardia to compensate for the decreased hemoglobin concentration eventually leads to left ventricular failure. The most common types of anemia in adults are iron-deficiency anemia, hemolytic anemia, pernicious anemia, and anemia related to chronic diseases (Goodnough & Schrier, 2014).

Iron-deficiency anemia, classified as a microcytic anemia, is the most common cause of anemia worldwide and is due to inadequate absorption of iron or excessive blood loss. Predisposing factors for the development of this anemia are diets poor in iron-rich foods, history of gastric surgery, chronic aspirin or nonsteroidal anti-inflammatory drug (NSAID) use, chronic blood loss, and menorrhagia. An unusual symptom of iron-deficiency anemia is pica, the compulsive eating of nonfood substances such as clay, dirt, and ice.

In hemolytic anemias, the life span of the RBC, usually 120 days, is shortened resulting in an increase in circulating reticulocytes related to bone marrow compensation. This anemia is classified as a microcytic anemia seen in persons with hemoglobinopathies, thalassemias, hereditary spherocytosis, glucose-6-phosphate dehydrogenase (G6PD), and blood transfusion reactions.

Pernicious anemia, also called *megoblastic anemia*, is classified as a macrocytic anemia and is characterized by large, immature, poorly functioning RBCs. The two most common causes are vitamin B_{12} deficiency and folate deficiency. This anemia is more prevalent in the fifth and sixth decade of life and in persons of Northern European descent. There is a progressive decrease in parietal cell function in the stomach, resulting in decreased production of intrinsic factor necessary for the absorption of vitamin B_{12}. Predisposing factors for pernicious anemia are a history of gastric surgery, chronic gastritis, chronic alcoholism, malnutrition, and use of certain drugs such as hydroxyurea, trimethoprim, zidovidine, and methotrexate. In addition to the common clinical manifestations seen in anemia, persons with pernicious anemia may present with a sore, beefy red tongue; angular cheilosis; parethesias in the extremities; and edema of the lower extremities.

Anemia of chronic disease (ACD), also referred to as *anemia of inflammation*, can be classified as normocytic or microcytic and is a result of decreased proliferation and shortened life span of RBCs. The reduction in RBCs is thought to be due to decreased erythropoietin and the release of proinflammatory cytokines. ACD is most commonly seen in the elderly and is associated with chronic kidney disease, autoimmune disease, malignancies, and inflammatory disorders such as rheumatoid arthritis and systemic lupus erythematosus.

Clinical Aspects

ASSESSMENT

History, physical exam, and laboratory testing are essential in evaluating the patient with anemia. Anemia is indicative of an underlying pathology and is never a normal finding. A thorough patient health history should include a comprehensive dietary history, current and past medical and surgical history, and a review of prescribed and over-the-counter medications. Specific questions should be directed toward a history of kidney or liver disease, malignancy, autoimmune disease, blood transfusions, weight loss, a decrease in appetite, color of stools, alcohol and NSAID use, and menstrual pattern. The aim of physical examination is to ascertain the severity and etiology of the anemia. The assessment should include the evaluation of the patient's general appearance, nutritional status, and observing the patient's skin, mucous membranes and conjunctiva for pallor or jaundice. Vital signs should be assessed for hypotension, tachycardia, dyspnea, and fever. In addition, a complete cardiac and abdominal exam noting the presence of murmurs or an enlarged liver or spleen should be performed.

The initial diagnostic workup for anemia should include a complete blood count (CBC) with differential, red cell indices, a peripheral smear, reticulocyte count, serum folic acid, serum vitamin B_{12}, serum iron, total iron-binding capacity (TIBC), ferritin level, and stool for occult blood (Cash & Glass, 2017). The reticulocyte count is of primary importance in diagnosis, as it reflects the early release of immature erythrocytes. The red cell indices and the peripheral smear include the mean corpuscular volume (MCV) measuring the average size of the RBC classifying the anemia as microcytic, macrocytic, or normocytic and the mean corpuscular hemoglobin (MCH) measuring the hemoglobin content per erythrocyte, classifying the color of the cell as hypochromic or normochromic. Serum iron studies, vitamin B_{12} and folate levels provide information to differentiate among the types of anemia. Stool for occult blood identifies blood loss contributing to anemia.

The treatment of anemia is tailored to the underlying cause. If anemia is the result of blood loss, the source must be identified. Iron-deficiency anemia and pernicious anemia require supplementation of iron, folate, or vitamin B_{12}. ACD will improve with recovery from the underlying disorder, although if recovery is not possible, transfusions and erythropoiesis-stimulating agents may be warranted (Goodnough & Schrier, 2014).

NURSING INTERVENTIONS, MANAGEMENT, AND IMPLICATIONS

Nursing-related problems include inadequate tissue perfusion related to decreased hemoglobin and activity intolerance related to fatigue. Nursing care should include monitoring of vital signs, monitoring of hemoglobin level, administering oxygen to maintain O_2 saturation greater than 90%, assessing skin color and capillary refill, providing frequent rest periods, administering prescribed medications, and patient teaching.

OUTCOMES

The major goal of medical management and nursing care is to identify and correct the underlying cause of the anemia and prevent tissue hypoxia leading to heart failure. The expected outcomes of nursing care are tolerance of normal daily activity, heart rate and blood pressure within normal parameters, maintaining adequate tissue perfusion, adherence to prescribed therapy, and the absence of complications.

Summary

The prognosis of anemia depends on its underlying cause. The severity, etiology, onset, and patient comorbidities play a significant role in the prognosis. Nursing care should focus on the prevention of the most serious complications due to tissue hypoxia, hypotension, and cardiac insufficiency.

Cash, J., & Glass, C. (2017). *Family practice guidelines* (4th ed.). New York, NY: Springer Publishing.

Goodnough, L. T., & Schrier, S. L. (2014). Evaluation and management of anemia in the elderly. *American Journal of Hematology, 89*(1), 88–96. doi:10.1002/ajh.23598

Le, C. H. (2016). The prevalence of anemia and moderate-severe anemia in the U.S. Population (NHANES 2003–2012). *PLOS ONE, 11*(11), e0166635. doi:10.1371/journal.pone.0166635

■ ATELECTASIS

Ashley L. Foreman

Overview

Atelectasis is a pulmonary complication that is the result of an injury, chronic disease process, or surgical intervention (Cabrera & Pravikoff, 2016). Atelectasis is defined as a reversible alveolar collapse typically resulting from obstruction of the airway serving the affected alveoli (Restrepo & Braverman, 2015; Schub, Uribe, & Pravikoff, 2016). More specific, it describes a decrease in the ability of alveolar spaces to inflate with oxygen, resulting in volume loss. The extent of involvement ranges from microatelectases that are undetectable on chest radiograph to complete lung collapse. Atelectasis can be acute or chronic. Chronic atelectasis is associated with chronic airway diseases, neuromuscular impairment, chest wall deformity, or lung cancer. Acute atelectasis is the most common complication of surgery. Postoperative atelectasis occurs in 90% of adults and children receiving anesthesia (Cabrera & Pravikoff, 2016). Prompt initiation of treatment is necessary to open the areas of obstruction and relieve symptoms. Techniques to mobilize secretions, improve ventilation, and reduce morbidity and mortality are priorities in the nursing management of patients with atelectasis.

Background

Atelectasis is defined as the collapse or incomplete expansion of the lung, and is classified into two broad categories, obstructive and nonobstructive (Ray, Bodenham, & Paramasivam, 2014). Although it is usually a benign finding, there is an inability of the alveoli to expand completely, leading to volume loss and progressive airway collapse. This affects systemic oxygenation by the loss of adequate ventilation to lung zones and inadequate gas exchange. Atelectasis caused by large airway obstruction is often linked to bronchial or metastatic tumors, inflammatory diseases (e.g., tuberculosis or sarcoidosis), or other foreign bodies. Atelectasis caused by small airway obstruction is associated with mucus plugging caused by inflammatory or infectious disease processes, including pneumonia, bronchitis, and bronchiectasis (Ray et al., 2014). Mechanisms associated with nonobstructive etiology or compressive atelectasis include large bullae (extensive air trapping), loss of contact between the visceral and parietal pleura (due to pleural effusion), or lack of surfactant production as seen in acute lung injury (ALI) or acute respiratory distress syndrome (ARDS).

Atelectasis affects up to 90% of patients undergoing major surgical procedures and can lead to postoperative pulmonary complications (PPCs). A PPC is any pulmonary abnormality that produces an "identifiable disease or dysfunction that negatively affects the clinical course after surgery" (Restrepo & Braverman, 2015, p. 97). Examples include aspiration pneumonias, interstitial/

alveolar edema, gas exchange abnormalities, respiratory failure, weaning failure, pleural effusion, or pneumothorax. Atelectasis has been recognized as a contributor to prolonged hospitalizations, admissions to the intensive care unit (ICU), and increased health expenditures (Restrepo & Braverman, 2015). Respiratory complications are the leading cause of morbidity and mortality in patients with impaired cough or neuromuscular disease (American Association for Respiratory Care [AARC], 2015).

Three important physiologic mechanisms found to cause or contribute to the development of atelectasis include "external compression (limitation of alveolar expansion), alveolar gas resorption and surfactant impairment" (Restrepo & Braverman, 2015, p. 97).

■ *External compression.* During general anesthesia (GA), mechanical ventilation forces the alveoli to collapse by disrupting the existing negative pressure that maintains them in the open state (Restrepo & Braverman, 2015). Dependent regions of the lung are then more prone to atelectasis secondary to decreased ventilation and insufficient spontaneous drainage of secretions with gravity (Ferri, 2014). In anesthetized patients, muscle relaxation displaces the diaphragm, which results in compression of adjacent lung tissue. Other factors influencing the development of compression atelectasis include chest anatomy and respiratory muscle changes (e.g., restrictive lung disease; Restrepo & Braverman, 2015).

■ *Alveolar resorption.* In alveolar resorption atelectasis, lower areas of ventilation (relative to perfusion) are susceptible to collapse due to mucus plugging in the bronchioles. In a normal state, "lung regions that have low ventilation compared with perfusion have low alveolar oxygen tension when the fraction of inspired oxygen is low" (Restrepo & Braverman, 2015, p. 99). Nitrogen helps to provide surface tension to prevent alveolar collapse. With GA, the fraction of inspired oxygen is increased with the addition of supplemental oxygen. Alveolar oxygen tension (partial pressure of arterial oxygen) then rises. Ultimately, the loss of nitrogen and increases in oxygen through GA result in diminished alveolar volume (Restrepo & Braverman, 2015).

■ *Surfactant impairment.* Pulmonary surfactant is a phospholipid that reduces alveolar surface tension, improves alveolar stability, and prevents collapse of the alveoli at end expiration. Anesthesia has been shown to diminish stabilizing properties of surfactant. Cyclical opening and closing of the alveoli during GA with mechanical ventilation leads to reduced availability of surfactant. Excessive alveolar surface tension reduces functional residual capacity (FRC) and pulmonary compliance.

In adults, atelectasis is commonly identified as a postoperative complication. Surgery greatly increases the risk for atelectasis due to supine positioning, chest wall splinting, abdominal distention, poor clearance of secretions, airway obstruction, and impaired cough reflex (Schub et al., 2016). Other major risk factors in the adult population include mucus plugs from obstructive lung disease, obesity, smoking, neuromuscular disease or chest wall injury (pneumothorax). Right middle lobe (RML) syndrome, a type of chronic atelectasis, usually results from bronchial compression and obstruction by surrounding lymph nodes or scarring (Sharma, 2015). The likelihood of PPCs increases in patients with pre-existing conditions.

Clinical Aspects

A thorough history and physical assessment should be performed to guide the nursing care of patients at risk for atelectasis. Evidence-based nursing interventions to prevent and treat atelectasis should be used to improve quality and safety outcomes.

ASSESSMENT

Physical assessment findings and clinical presentation may include decreased or absent breath sounds, cough, shortness of breath, tachycardia and diminished chest expansion, low-grade fever or hypoxia (Ferri, 2014). Patients may also present with concurrent history of recent surgery (anesthesia), chronic bronchitis, endobronchial neoplasm, chest infection, or injury. Imaging studies, including chest radiograph or CT scans, are commonly performed to investigate symptoms and narrow differential diagnoses. On chest radiograph, areas of atelectasis would be seen as volume loss, a linear or wedge-shaped density or loss of contour of the hemidiaphragm (Watters, 2014). Intravenous contrast may be required for appropriate differentiation of the types of atelectasis (Sharma, 2015). In selected patients, fiberoptic bronchoscopy may be helpful in removing foreign bodies, or mucus plugs unresponsive to conservative measures. Bronchoscopy is used to evaluate endobronchial or peribronchial lesions (Ferri, 2014). Arterial blood gases may be used to identify hypoxemia and bacterial cultures of sputum and blood are helpful in identifying sources of infection.

NURSING INTERVENTIONS, MANAGEMENT, AND IMPLICATIONS

Various nonpharmacologic therapies promote adequate pulmonary ventilation and airway clearance. Deep breathing/coughing, repositioning, and early ambulation after surgery are effective methods. Other mechanisms, such as incentive spirometry (ICS), tracheal suctioning (as appropriate), chest physiotherapy, and postural drainage, are also effective in mobilizing secretions. These techniques can be used in both acute and chronic atelectasis (Ferri, 2014). Nursing care should be focused on reducing the work of breathing and promoting optimal oxygenation. In more select cases, continuous positive airway pressure devices have also been used to promote positive end expiratory pressure (PEEP). Patients on mechanical ventilation may be given recruitment maneuvers to improve gas exchange, along with utilizing aggressive ventilator-weaning protocols as appropriate. These interventions help to reduce pulmonary complications, length of stay, and minimize readmissions to the hospital.

Aerosolized medications, including bronchodilators, expectorants, and mucolytic agents, have been used to improve airway clearance, but there is limited research to support the efficacy of these medications. AARC (2015) recommends nonpharmacological approaches to airway clearance, in combination with an individualized plan that may include pharmacological intervention as appropriate.

OUTCOMES

The use of bronchodilators and corticosteroids in symptomatic patients with chronic obstructive pulmonary disease (COPD) is highly recommended to reduce inflammation and mucus production (AARC, 2015). Inhaled dornase alfa (Pulmozyme), a mucolytic agent, in combination with hypertonic saline is an approved treatment for patients with cystic fibrosis for sputum clearance (Bilton & Stanford, 2014). This medication can also be used for mechanically ventilated patients with atelectasis.

Summary

Although atelectasis is usually a benign finding, it is important that practicing nurses understand the background, clinical presentation, and nursing implications of atelectasis. Early identification of symptoms is key in the management of atelectasis. To improve patient safety and quality, approaches to care should be tailored to meet individual patient needs based on clinical presentation and risk factors. Continued research in this area is needed to determine efficacy of treatment options and to improve health outcomes for patients.

American Association for Respiratory Care. (2015). AARC clinical practice guideline: Effectiveness of pharmacologic airway clearance therapies in hospitalized patients. *Respiratory Care, 60*(7), 1073–1077.

Bilton, D., & Stanford, G. (2014). The expanding armamentarium of drugs to aid sputum clearance: How should they be used to optimize care? *Current Opinion in Pulmonary Medicine, 20*(6), 601–606. doi:10.1097/MCP.0000000000000104

Cabrera, G., & Pravikoff, D. (2016). Quick lesson: Atelectasis, postoperative. *CINAHL Nursing Guide.* Ipswich, MA: EBSCO Publishing.

Ferri, F. F. (2014). *Ferri's clinical advisor 2014.* Philadelphia, PA: Elsevier/Mosby.

Ray, K., Bodenham, A., & Paramasivam, E. (2014). Pulmonary atelectasis in anaesthesia and critical care. *Critical Care & Pain, 4*, 236–244.

Restrepo, R. D., & Braverman, J. (2015). Current challenges in the recognition, prevention and treatment of perioperative pulmonary atelectasis. *Expert Review of Respiratory Medicine, 9*(1), 97–107. doi:10.1586/17476348.2015.996134

Schub, T., Uribe, L. M., & Pravikoff, D. (2016). Quick lesson: Atelectasis, in children. *CINAHL Nursing Guide.* Ipswich, MA: EBSCO Publishing.

Sharma, S. (2015). Lobar atelectasis imaging. *Medscape.* Retrieved from http://emedicine.medscape.com/article/353833-overview

Watters, J. R. (2014). A systematic approach to basic chest radiograph interpretation: A cardiovascular focus. *Canadian Journal of Cardiovascular Nursing, 24*(2), 4–10.

■ ATHEROSCLEROSIS

Kari Gali

Overview

Atherosclerosis is a progressive, inflammatory disease characterized by the formation of a fatty plaque in the intimal layer of medium- and large-size arteries. Derived from the Greek terms, "athero," which means gruel or wax, describing the fatty luminal plaque and "sclerosis," which means hardening corresponding to the fibrous cap on the plaque's edge. Atherosclerosis is considered one of the most lethal diseases in the world today (Ladich & Burke, 2016). Starting from childhood, fatty streaks develop and over time grow into atheromas (plaques) narrowing arteries and impairing blood flow. Clinical manifestations generally do not occur until at least 75% of the arterial lumen is blocked. Presenting in three general ways, atherosclerosis progresses into cardiovascular diseases, peripheral artery disease (PAD), and chronic kidney disease associated with renal stenosis.

According to the 2017 Heart Disease and Stroke Statistic Update, cardiovascular disease accounts for 33% of the deaths in the United States, killing over 800,000 Americans annually (American Heart Association [AHA], 2017). With more than 92 million Americans affected by cardiovascular heart disease or stroke, estimated care costs currently exceed $316 billion annually. Peripheral vascular disease affects 8 to 12 million Americans and renal artery disease affects 6.8% of the population older than 60 years, or approximately 2 million people. The disease burden of atherosclerosis as reflected by the associated diseases (cardiovascular disease including stroke, renal artery disease and PAD) is not sustainable in today's health care environment. Health care reform and the move toward value-based health care are requiring more cost-effective and quality outcomes. This entry presents evidence to direct the nursing care of individuals with atherosclerosis.

Background

Atherosclerosis is a preventable disease; however, the associated disease burden that is measured by cost, morbidity, and mortality has exceeded epidemic proportions. Atherosclerosis prevalence and incidence rates are generally reported according to the disease with which they are associated and not reported solely under atherosclerosis. The AHA reports that heart disease (coronary heart disease, hypertension, and stroke) is currently the number one killer in the United States (AHA, 2017). Although there has been a gradual decline in cardiovascular-related mortality in higher income countries between 1990 and 2010, cardiovascular disease still accounts for one in three deaths in U.S. citizens who are older than 35 years of age. Prevalence increases with age, male gender, and ethnicity. Fifty percent of Black American adults have some form of cardiovascular disease. The lifetime risk of developing cardiovascular disease for people 40 years old is 49% in men and 32% in females compared to people reaching 70 years, when the lifetime risk is 35% and 24%, respectively (Centers for

Disease Control and Prevention [CDC] & National Center for Health Statistics [NCHS], 2015; Sanchis-Gomar, Perez-Quillis, Leischik, & Lucia, 2016). Stroke is the fifth leading cause of death in the United States, killing more than 130,000 Americans annually, or one death every 4 minutes (CDC & NCHS, 2015).

Stroke, the fifth leading cause of death in the United States, accounts for 5% of all deaths and is the second cause of death globally. Annually 795,000 Americans suffer from a stroke, with 76% of those being a first-time attack. Poststroke disability occurs in 90% of stroke victims, which can impact both physical and cognitive ability.

PAD is another high-burden disease with a predominant association to atherosclerosis. Atherosclerotic plaque impairs blood flow to the arms, legs, or pelvic region and affects nearly 8.5 million Americans, 12% to 20% of whom are 60 years or older. A major challenge for PAD is that only 25% of individuals have a general awareness of the disease, prolonging diagnosis and treatment (CDC, 2016; Davies et al., 2017).

The pathogenesis of atherosclerosis begins with chronic endothelial injury, damage, and adaptive thickening. Atherogenic triggers include one or more of these insults: (a) physical injury, direct trauma, or turbulent blood flow (hypertension); (b) free radical and toxins in circulation (smoking, infection, inflammation); (c) hypercholesteremia (elevated low-density lipoprotein [LDL] or very low density lipoprotein [VLDL]); (d) chronically elevated blood glucose (insulin resistance or poor diet); or (e) high levels of homocysteine, which is toxic to the endothelium.

Once the endothelium is damaged, cytokines attract leukocytes (monocytes and t-lymphocytes) that adhere to the endothelium, squeezing underneath the endothelial cells. The endothelial cells change shape, the tight junctions relax and leaking fluid, lipoproteins, macrophages, and enzymes accumulate in the intima. The accumulation of lipids on the endothelium identified as the fatty streak development begins the atherosclerotic process, yet is considered reversible. As the plaque continues to increase in size an atheroma forms, followed by the addition of a fibrous cap resulting in a fibroma. Lipids, fibrous tissue, calcium, cellular debris, and capillaries form these complex lesions, which can hemorrhage, calcify, or ulcerate stimulating thrombotic lesion development. Plaques can either form in an asymmetric pattern or cover the entire vessel circumference and often develop where arteries bifurcate. Some arteries have a high propensity for atherosclerosis development, including the left ascending coronary artery, renal arteries, and branching areas of carotid arteries. Atherosclerotic plaque also weakens artery walls, increasing the risk of aneurysms. Clinical manifestations result from restricted flow of oxygen-rich blood and vary depending on the location, severity, and speed of occlusion from these plaques.

Clinical Aspects

ASSESSMENT

In coronary artery disease, also called coronary heart disease, atherosclerosis interrupts normal blood flow through the coronary arteries. Plaque can lead to the development of blood clots that can break off and partially or completely block blood supply to an area of the heart muscle. Angina pectoris is characterized by transient chest pain, which occurs from an imbalance in oxygen demand and supply to the coronary artery. Myocardial infarction (MI) occurs when blood flow is interrupted and the heart muscle is deprived of oxygen for a period of time, resulting in a cardiac muscle ischemia and necrosis. Symptoms characterizing an MI include chest pain, which may or may not radiate, shortness of breath, dizziness, nausea, diaphoresis, and anxiety. Nursing implications center on hemodynamic evaluation, including cardiac output monitoring and tissue perfusion assessment and pain management, including evaluating, documenting, and administering measures to reduce pain. Nursing care should focus on reducing knowledge deficits, promoting self-care, and self-efficacy to engage in self-care behaviors as evidenced by the maintenance of a therapeutic regimen.

A comprehensive approach to atherosclerosis is key to reducing death, disability, and the associated global economic burden. Prevention strategies aimed at minimizing risk have been identified and refined by large prospective observational studies such as the Framingham study. Targeting risk factors for both symptomatic and asymptomatic patients is the first step and a shift from traditional management, which focused on preventing recurrence. Enhanced understanding of nonmodifiable and modifiable risk factors provides an opportunity to modify disease progression. Nonmodifiable factors include age, gender, and family history, whereas modifiable factors can be both pathologic and lifestyle oriented. Population health focuses on addressing lifestyle factors and behavior modification in regard to smoking, diet, activity, obesity, and medication use in women (oral contraceptive pills and hormone replacement therapy). Pathologic modifiable factors are associated with specific diseases, including hyperlipidemia, diabetes mellitus, and hypertension and improving clinical outcomes.

Nursing care for atherosclerosis entails primary, secondary, and tertiary prevention strategies. Atherosclerosis may be asymptomatic, based on the percentage of blockage in an artery and the development of collateral circulation, or symptomatic, as seen in a specific disease such as occurs after myocardial infarction (MI). Applicable to populations, promotion of healthy lifestyle behaviors, including not smoking, consumption of a healthy diet, adequate physical exercise, and weight management play a role in each stage. Learning readiness, learning support, decision-making support, and self-management are all aspects of nursing care. Addressing knowledge deficits with evidence-based education can help minimize the negative consequence associated with negative lifestyle behaviors.

Improving cholesterol levels with lifestyle modifications is the first step in management of atherosclerosis in patients with known disease, targeting the levels of both LDLs and high-density lipoproteins (HDLs). New atherosclerotic cardiovascular disease (ASCVD) American College of Cardiology and American Heart Association (ACC/AHA) guidelines in 2013 recommend (a) secondary prevention by targeting patients with any known form of ASCVD, (b) secondary prevention by targeting patients with LDL levels greater than 190, (c) primary prevention in patients with diabetes mellitus (40–75 years of age) with LDL levels 70–189, and (d) primary prevention in a patient without diabetes but with a slightly elevated hemoglobin A1c (less than 7.5%; Stone et al, 2013). Diabetes and poor glucose control, hyperinsulinemia, and altered functioning of platelets affecting arterial endothelium contribute to the inflammatory process and the development of atherosclerosis. Diabetes is also associated with high lipid levels, obesity, and hypertension, which also impact the progression of atherosclerosis. Nursing care includes addressing knowledge deficits through education, facilitating adherence to a therapeutic regime, and minimizing the effects of hyperglycemia.

Summary

Atherosclerosis is a progressive disease at the root of many lethal diseases that cause significant disease burden across the globe. Nevertheless, atherosclerosis is preventable. Incorporating primary prevention strategies or modifiable in secondary and tertiary prevention strategies when providing nursing care can shift the paradigm toward reducing disease-related illness and suffering. Through the use of evidence-based guidelines to inform practice, nursing collaboratively can improve clinical outcomes associated with the management of atherosclerosis, facilitating lifestyle changes at both the individual and population level.

American Heart Association. (2017). Heart disease and stroke 2017 statistic updates. Retrieved from https://www.heart.org/idc/groups/ahamah-public/@wcm/@sop/@smd/documents/downloadable/ucm_491265.pdf

CDC. (2016). Peripheral Artery Disease (PAD) Fact Sheet. Retrieved from https://www.cdc.gov/dhdsp/data_statistics/fact_sheets/fs_pad.htm

CDC, NCHS. (2015). Underlying cause of death 1999–2013. Retrieved from https://wonder.cdc.gov

Davies, J. H., Richards, J., Conway, K., Kenkre, J. E., Lewis, J. E., & Mark Williams, E. (2017). Primary care screening for peripheral arterial disease: A cross-sectional observational study. *British Journal of General Practice, 67*(655), e103–e110. doi:10.3399/bjgp17X689137

Ladich, E., & Burke, A. (2016). Atherosclerosis pathology: The heart. *Medscape.* Retrieved from http://reference.medscape.com/article/1612610-overview

Sanchis-Gomar, F., Perez-Quillis, C., Leischik, R., & Lucia, A. (2016). Epidemiology of coronary heart disease and acute coronary syndrome. *Annals of Translational Medicine, 4*(13), 256.

Stone, N., Robinson, J., Lichtenstein, A., Merz, C. N., Blum, C., Eckel, R., . . . Wilson, P. (2013). 2013 ACC/AHA guidelines on the treatment of blood cholesterol to reduce atherosclerotic cardiovascular risk in adults. *Circulation,* 1–85. doi:10.1161/01.cir.0000437738.63853.7a

■ BENIGN PROSTATIC HYPERPLASIA

Kelly Ann Lynn

Overview

Benign prostatic hyperplasia (BPH) is a medical condition characterized by non-cancerous overgrowth of prostatic tissue. Men with BPH often present with complaints of significant lower urinary tract symptoms (LUTS), which include a weak urinary stream, frequency and urgency of urination, and nocturia (Vuichoud & Loughlin, 2015). Patients suffering from BPH may be at risk for significant morbidity, including urinary retention, the formation of bladder stones, sepsis, and renal insufficiency. Nursing care for patients with BPH focuses on early diagnosis, education, psychosocial support, and management of symptoms and the medications prescribed to treat the symptoms.

Background

BPH is one of the most common conditions affecting older men. The incidence of BPH increases as men age. Moreover, it is associated with considerable morbidity that can adversely affect quality of life. According to the National Institute of Health, BPH can start as early as 40 years of age and is estimated to affect about 50% of men between the ages of 51 and 60 years. Approximately 90% of men will develop histologic evidence of BPH by age 80 years (Lepor, 2005). Symptomatic BPH and LUTS affects 50% to 75% of men aged 50 years and older, and 80% of men older than 70 years (Egan, 2016).

BPH treatment in the United States costs approximately $4 billion per year (Vuichoud & Loughlin, 2015). Given the progressive nature of BPH and the increase in average life expectancy, it is presumed that the cost of managing the symptoms of BPH will only rise.

The exact cause of BPH remains unclear. However, there are some indications that aging and the long-time exposure to male hormones play a significant role. According to the National Institute of Diabetes and Digestive and Kidney Diseases (NIDDK), part of the National Institutes of Health (NIH; 2014), men whose testicles are removed before they reach puberty do not develop BPH. This indicates that aging and hormone levels (testosterone, estrogen, dihydrotestosterone) may have a causative role in the development of BPH. Black and Hispanic men are at increased risk for developing BPH compared to White men (Kristal et al., 2007). Other factors that appear to increase the incidence of BPH include a history of prostatitis and obesity, indicating that inflammation may also play a role. Moreover, increased levels of physical activity appears to be associated with a decreased risk for clinical BPH.

Various terms are used to describe BPH and the resulting symptoms. BPH is often interchanged with "benign prostatic enlargement" (BPE). However, it is important to note that BPH is a histologic diagnosis that refers to a progressive increase in the number of stromal and epithelial cells in the prostate. This proliferative process is most prevalent in the prostate region adjacent to the urethra, known as the *transitional zone* (T-zone; Egan, 2016). Given its proximity to the urethra, BPH in the T-zone may be associated with significant urinary obstruction to the flow of urine. BPE, by contrast, describes increased volume of the gland. It is important to note that the size of the prostate does not always determine the severity of the symptoms.

BPH-associated symptoms are categorized into (a) voiding or obstructive symptoms and (b) storage or irritative symptoms. Voiding symptoms include hesitancy, a delay in the start of urine flow; weak urinary stream; straining to urinate; postvoid dribbling; urinary retention and overflow incontinence. Storage symptoms include those clinical indications related to instability of the detrusor muscle. That is, that the detrusor contracts without our consent, manifesting in bladder instability with complaints of frequency, urgency, and nocturia.

As the prostate increases in size, it can obstruct the flow of urine as it exits the bladder and passes through the prostatic urethra. If the patient is not treated for this progressive bladder outlet obstruction, he may develop acute or chronic urinary retention. Chronic urinary retention can quietly lead to the development of renal insufficiency, ultimately resulting in renal failure. Another adverse effect of chronic urinary retention is the deterioration of bladder muscle function. When the bladder is unable to empty adequately, impaired detrusor contractility will occur. Moreover, in time, functional deterioration of the detrusor muscle can contribute to chronic bladder outlet obstruction. Long-term impairment of the detrusor muscle may be irreversible. Untreated, chronic obstruction can also lead to the development of bladder diverticula as a result of the high pressure in the bladder. Additionally, hydronephrosis, hydroureter, and vesicoureteral reflux can result from prolonged, untreated prostatic obstruction.

The clinical significance of BPH and LUTS cannot be understated. BPH and LUTS symptoms (i.e., urgency and nocturia) are associated with increased incidence of falls in the elderly (Schimke & Schimke, 2014). Elderly patients with decreased mobility are particularly susceptible to falling while rushing to use the bathroom. Moreover, skin integrity can be compromised by urinary incontinence. Electrolyte imbalances may result from chronic obstruction. There is also considerable emotional distress associated with the BPH and LUTS symptom complex.

Clinical Aspects

ASSESSMENT

A thorough nursing assessment is essential to identify and characterize a patient's symptoms associated with BPH. This includes a comprehensive patient history with targeted questions related to voiding patterns (urinary stream, frequency, straining to void), history of urinary tract infections, bladder stones, and the incidence of incontinence and nocturia. The International Prostate Symptom Score (IPSS) is a quick, inexpensive, and effective screening tool that can help diagnose and track progress of BPH. Physical assessment should be thorough and address vital signs, particularly blood pressure. It is also essential to examine the patients' ankles and feet for signs of fluid retention. Percussion and palpation of the suprapubic area allow for the detection of significant bladder overdistention. Obtaining a postvoid residual to assess bladder emptying will further clarify the efficacy of bladder emptying for a given patient. Uroflowmetry can be used to measure the urine flow rate. Moreover, a review of essential laboratory values relating to the health of the urinary system is of great value. The urinalysis will help detect the presence of WBCs and RBCs in the urine; serum chemistry will assess for electrolyte imbalances and serum blood urea nitrogen (BUN) and creatinine levels, thus helping to evaluate renal function; prostate-specific antigen (PSA). PSA is often used to detect prostate cancer, an elevated PSA level may also be indicative of BPH or acute bacterial prostatitis.

The review of medications is an essential part of the nursing assessment. Some medications (i.e., diuretics) can cause urinary frequency and increase distress for patients with BPH. Medications can contribute to acute urinary retention. Oral decongestants and antihistamines can cause constriction in the bladder neck and should be avoided in men with BPH. Other medications can affect detrusor muscle contractility and should be used cautiously in patients with BPH. These medications include anticholinergic agents (e.g., tricyclic antidepressants, selective serotonin reuptake inhibitors (SSRIs), antispasmodics), calcium channel blockers, nonsteroidal anti-inflammatory drugs (NSAIDs), opioids, and anti-Parkinsonian agents.

Nursing assessment of BPH must include all three components: comprehensive, in-depth history; a physical examination with evaluation and interpretation of laboratory and diagnostic tests; and medication review. Any encounter with a male patient older than the age of 50 years (regardless of whether he reports a history of BPH) should address all of these issues.

NURSING INTERVENTIONS, MANAGEMENT, AND IMPLICATIONS

Nursing care of patients with BPH should be tailored to the patients' symptoms and clinical status. The focus of care should be the prevention of the serious consequences related to BPH, such as renal failure, urinary retention, and urinary sepsis. Optimizing urinary elimination will reduce incidence of stasis, urinary tract infections (UTIs), bladder stones, detrusor instability, and electrolyte imbalances. Nursing care must include comprehensive education and emotional support for patients and their families.

Nursing interventions will vary, based on the clinical presentation, the treatment course, and the long-term objectives for a given patient.

Patients with BPH need considerable education about their disease process, treatment options, and the side effects of medications that may be offered. Newly diagnosed patients will need considerable education surrounding the disease process, the treatment options, and symptom management. Many patients are diagnosed with BPH only after they present in acute urinary retention. Patients in acute urinary retention will need to be catheterized to drain the urine out of the bladder. Some patients will be discharged home with an indwelling Foley catheter and leg bag for several days to allow the bladder to recover and to give medications a chance to work. Other patients may be taught to self-catheterize. Both groups will rely on comprehensive nursing education to manage their catheters and urine output.

Patients who are unresponsive to medical management, or those who have frequent UTIs, develop bladder stones, and/or renal insufficiency may be referred for consideration for surgical intervention. These patients will need education about the planned surgery and specific issues related to the various surgical options (TURP, laser ablation). The details of the management of the indwelling catheter, and the signs and symptoms of infection need to be reviewed in detail. Moreover, patients should be advised that they will, most likely, experience retrograde ejaculation as a consequence of the surgery. This is not dangerous, but it can be alarming for patients who may not be aware of it before they experience it.

Patients opting for medical management of their symptomatic BPH will need education focusing on the various medications and their possible interactions. Caffeine, spicy foods, alcohol, and chronic constipation are all associated with an increase in the severity of LUTS that may be experienced. Nurses should counsel patients to avoid these items. Warm sitz baths may temporarily relieve symptoms of LUTS. Also, avoiding constipation tends to decrease lower urinary tract discomfort, in general.

Patients with BPH or LUTS are encouraged to empty their bladders every 2 to 4 hours. They are advised to restrict fluids after 6 p.m. to reduce the incidence of nocturia. Also, patients with dependent edema are encouraged to wear compression stockings and to elevate their lower extremities well before they go to bed. These maneuvers will help sleep quality.

BPH affects not only patients, but also their partners and families. Chronic illness can be a significant stressor. Nurses must offer patients and families an opportunity to process the complex emotions surrounding this disease.

OUTCOMES

The expected outcomes of evidence-based nursing care for patients with BPH are the prevention of serious consequences associated with the progression of this disease (renal failure, urinary retention, urinary sepsis) so as to increase the patient's quality of life, and decrease the incidence of adverse events, like falls related to nocturia.

Summary

BPH is recognized as a chronic health issue for many men aged 50 years and older. Early intervention and initiation of appropriate nursing care can prevent significant morbidity and result in better quality of life. As the population ages, the incidence of BPH will continue to rise. The symptoms associated with BPH are considerable and contribute to unnecessary suffering. Nursing support and education can help patients to better manage their symptoms to ease their distress and promote compliance with their care plans.

The clinical ramifications of BPH extend far beyond the prostate. In fact, prostate health is essential to men's overall health. Nursing plays a significant role in the successful management of BPH.

Egan, K. B. (2016). The epidemiology of benign prostatic hyperplasia associated with lower urinary tract symptoms: Prevalence and incident rates. *Urologic Clinics of North America, 43*(3), 289–297. doi:10.1016/j.ucl.2016.04.001

Kristal, A. R., Arnold, K. B., Schenk, J. M., Neuhouser, M. L., Weiss, N., Goodman, P., . . . Thompson, I. M. (2007). Race/ethnicity, obesity, health related behaviors and the risk of symptomatic benign prostatic hyperplasia: Results from the prostate cancer prevention trial. *Journal of Urology, 177*(4), 1395–400; quiz 1591. doi:10.1016/j.juro.2006.11.065

Lepor, H. (2005). Pathophysiology of lower urinary tract symptoms in the aging male population. *Reviews in Urology, 7*(Suppl. 7), S3–S11.

Schimke, L., & Schinike, J. (2014). Urological implications of falls in the elderly: Lower urinary tract symptoms and alpha-blocker medications. *Urologic Nursing, 34*(5), 223–229.

Vuichoud, C., & Loughlin, K. R. (2015). Benign prostatic hyperplasia: Epidemiology, economics and evaluation. *Canadian Journal of Urology, 22*(Suppl. 1), 1–6.

■ BLADDER CANCER

Dianna Jo Copley

Overview

Bladder cancer is classified by histological type. The most common type is urothelial carcinoma (previously known as *transitional cell carcinoma*), which is further divided into papillary and flat carcinomas based on the pattern of growth. Other less common types of bladder cancer include adenocarcinoma and squamous cell carcinoma. Bladder cancer is the sixth most common cancer in the United States with men three to four times more likely to develop it in their lifetime than women (American Cancer Society, 2017). Like many other types of cancers, both modifiable and nonmodifiable risk factors can increase a person's likelihood of developing bladder cancer. Nursing care can vary depending on the stage of the cancer and planned interventions. An individual's emotional and psychological well-being, in addition to physiological symptoms related to the bladder cancer and treatments, should be considered.

Background

According to the American Cancer Society, there will be approximately 79,030 new cases and 16,870 deaths related to bladder cancer in 2017. Incidence rates have been declining for both men and women, although bladder cancer deaths decline in women and remain stable in men (American Cancer Society, 2017). Women have a higher mortality rate and are more likely to experience recurrence after treatment (Pozzar & Berry, 2017). Caucasians are diagnosed at a rate twice as often compared to African Americans or Hispanic Americans (American Cancer Society, 2017). Age is another nonmodifiable risk factor, with approximately nine in 10 individuals with bladder cancer older than 55 years (American Cancer Society, 2017).

Smoking tobacco is the most significant modifiable risk factor contributing to an estimated 50% of bladder disease, especially urothelial carcinoma (Chang et al., 2017). Chang et al. (2017) note that current smoking impacts the risk of bladder cancer by a factor of 4.1 and former smokers by a factor of 2.2 compared to individuals who have never smoked. Risk factors, such as second-hand smoke and occupational exposure to carcinogens, contribute to bladder cancer risk (Chang et al., 2017). A history of bladder or other urothelial cancers, family history, and previous exposure to chemotherapy and/or radiation, especially pelvic, can also increase one's risk for bladder cancer (American Cancer Society, 2017). Prevention is aimed at reducing modifiable risk factors. The American Cancer Society (2017) notes that increasing fluids and a diet high in fruits and vegetables may reduce the risk of bladder cancer. Exposure to *Schistosoma haematobium* infection can increase an individual's risk for squamous cell carcinoma of the bladder, but is not common in the United States (Chang et al., 2017).

Staging is separated into clinical and pathological stage and the tumor-node-metastases (TNM) classification that is outlined by the American Joint Committee on Cancer (AJCC) is used (Chang et al., 2016). The clinical stage is based on the physical exam, histologic findings at the time of the transurethral resection of the bladder tumor (TURBT), and radiologic imaging (Chang et al., 2016). Pathological staging is also known as surgical staging and is based on the extent of the disease after surgical removal of the bladder and surrounding lymph nodes (Chang et al., 2016). Stage 0 is noninvasive carcinoma with no lymph node involvement; stage I means that the cancer has grown to the connective tissue, but not the muscle with no lymph node involvement; stage II indicates cancer has penetrated the muscle of the bladder wall with no lymph node involvement; and stage III means the cancer has penetrated the fatty tissue around the bladder and may have spread into the surrounding genitourinary structures, including the prostate, uterus, and vagina but not the pelvic or abdominal wall (American Cancer Society, 2017). Stage IV includes cancer that has penetrated into the pelvic and abdominal wall with or without lymph node involvement and cancer that has metastasized to distant lymph nodes or other organs (American Cancer Society, 2017). Of newly diagnosed bladder cancers, approximately 30% are muscle-invasive (Chou et al., 2016).

Bladder cancer, depending on stage and treatment, can greatly impact an individual's quality of life. Interventions and treatment can impact urinary and bowel function, sexual function, body image, and emotional/mental well-being. Bladder cancer treatment can impact fertility, which should be considered when an individual is making treatment decisions. Individuals with bladder cancer may experience anxiety, fear, and hopelessness related to the diagnosis and prognosis. Survival rate for all stages of bladder cancer at 5 years is approximately 77%; 5-year survival rate for stage 0 is 98%; I is 88%; II is 63%; III is 46%; and IV, which indicates metastasis has occurred, is 15% (American Cancer Society, 2017).

Treatment for bladder cancer varies depending on the stage. Nonmuscle invasive bladder cancer (NMIBC) may be treated with TURBT and/or intravesical therapy (Dunn, 2015). Frequently used medications for intravesical therapy include bacillus Calmette-Guerin (BCG), mitomycin C, and epirubicin (Chang et al., 2016). Muscle-invasive bladder cancer (MIBC) may be treated with a variety of treatment modalities, including surgery, radiation, chemotherapy, or a combination of modalities (Dunn, 2015). Surgical interventions include partial cystectomy, radical cystectomy (removal of bladder, prostate, seminal vesicles in males; bladder, uterus, fallopian tubes, ovaries, and anterior vaginal walls in females), and lymphadenectomy (Chang et al., 2017).

Patients who undergo a radical cystectomy will require a urinary diversion. Urinary diversions include incontinent conduit, continent cutaneous, or orthotopic neobladder. An ileal conduit, the most commonly performed incontinent conduit, consists of a stoma constructed of small intestine with the ureters transplanted into the ileal segment. The urine drains through the stoma created on the abdominal wall and is collected in an external drainage bag. A continent cutaneous diversion requires intermittent catheterization of a stoma on the abdominal wall. The orthotopic neobladder consists of forming a new reservoir for urine with a segment of small intestine; the urethra and ureters are anastomosed to the neobladder allowing normal urination after healing (Merandy, Morgan, Lee, & Scherr et al., 2017).

Individual decision making should be supported when treatments are discussed. Pozzar and Berry (2017) highlight that women are less likely to receive a continent urinary diversion and less likely to undergo lymph node dissection than men with bladder cancer. Including the patient's family and support network as appropriate is an important consideration during the patient's decision-making process (Pozzar & Berry, 2017).

Clinical Aspects

ASSESSMENT

Nursing assessment should begin with a thorough patient history. Signs and symptoms of bladder cancer include microscopic or macroscopic hematuria, frequency, urgency, dysuria, inability to empty the bladder, and pain in more advanced stages. Bladder cancer signs and symptoms can mimic other genitourinary diseases.

Diagnostic tests include urine cytology, urine culture, urine tumor markers, and imaging of the urinary tract (American Cancer Society, 2017). Imaging may include MRI, ultrasound, radiographs, CT, and an intravenous or retrograde pyelogram. A cystoscopy will be performed examining the patient's urethra and bladder (Chang et al., 2016). Nurses should ask patients about their baseline sexual function before treatment is started (Dunn, 2015).

Focused nursing assessment is dependent on the patient's treatment plan. For patients receiving chemotherapy, assessment should include monitoring for infection, including reduced white blood cell (WBC) counts and any adverse reactions to the chemotherapy. Patients who have undergone surgical interventions should be monitored for infection, delays in wound healing, and stoma viability.

NURSING INTERVENTIONS, MANAGEMENT, AND IMPLICATIONS

Nursing-related problems may include acute and/or chronic pain, anxiety, deficient patient knowledge, nausea, risk for bleeding and/or infection, impaired skin integrity, risk for sexual dysfunction, risk for disturbed body image, and risk for dysfunctional gastrointestinal motility. Considerations should always be made for enhanced coping and psychosocial support of the patient and family.

Nursing interventions always include providing support and encouraging verbalization of feelings related to the diagnosis of bladder cancer and treatments. Nurses should support the patient's preference regarding discussing sexual function and sexuality with his or her partner (Dunn, 2015).

OUTCOMES

Patient and family education should focus on the individual's treatment and adapted to accommodate any barriers in learning. For patients undergoing surgical intervention, the nurse should assess the patient's ability for self-care and discharge needs at the preoperative visit. Education should begin immediately as demonstration of self-care is essential to promote independence and reduce risk for readmission.

Summary

Bladder cancer is a diagnosis that individuals need to monitor for the rest of their lives, regardless of the treatment method. Nurses have long been trusted to educate and advocate for patients and are critical for individuals being evaluated for bladder cancer, during treatment, and into survivorship.

American Cancer Society. (2017). Bladder cancer. Retrieved from https://www.cancer .org/cancer/bladder-cancer.html

Chang, S. S., Bochner, B. H., Chou, R., Dreicer, R., Kamat, A. M., Lerner, S. P., . . . Holzbeierlein, J. M. (2017). Treatment of non-metastatic muscle-invasive bladder cancer: AUA/ASCO/ASTRO/SUO guideline. *Journal of Urology, 198*(3), 552–559. doi:10.1016/j.juro.2017.04.086

Chang, S. S., Boorjian, S. A., Chou, R., Clark, P. E., Daneshmand, S., Konety, B. R., . . . McKiernan, J. M. (2016). Diagnosis and treatment of non-metastatic muscle-invasive bladder cancer: AUA/SUO guideline. *Journal of Urology, 196*(4), 1021–1029. doi:10.1016/j.juro.2016.06.049

Chou, R., Selph, S. S., Buckley, D. I., Gustafson, K. S., Griffin, J. C., Grusing, S. E., & Gore, J. L. (2016). Treatment of muscle-invasive bladder cancer: A systematic review. *Cancer, 122*(6), 842–851. doi:10.1002/cncr.29843

Dunn, M. W. (2015). Bladder cancer: A focus on sexuality. *Clinical Journal of Oncology Nursing, 29*(1), 68–73.

Merandy, K., Morgan, M. A., Lee, R., & Scherr, D. S. (2017). Improving self-efficacy and self-care in adult patients with a urinary diversion: A pilot study. *Oncology Nursing Forum, 44*(3), E90–E100. doi:10.1188/17.ONF.E90-E100

Pozzar, R. A., & Berry, D. L. (2017). Gender differences in bladder cancer treatment decision making. *Oncology Nursing Forum, 44*(2), 204–209. doi:10.1188/ 17.ONF.204-209

■ BOWEL OBSTRUCTION

Kelly Ann Lynn
Jane F. Marek

Overview

Bowel obstruction is a complete or partial blockage in either the small or large intestine that prevents the passage of intestinal contents. Patients with bowel obstruction usually have other underlying comorbidities and may present with acute, constant, or intermittent abdominal pain; vomiting; and decrease or absence of bowel activity (flatus and bowel movement). Small bowel obstruction (SBO) accounts for 12% to 16% of U.S. hospital admissions for acute abdominal pain (Paulson & Thompson, 2015). Most patients with SBO are treated conservatively by inserting a nasogastric tube to decompress the bowel. Patients with adhesive SBO who are managed conservatively have a shorter length of stay, but also have a higher recurrence of SBO and higher readmission rates than patients treated surgically (Di Saverio et al., 2013). Failure to promptly diagnose and treat bowel obstruction may result in serious complications, including ischemic bowel, short-gut syndrome, perforation, intra-abdominal abscess, peritonitis, sepsis, and death. Mortality rates associated with SBO are dependent on early recognition and treatment and may be as high as 25% with ischemic bowel or if surgical intervention is delayed (Paulson & Thompson, 2015).

Background

Bowel obstruction can be classified as either nonmechanical/functional or mechanical/physical. Mechanical obstructions occur either inside (intraluminal) or outside of the bowel (extraluminal). Extraluminal obstructions can be due to scar tissue or an intra-abdominal mass compressing the bowel and obstructing the lumen. Functional obstructions result from disruption of the neurovascular supply to the bowel, preventing peristalsis or causing ischemia. Examples of functional bowel obstruction include ileus (most commonly postoperative), use of opioid analgesics, electrolyte imbalances, and mesenteric infarct. Physiologic ileus following abdominal surgery is a normal finding and typically resolves within 48 to 72 hours. Delayed return of gastrointestinal function (over 72 hours) following abdominal surgery is referred to as *postoperative adynamic* or *paralytic ileus* and is due to a variety of factors, including bowel manipulation, surgical trauma, stress response, opioid use, and perioperative interventions (Ge, Chen, & Ding, 2015). Chronic functional bowel obstruction can be caused by a neuromuscular disorder such as Parkinson's disease, diabetes, or Hirschsprung's disease (aganglionic megacolon).

The most common cause of SBO is postoperative intra-abdominal adhesions, accounting for 60% and 70% of all SBO (Di Saverio et al., 2013). Adhesion formation is more common in open than in laparoscopic procedures; other risk factors for abdominal adhesions include colorectal and gynecologic procedures, age older than 60 years, laparotomy within 5 years, and history of abdominal trauma, previous adhesions, or emergency surgery (Loftus et al., 2015). Abdominal adhesions can begin to form within a few hours following surgery. Other causes include hernia, inflammatory bowel disease, volvulus, intussusception, tumor, and adhesions resulting from pelvic inflammatory disease. Large bowel obstruction (LBO) is most frequently related to a neoplastic process, usually colon or ovarian cancer; other causes include strictures, diverticulitis, volvulus, or fecal impaction.

Patients typically present with cramping, intermittent abdominal pain, abdominal distention, nausea, vomiting, and inability to pass stool or flatus. Fever, tachycardia, and peritoneal signs (abdominal rigidity, rebound tenderness) are usually indicative of strangulation and ischemic bowel. Percussion may reveal tympany due to trapped air; bowel sounds are typically hyperactive in the early stages of obstruction as peristalsis attempts to overcome the obstruction; hypoactive or absent bowel sounds occur in the later stages of obstruction. Patients presenting with these symptoms, particularly in combination with history of abdominal or pelvic surgery, malignancy, or treatment with abdominal radiation, need immediate workup to determine the cause and location of the obstruction.

Prompt treatment is essential to prevent complications, particularly ischemic bowel, perforation, peritonitis, and dehydration. Patients without strangulation or ischemia can be managed conservatively with intravenous fluid resuscitation, nasogastric tube decompression, and bowel rest (Loftus et al., 2015). If the obstruction is not relieved within 48 to 72 hours, surgical intervention is recommended. Surgical intervention is indicated for strangulation, ischemia, or tumor; laparoscopic approach is preferred over open technique (Paulson & Thompson, 2015). Conservative management is not indicated for patients with signs of strangulation or peritonitis; these patients should be treated promptly with surgical intervention.

Clinical Aspects

ASSESSMENT

Nursing assessment of patients with a bowel obstruction begins with a comprehensive assessment of the history of present illness and presenting symptoms, surgical history, bowel function, and medication and dietary history. Physical assessment includes assessing vital signs, specifically temperature, blood pressure, and heart rate, to identify early signs of infection and volume depletion and a thorough abdominal assessment, including palpation and percussion of the abdomen. Measuring abdominal girth may be useful to monitor the degree of abdominal distention. It is important to note that flatus or bowel movement may occur before the obstruction is relieved if the stool or gas is below the level of obstruction. Therefore, one must not take bowel movement or flatus as sign of resolution of obstruction; the complete clinical picture must be considered.

Nurses should be alert for signs and symptoms of acute abdomen, including pain upon palpation, tension, rigidity, and increasing distension. Laboratory studies include assessment of the complete blood cell count; the white blood cell count may be elevated with strangulation and the hematocrit may be elevated due to dehydration. Serum lactate levels may be elevated due to dehydration or ischemia; serum chemistry panels should be assessed for electrolyte imbalances and metabolic acidosis. Abdominal x-rays are performed to evaluate for air/fluid levels, free air, distended bowel loops, and gas patterns; CT scan with water-soluble contrast can identify the location of the obstruction and characterize the degree of obstruction.

NURSING INTERVENTIONS, MANAGEMENT, AND IMPLICATIONS

Delayed return of gastrointestinal function following abdominal surgery is a major cause of increased length of stay and morbidity. Nurses can play a key role in preventing postoperative ileus by implementing interventions to promote return of bowel function and identifying patients at risk for developing postoperative ileus. Early ambulation; cautious use of opioid analgesics; frequent abdominal assessment, including auscultating for bowel sounds; and gradual resumption of diet are effective interventions to enhance recovery of GI function. Chewing gum after surgery is thought to enhance return of GI function by cephalic–vagal stimulation, but there is insufficient evidence to support this intervention.

Nursing care of patients with bowel obstruction should focus on resolution of the issue and prevention of serious consequences related to obstruction, specifically dehydration, perforation, peritonitis, and sepsis. Patients should receive information on the available treatment options, including conservative management with nasogastric (NG) tube and bowel rest, endoscopic management, including stenting for LBO, and surgery to relieve the cause of the obstruction. Patients are at risk for developing another bowel obstruction and should receive education to monitor their bowel habits and recognize early signs of recurrence. Education regarding signs of bowel obstruction should be included in the discharge teaching for patients following abdominal and pelvic surgery due to the risk of developing postoperative adhesions.

Nursing interventions will vary, based on the clinical presentation, location, and extent of the obstruction, treatment course, and the long-term objectives for a given patient. All patients will need education about the underlying conditions and various treatment options. It is essential that nurses partner with patients and their families to allow patients to make decisions regarding their treatment options. This is particularly important when caring for patients with bowel obstruction caused by malignancies. Nurses should allow patients and their families the opportunity to express their treatment goals and facilitate the decision-making process to maximize quality of life.

Initial treatment of patients with bowel obstruction begins with conservative symptom management while the diagnostic workup is completed. Patients are not permitted anything by mouth and an NG tube is usually passed and placed to intermittent suction to relieve distention and decompress the bowel. NG tubes should be assessed for placement and patency and oral care is imperative due to nothing per os (NPO) status. Patients are at risk for developing respiratory complications due to increased intra-abdominal pressure, and reluctance to cough and deep breathe often related to abdominal pain. Assessing and monitoring respiratory status and interventions to promote optimal respiratory function is a nursing priority.

Patients with bowel obstruction are at risk for fluid volume and electrolyte imbalance due to dehydration. Dehydration and electrolyte imbalances occur as a result of fluid loss from emesis, bowel edema, and loss of absorptive capacity. Careful assessment and documentation of intake and output (I&O) are essential as patients will require intravenous fluid resuscitation and electrolyte replacement.

Monitoring for infection and peritonitis is another important nursing intervention. Stasis of intestinal contents can result in overgrowth of intestinal flora and may lead to peritonitis. Other nursing interventions include pain management. A comprehensive assessment of symptoms and response to medications and interventions is essential.

OUTCOMES

The expected outcomes of evidence-based nursing care for patients with bowel obstruction are the return of bowel function and prevention of complications.

Summary

Bowel obstruction is a serious health issue that requires prompt intervention and comprehensive nursing care to prevent significant morbidity and adverse outcomes. Nurses must partner with their patients to develop customized care plans to improve health and to prevent complications and recurrence.

Di Saverio, S., Coccolini, F., Galati, M., Smerieri, N., Biffl, W. L., Ansaloni, L., . . . Catena, F. (2013). Bologna guidelines for diagnosis and management of adhesive small bowel obstruction (ASBO): 2013 update of the evidence-based guidelines from the world society of emergency surgery ASBO working group. *World Journal of Emergency Surgery, 8*(1), 42. doi:10.1186/1749-7922-8-42

Ge, W., Chen, G., & Ding, Y.-T. (2015). Effect of chewing gum on the postoperative recovery of gastrointestinal function. *International Journal of Clinical and Experimental Medicine, 8*(8), 11936–11942.

Loftus, T., Moore, F., VanZant, E., Bala, T., Brakenridge, S., Croft, C., . . . Jordan, J. (2015). A protocol for the management of adhesive small bowel obstruction. *Journal of Trauma and Acute Care Surgery, 78*(1), 13–19; discussion 19. doi:10.1097/TA.0000000000000491

Paulson, E. K., & Thompson, W. M. (2015). Review of small bowel obstruction: The diagnosis and when to worry. *Radiologic Society of North America: Radiology, 2*(275), 332–342, doi:10.1148/radiol.15131519

■ BRAIN TUMORS

Peter J. Cebull

Overview

The tissue found in the central nervous system (CNS) is complex and at times is the site of abnormal cellular growth. For many patients, brain tumors represent a feared and often unexpected diagnosis. In 2012, there were 688,000 people living with a primary brain or CNS tumor in the United States. Although the diagnosis of tumor often incites fear of malignancy, the majority of tumors were benign, with only 37% of primary brain tumors in the United States diagnosed as malignant (Ostrom et al., 2015). Providing nursing care for a patient with a brain tumor can be a challenging endeavor that requires an understanding of the prevalence and background behind the diagnosis, as well as a familiarity with the key clinical aspects of this condition.

Background

A brain tumor is tissue in the brain or central spine that has undergone abnormal growth and has the potential to disrupt normal brain function. In 2016, the World Health Organization (WHO) revised the 2007 classification system for CNS tumors. Before this reclassification, tumors were generally defined based on histology. The most recent classification system recommends considering the genetic composition of the tissue through the identification of molecular markers in addition to the histological features. This current system identifies over 120 different types and subtypes of brain and spinal tumors (Louis et al., 2016).

Another important aspect of defining a brain tumor is relative malignancy. Brain tumors that originate from cells found in or near the brain and do not contain cancerous cells are considered benign. Well-defined borders with a lack of involvement of surrounding tissue also characterize benign tumors. The most common nonmalignant brain tumor is meningioma, representing 53.4% of all benign brain tumors diagnosed between 2008 and 2012 (Ostrom et al., 2015). Malignant brain tumors grow more quickly than benign tumors due to the rapid division of cancer cells. The borders of malignant tumors are typically less defined and often spread into surrounding tissue as the tumor grows, rapidly becoming life-threatening (National Brain Tumor Society [NBTS], 2017). The most common malignant brain tumor is glioblastoma (GBM) representing 46.1% of all malignant brain tumors diagnosed between 2008 and 2012 (Ostrom et al., 2015).

Finally, when classifying a brain tumor, it is essential to identify the origin of the cells. Primary brain tumors begin from abnormal cellular growth in brain cells. When malignant, these often spread to other parts of the brain though rarely metastasize to areas outside of the CNS. Secondary brain tumors, also called *metastatic tumors* are the most common type of brain tumor. They begin in cells outside of the CNS and are referred to by their location of origin (National Brain Tumor Society [NBTS], 2017).

In 2016, The Central Brain Tumor Registry of the United States reported a primary CNS tumor incidence rate of 22.36 cases per 100,000 persons in the United States. Of those cases, 7.18 represented malignant tumors. When isolated by gender, females have a higher incidence at 24.46/100,000. In 2017, an estimated 26,070 cases of primary malignant CNS tumors will be diagnosed and an estimated 16,947 deaths will occur (Ostrom et al., 2015).

Five-year survival rates are impacted by several factors. For men with a primary malignant CNS tumor diagnosed between 1995 and 2013, 33.5% survived 5 years following diagnosis, whereas 36.1% of women survived 5 years following the same diagnosis. For nonmalignant CNS tumors diagnosed during this time frame, there was a 90.4% 5-year survival rate (Ostrom et al., 2015). The age of a patient at the time of diagnosis also factors heavily into the likelihood of 4-year survival. There is an inverse correlation between 5-year survival and age of diagnosis of primary malignant CNS tumor. Of patients with primary CNS malignancies, approximately 73.8% of patients aged 0 to 19 years survived to 5 years, whereas 33.5% of patients aged 45 to 54 years survived 5 years following diagnosis. The prevalence of any primary CNS tumor is considerably lower in the 0 to 19 age group, at 35.4 per 100,000 compared to an overall prevalence of 221.8 per 100,000 (Ostrom et al., 2015).

Clinical Aspects

ASSESSMENT

One of the most valuable portions of any assessment is the patient's history. When providing nursing care for a patient diagnosed with a brain tumor, it is beneficial to obtain a history from both the patient and his or her primary caregiver, who is familiar with the patient's most recent signs and symptoms. After the history, the most essential portion of the nurse's assessment is a complete neurologic examination. This establishes critical baseline information on the patient's deficits and aids in identifying the evolution or addition of neurologic deficits.

Neurologic deficits will vary based on the size and location of the brain tumor in relation to the physiologic functions of the affected brain tissue. For example, destruction or distortion of cerebral tissue in the supratentorial (cerebral) region can cause deficits such as memory loss, aphasia, and cognitive impairment. Tumors affecting tissue in the infratentorial (cerebellar) region can cause ataxia and autonomic dysfunction. As a tumor grows and occupies space in the cranial vault, the increase in intracranial pressure (ICP) worsens the deficits. In addition to these specific assessments, appropriate nursing assessment also includes screening for common findings associated with the presence of a brain tumor: visual disturbances such as blurriness, double vision and cuts in the visual fields; alteration of mental status or personality not otherwise explained; nausea and vomiting not explained by other illness or gastrointestinal irritants; onset of seizures; and headaches rated as most severe in the morning with improvement or resolution as the day progresses.

The diagnosis of a brain tumor relies heavily on high-quality neuroimaging. MRI following injection of IV contrast is typically the initial diagnostic choice, to identify the presence or absence of vasculature in a questionable lesion. After diagnosis, CT is often used to evaluate progression of disease and response to interventions. Surgical biopsy is often indicated to gain the necessary histological information needed to make an exact diagnosis and classification based on the WHO grading criteria.

NURSING INTERVENTIONS, MANAGEMENT, AND IMPLICATIONS

Medical interventions for brain tumors can include nonsurgical options, such as chemotherapy and radiation for malignancies, as well as more invasive surgical approaches, for example, craniotomy, tumor excision, or stereotactic radiosurgery. Similarly, nursing-related problems can vary based on the elected medical interventions.

Examples of nursing-related problems associated with the disease process can include communication barriers resulting from aphasia, risk for falls and injuries related to gait ataxia, and maladaptation complicated by changes in cognitive function and personality. Examples of nursing-related problems associated with nonsurgical treatment can include managing the adverse effects of chemotherapy. Surgical treatment can present nursing problems, including risk of infection, postoperative intracranial bleeding, and complications due to swelling of brain tissue.

When addressing the potential problems facing a patient with a brain tumor, there are multiple interventions for nurses to implement. The following are several examples of common problems and appropriate interventions. Aphasia resulting from a tumor affecting the speech centers of the brain can become a barrier to communication. Depending on the expressive or receptive nature, a written-communication board and other nonverbal forms of expression can be offered by a nurse.

High risk for falls is a common complication of gait disturbance with infratentorial tumors. Assistive devices and gait belts reduce this risk, improving safety for both the patient and nurse.

Nausea and vomiting related to chemotherapy are a common, uncomfortable, and even dangerous side effect when uncontrolled. There are many medications used to manage nausea and vomiting associated with chemotherapy, including serotonin receptor (5-HT3) antagonists, steroids, and neurokinin-1 receptor antagonists. Dietary modifications can also be beneficial.

Risk of infection is associated with any surgical procedure, including craniotomy. Postoperatively, the nurse needs to attentively monitor for signs of local and systemic infection in addition to administering prophylactic parenteral antibiotics such as cefazolin (Ancef).

OUTCOMES

Cerebral edema is a common complication of both brain tumors and treatment modalities such as tumor excision or debulking. A nurse must be vigilant in assessing the patient to identify early signs of increased ICP and administering parenteral or oral corticosteroids such as dexamethasone (Decadron) to decrease inflammation.

Summary

The diagnosis of brain tumor can present many challenges to patients and their caregivers. It is important to understand the key features that differentiate benign, malignant, primary, and secondary CNS tumors. Recognizing the relative incidence of this diagnosis as well as the significant mortality associated with primary malignant tumors can inform the nursing process. As a nurse, performing a high-quality assessment is essential to both identify and anticipate the nursing problems associated with this diagnosis.

Louis, D. N., Perry, A., Reifenberger, G., von Deimling, A., Figarella-Branger, D., Cavenee, W. K., . . . Ellison, D. W. (2016). The 2016 World Health Organization classification of tumors of the central nervous system: A summary. *Acta Neuropathologica*, *131*(6), 803–820. doi:10.1007/s00401-016-1545-1

National Brain Tumor Society. (2013). Understanding brain tumors. Retrieved from http://braintumor.org/brain-tumor-information/understanding-brain-tumors

Ostrom, Q. T., Gittleman, H., Fulop, J., Liu, M., Blanda, R., Kromer, C., . . . Barnholtz-Sloan, J. S. (2015). CBTRUS statistical report: Primary brain and central nervous system tumors diagnosed in the United States in 2008–2012. *Neuro-oncology*, *17*(Suppl. 4), iv1–iv62. doi:10.1093/neuonc/nov189

■ CARDIOMYOPATHY

Elsie A. Jolade

Overview

Cardiomyopathies are a diverse group of diseases affecting the myocardium in which the heart muscle becomes abnormally enlarged, thick or rigid, thereby losing the ability to contract effectively with each heartbeat. In rare cases, the myocardium is replaced with scar tissue. As the disease progresses, the heart weakens, leading to heart failure, arrhythmias, and valvular problems (American Heart Association [AHA], 2017). Many cases of cardiomyopathies are idiopathic. The disease can also be secondary to genetic predisposition, infectious diseases, exposure to toxins, systemic connective tissue disease, infiltrative and proliferative disorders, or nutritional deficiencies (McCance & Huether, 2014).

Background

A more thorough understanding and classification system for cardiomyopathy has evolved in the past 50 years. The term was first proposed by Bridges in 1957 as an uncommon, noncoronary heart muscle disease. In 2006, the American Heart Association (AHA) categorized the disease as primary and secondary cardiomyopathies. Primary cardiomyopathies predominantly involve the heart, whereas secondary cardiomyopathies are accompanied by other organ system involvement. Most recent in 2016, the National Heart, Liver, and Blood Institute (NHLBI) placed cardiomyopathy in five categories: as hypertrophic, dilated, restrictive, arrhythmogenic right ventricular, and unclassified cardiomyopathy (NHLBI, 2016).

Hypertrophic cardiomyopathy (HCM) is characterized by enlargement of the myocardial cells and thickening of the walls of the ventricles. Usually the ventricles and septum thicken, creating narrowing or blockages in the ventricles, making it harder for the heart to effectively pump blood. HCM can also cause stiffness of the ventricles, changes in the mitral valve, and cellular changes in the heart tissue (NHLBI, 2016).

HCM is a very common condition and can occur without an obvious cause. It is usually inherited and affects men and women of any age equally (AHA, 2016). Clinical manifestations of HCM include dyspnea and chest pain in the absence of coronary artery disease. Postexertional syncope due to diminished diastolic filling and increased outflow obstruction is also common. Ventricular arrhythmias are common and sudden death may occur, often in athletes after extensive exertion (Porth, 2015).

Dilated cardiomyopathy (DCM) is characterized by progressive cardiac dilation and contractile (systolic) dysfunction (Porth, 2015). DCM occurs in adults 20 to 60 years old; it is more common in men than in women. The disease frequently starts in the left ventricle, where the heart muscle begins to stretch, dilate, and thin, leading to enlargement of the chamber (AHA, 2016). DCM is a common cause of heart failure and the leading indication for heart transplantation. Clinical manifestations include dyspnea, orthopnea, and reduced exercise capacity. As the disease progresses, people in late-stage DCM often have ejection fractions (EF) of less than 25% (normal EF 50%–66%). Thrombosis can form within the chambers of the heart and systemic emboli can occur in late stages of the disease (Porth, 2015).

Restrictive cardiomyopathy (RCM) is a rare form of myocardial disease in which ventricular filling is restricted due to excessive rigidity, but without thickening of the ventricular wall (Porth, 2015). The ventricles are nondilated, though there is impaired ventricular filling. RCM is less common than DCM and HCM and is idiopathic or associated with other disorders such as scleroderma, endomyocardial fibrosis, amyloidosis, and sarcoidosis. The most common clinical manifestation of RCM is right heart failure with systemic venous congestion, cardiomegaly, and dysrhythmias (McCance & Huether, 2014).

Arrhythmogenic right ventricular cardiomyopathy (ARVC), also called *arrhythmogenic right ventricular dysplasia (ARVD)*, is a rare type of cardiomyopathy that occurs when the muscle tissue in the right ventricle is replaced with fatty or fibrous tissue leading to various rhythm disturbances, particularly ventricular tachycardia and, potentially, heart failure. More than 50% of ARVD cases are inherited as an autosomal dominant trait. ARVD ranks second to HCM as the leading cause of sudden cardiac death in young athletes. Clinical manifestations include palpitations, syncope, or cardiac arrest, usually in young- or middle-aged men (McCance & Huether, 2014; NHLBI, 2016).

Other types of cardiomyopathy include peripartum cardiomyopathy (PPCM) and Takotsubo cardiomyopathy. PPCM is a DCM that occurs in an otherwise healthy woman without a previously diagnosed cardiac disorder in the last month of pregnancy and up to 5 months postpartum. PPCM is manifested by signs of systolic dysfunction and heart failure for which there is no identifiable cause or evidence before the last month of pregnancy. It is the fifth leading cause of mortality during pregnancy. Diagnosis of PCCM is often delayed due to overlapping signs and symptoms of other pregnancy-related problems. Incidence is greater in Black, multiparous, or older women with twin fetuses or preeclampsia (McCance & Huether, 2014; Troiano, 2015).

Takotsubo cardiomyopathy, also called *broken heart syndrome*, is a transient reversible left ventricular dysfunction in response to profound psychological or emotional stress characterized by ventricular apical ballooning (McCance & Huether, 2014).

The mean age for onset is older than 60 years, with about 90% of cases occurring in postmenopausal women. Patients present with chest pain, electrocardiographic evidence of ST segment elevation myocardial infarct (STEMI), and impaired myocardial contractility without evidence of coronary disease.

Clinical Aspects

ASSESSMENT

An in-depth history and physical assessment are imperative to recognize, diagnose, and implement appropriate medical interventions early in the disease process. Clinical presentation of cardiomyopathies varies depending on the etiology and severity of the disease. Clinical manifestation, such as dyspnea, ventricular arrhythmias, orthopnea, reduced exercise capacity, syncope, and signs of right heart failure such as elevated jugular venous distension (JVD) and lower extremity edema, tend to occur in most types of the disease. Patients with ARVD typically present with palpitations, syncope, or cardiac arrest in young athletes. A systematic approach to family screening has contributed to better assessment of familial cardiomyopathies and allowed the identification of family members predisposed to disease based on the inheritance of cardiomyopathy-associated genes (Arbustini et al., 2014).

Diagnostic tests for cardiomyopathy include EKG to assess for heart rhythm abnormalities, 2D echocardiography to assess left ventricular EF, and Holter or event monitors to allow continuous monitoring of the heart's electrical activity for a full 24 to 48 hours. Other diagnostics include cardiac MRI to assess the shape and size of the heart, cardiac catheterization, and genetic testing through bidirectional DNA sequence analysis to identify specific gene mutations. Stress testing, chest radiography, and serum blood analysis for cardiac biomarkers are also performed (Porth, 2015).

OUTCOMES

Treatment goals for cardiomyopathy include managing any contributing factors, controlling signs and symptoms, slowing the progression of the disease, and reducing complications and the risk of sudden cardiac death. Methodologies include lifestyle changes, medications, surgical interventions, and implanted devices to prevent or treat arrhythmias.

Patient education focusing on lifestyle changes, such as smoking cessation, weight loss, avoidance of alcohol, stress management strategies, and compliance with the prescribed medication regimen for underlying diseases such as hypertension and diabetes mellitus, are also essential. Nurses traditionally take the lead in patient education; nurse-led interventions can result in a significant improvement in self-management and cardiac knowledge scores (Mackie et al., 2014).

Classes of medications used to treat cardiomyopathy include diuretics to remove excess fluid and reduce preload as well as beta-blockers, calcium channel blockers, and angiotensin-converting enzyme (ACE) inhibitors to control heart rate, reduce blood pressure, and slow the progression of the disease. Patients may be prescribed antiarrhythmics and anticoagulants (AHA, 2016). Some patients may need an automatic implantable cardioverter-defibrillator (AICD), which delivers an electrical impulse or shock to the heart when it senses a life-threatening change in the heart rhythm.

Summary

In conclusion, cardiomyopathy is a very complex disease with various etiologies that affect all ages. Advances in early recognition, diagnosis, and management of cardiomyopathy have resulted in better patient outcomes. An evidence-based approach to care is continually evolving and has improved the quality of life of patients with cardiomyopathy. Because cardiomyopathy often manifests with symptoms similar to heart failure, nurses have and will continue to play a leading role in patient education and other interventions for optimal heart failure management, which are known to contribute to better patient outcomes.

American Heart Association. (2016). What is cardiomyopathy in adults? Retrieved from http://www.heart.org/HEARTORG/Conditions/More/Cardiomyopathy/What -Is-Cardiomyopathy-in-Adults_UCM_444168_Article.jsp#.WIVgVxsrLIU

Arbustini, E., Narula, N., Tavazzi, L., Serio, A., Grasso, M., Favalli, V., . . . Narula, J. (2014). The MOGE(S) classification of cardiomyopathy for clinicians. *Journal of the American College of Cardiology, 3*(64), 304–318.

Mackie, A. S., Islam, S., Magill-Evans, J., Rankin, K. N., Robert, C., Schuh, M., . . . Rempel, G. R. (2014). Healthcare transition for youth with heart disease: A clinical trial. *Heart, 100*(14), 1113–1118. doi:10.1136/heartjnl-2014-305748

McCance, K., & Huether, S. (2014). *Pathophysiology: The biologic basis for disease in adults and children* (7th ed.). New York, NY: Mosby.

National Heart, Lung, and Blood Institute. (2016). Types of cardiomyopathy. Retrieved from https://www.nhlbi.nih.gov/health/health-topics/topics/cm/types#

Porth, C. (2015). *Essentials of pathophysiology* (4th ed.). Philadelphia, PA: Lippincott Williams & Wilkins.

Troiano, N. H. (2015). Cardiomyopathy during pregnancy. *Journal of Perinatal & Neonatal Nursing, 29*(3), 222–228. doi:10.1097/JPN.0000000000000113

■ CHRONIC KIDNEY DISEASE

Mary de Haan

Overview

Chronic kidney disease (CKD) is defined as an abnormality in kidney function or structure lasting longer than 3 months that negatively impacts a person's health (Garcin, 2015; Smith, 2016). Most adults with CKD experience a progressive decrease in kidney function along with kidney damage, ultimately resulting in life-threatening kidney failure. Interdisciplinary management focuses on preventing kidney dysfunction in high-risk populations and delaying disease progression, while preventing or managing complications, in adults diagnosed with CKD (Vassalotti et al., 2016). Nursing care involves timely assessment, evidence-based interventions, health-promoting activities, and self-management education designed to support adults with CKD and members of their support system over the course of their disease.

Background

It is estimated that 26 million adults in the United States have CKD, with over 660,000 requiring life-sustaining renal replacement therapy (RRT), which involves hemodialysis (HD) or peritoneal dialysis (PD) or renal transplantation due to kidney failure (National Kidney Foundation [NKF], 2016; U.S. Renal Data System [USRDS], 2016). Each year in the United States, more deaths are attributed to kidney disease than either breast or prostate cancer (USRDS, 2016). In addition to morbidity and mortality, CKD disease creates a financial burden as well. In 2014, Medicare spending for persons aged 65 years or older with CKD exceeded $50 billion, or 20% of all Medicare spending in that age group (USRDS, 2016). The two principal causes of CKD in adults are diabetes mellitus and hypertension, with nearly half of all adults with CKD experiencing one or both disorders (NKF, 2016). The Centers for Disease Control and Prevention (CDC) estimate that more than 70% of all new cases of kidney failure can be attributed to diabetes and/or hypertension (CDC, 2015). Other disorders that can lead to CKD include chronic glomerulonephritis, polycystic kidney disease, systemic lupus erythematosus, congenital kidney malformations, and repeated acute kidney injury (CDC, 2015; NKF, 2016). Populations at increased risk for developing CKD include older adults (older than 60 years), persons with a family history of kidney disease, and select racial/ethnic groups (African Americans, Hispanics, Native Americans, and Pacific Islanders; CDC, 2015; NKF, 2016).

The diagnosis of CKD is made based on the presence of one or more markers of kidney damage and/or a decrease in estimated glomerular filtration rate (eGFR less than 60 mL/min/1.73 m^2; National Kidney Disease Education Program [NKDEP], 2014; Vassalotti et al., 2016). Markers of kidney damage include albuminuria (defined as greater than 30 mg or urine albumin/gram of urine creatinine for more than 3 months), abnormal urine sediment, disruption of electrolyte and fluid balance, and kidney abnormalities discovered by histology or imaging (NKDEP, 2014; Vassalotti et al., 2016). Although approximately one in 10 adults have some degree of CKD, not all progress to kidney failure (eGFR less than 15 mL/min/1.73 m^2). Adults with high-grade albuminuria, steady decline in eGFR, and poorly controlled blood pressure are more likely to experience disease progression (NKDEP, 2014).

Medical management of adults with CKD focuses on implementing appropriate treatment, monitoring the patient's progress and disease progression, screening for CKD complications, and providing self-management education (NKDEP, 2014). Specific interventions aimed at reducing CKD progression include blood pressure control (lesser than 140/90 mmHg), use of angiotensin-converting enzyme inhibitors (ACEIs) or angiotensin receptor blockers (ARBs) to control hypertension and reduce albuminuria, glycemic control (HbA$_1$C ~7%), and avoidance of nephrotoxic substances, such as nonsteroidal anti-inflammatory drugs (NSAIDs) and iodinated contrast dye (Smith, 2016; Vassalotti et al., 2016). Because cardiovascular disease is the leading cause of death for adults with CKD, cardiac risk factors also need to be addressed and health-promoting interventions initiated (CDC, 2015). These interventions include weight management, diet therapy, implementation of an exercise routine, and, in select cases, the administration of statins (Smith, 2016; Vassalotti et al., 2016).

Adults with severely decreased kidney function (eGFR 15–29 mL/min/1.73 m^2) should receive education regarding approaching kidney failure and treatment options such as RRT, renal transplantation, or conservative treatment, including palliative care (NKF, 2015; Smith, 2016). The decision to initiate RRT (HD or PD) is based on the presence of signs and symptoms of uremia, evidence of protein-energy wasting, and the ability to safely manage complications with medical therapy alone (NKF, 2015).

Patient preference and lifestyle, along with risks and benefits of each form of therapy, should also be considered. HD is the most common form of RRT. It involves the use of a machine to filter a patient's blood through an artificial semipermeable membrane for the purpose of removing waste products and excess fluid and restoring electrolyte balance (National Institute of Diabetes and Digestive and Kidney Diseases [NIDDK], 2016; Winkelman, 2016). HD can be administered at a dialysis center (three times per week for 3 to 5 hours per session) or in the patient's home (five to seven times per week for 2 to 3 hours per session).

Although HD is the most efficient mode of RRT, it does require specially trained personnel to maintain and operate the dialysis machine; patients also need vascular access via a temporary dialysis catheter or arteriovenous (AV) fistula (NIDDK, 2016; NKF, 2015). Potential HD complications include hypotension, blood-borne infections, thrombosis of the AV fistula, and peripheral ischemia (Winkelman, 2016).

PD is used to filter fluids, electrolytes, and waste products from the peritoneum (similar to a semipermeable membrane) into dialysis fluid. This fluid (dialysate) is infused into the peritoneal space via a surgically implanted intra-abdominal silicone catheter.

The fluid is allowed to "dwell" for a prescribed period of time before being drained from the peritoneal space (NIDDK, 2016; Winkelman, 2016). This process is repeated several times within a 24-hour period. Exchanges can be done using continuous ambulatory PD (four to six exchanges with dwell times of 4 to 8 hours occurring 7 days/week) or continuous cycling PD (exchanges occur overnight while the patient is sleeping via an automated cycling machine; NIDDK, 2016). PD allows for greater flexibility of lifestyle and diet, as compared to HD, yet fewer than 10% of adults with kidney failure use this form of RRT.

Potential PD complications include abdominal discomfort, exit site and tunnel infections, and peritonitis (Winkelman, 2016; NIDDK, 2016).

Clinical Aspects

ASSESSMENT

Nursing plays an important role in screening high-risk populations for CKD, especially since kidney disease in its early stages is often asymptomatic (USRDS, 2016). A thorough history from adults at risk for or diagnosed with CKD is critical. It should include personal and family history of kidney injury or disease, cardiovascular disease, diabetes, and/or hypertension. The history should also address medication use (both prescribed and over-the-counter products), dietary habits, tobacco and alcohol usage, and exercise. Physical assessment should focus on cardiopulmonary status (presence of extra heart sounds and/or adventitious breath sounds, presence of dependent edema, reports of dyspnea and/or activity intolerance) and renal function.

Additional symptoms that may be reported in adults with CKD include fatigue, lethargy, difficulty concentrating, anorexia, muscle cramping, and pruritus (NKF, 2016; Smith, 2016). Laboratory testing includes an eGFR, urine albumin-to-creatinine ratio (UACR), serum blood urea nitrogen (BUN) and creatinine, and serum electrolytes (Smith, 2016). Because CKD impacts all body systems, screening for complications such as anemia (complaints of fatigue and dyspnea, decreased red blood cells [RBCs], hemoglobin, hematocrit, and iron stores), malnutrition (unintentional weight loss, muscle wasting, decreased serum albumin), mineral and bone disorders (calcium and phosphorus imbalance), depression, and decreased functional status is also warranted (NKDEP, 2014; Vassalotti et al., 2016).

NURSING INTERVENTIONS, MANAGEMENT, AND IMPLICATIONS

The focus of nursing care for adults with CKD is to manage problems and reduce the effects of complications (Garcin, 2015). Nursing-related problems that need to be addressed include excess fluid volume due to decreased kidney function; decreased cardiac function related to fluid overload and increased peripheral resistance; risk for infection and injury related to skin break-down, falls, vascular access occlusion, or PD catheter site contamination; fatigue related to uremia, anemia, and malnutrition; and impaired psychosocial integrity related to anxiety, depression, and hopelessness associated with the diagnosis of a progressive chronic illness (Winkelman, 2016).

Fluid balance, respiratory status, and cardiac function need to be assessed due to the potential for fluid volume overload, pulmonary edema, and/or heart failure. Interventions should include monitoring intake, output, and patient weight; assessing cardiopulmonary status; maintaining a position of comfort to facilitate adequate ventilation; and administering prescribed medications (diuretics, ACEIs, ARBs) to control blood pressure. Electrolyte imbalances, such as hypo/hypernatremia and hyperkalemia, are common and require diligent monitoring of laboratory values, heart rate and rhythm, and neurological status (Smith, 2016; Winkelman, 2016).

Infection is a potentially life-threatening occurrence for adults with CKD. Uremic pruritus can lead to excoriation and skin breakdown, whereas dialysis access devices offer routes of entry to pathogens. Patients need to be monitored for fever, malaise, and evidence of skin breakdown, redness, or edema—particularly at the dialysis access insertion sites. Sterile technique should be used whenever an HD vascular access device or PD catheter is in use.

Nutritional needs, including fluid balance, glycemic control, protein and phosphorus intake, and sodium/potassium balance, should be discussed in collaboration with a registered dietician (Garcin, 2015; Winkelman, 2016).

Psychosocial support and self-management education should be offered to all adults with CKD and members of their immediate support system. Support should include providing information regarding the CKD diagnosis, anticipated disease progression, and treatment options, as well as referral to counseling services and support groups (Winkelman, 2016; NKDEP, 2014).

OUTCOMES

Adults with CKD should maintain adequate cardiac function and optimal fluid and electrolyte balance. Nutritional needs should be met in order to maintain an adequate protein–calorie intake, regardless of the dietary restrictions that may be recommended based on their degree of kidney function. Adults with CKD should avoid injury and infection and should be involved in health-promoting activities designed to prevent or delay the progress of CKD and its complications.

Psychosocial and educational needs should be evaluated and effective coping mechanisms supported by all members of the interdisciplinary care team. Effective nursing care applies principles of patient-centered care, teamwork, collaboration, and communication to address each of these evidence-based expected outcomes (NKDEP, 2014; Winkelman, 2016).

Summary

Adults diagnosed with CKD must cope with a number of uncertainties in terms of physical, psychosocial, and lifestyle changes they will face. Nurses, as members of the interdisciplinary team focused on preventing or delaying the progression of CKD and its associated complications, play a vital role in providing evidence-based care, health-promoting activities, and education to provide support throughout the course of the disease.

Centers for Disease Control and Prevention. (2015). Chronic kidney disease issue brief. Retrieved from http://www.cdc.gov/diabetes/pdfs/progress/CKDBrief.pdf

Garcin, A. (2015). Care of the patient with chronic kidney disease. *MedSurg Matters, 24*(5), 4–7.

National Institute of Diabetes and Digestive and Kidney Diseases. (2016). Kidney disease education lesson builder: Choices for treatment of kidney failure. Retrieved from https://www.niddk.nih.gov/health-information/health-communication-programs/nkdep/a-z/Documents/ckd-primary-care-guide-508.pdf

National Kidney Disease Education Program. (2014). *Making sense of chronic kidney disease: A concise guide for managing CKD in the primary care setting* (NIH pub No. 14-7989).

National Kidney Foundation. (2015). KDOQI clinical practice guideline for hemodialysis adequacy: 2015 update. *American Journal of Kidney Disease, 66*(5), 884–930.

National Kidney Foundation. (2016). About chronic kidney disease. Retrieved from http://kidney.org/kidneydisease/aboutckd

Smith, C. A. (2016). Evidence-based treatment of chronic kidney disease. *Nurse Practitioner, 41*(11), 42–48. doi:10.1097/01.NPR.0000502790.65984.61

U.S. Renal Data System. (2016). *2016 USRDS annual data report: Epidemiology of kidney disease in the United States.* Bethesda, MD: National Institutes of Health, National Institute of Diabetes and Digestive and Kidney Diseases.

Vassalotti, J., Centor, R., Turner, B., Greer, R., Choi, M., Sequist, T.; National Kidney Foundation Kidney Disease Outcomes Quality Initiative. (2016). Practical approach to detection and management of CKD for the primary care clinician. *American Journal of Medicine, 129*(2), 153–162.

Winkelman, C. (2016). Care of patients with acute kidney injury and chronic kidney disease. In D. Ignatavicius & M. Workman (Eds.) *Medical surgical nursing: Patient-centered collaborative care* (8th ed., pp. 1411–1447). Philadelphia, PA: Elsevier.

■ CHRONIC OBSTRUCTIVE PULMONARY DISEASE

Christina M. Canfield

Overview

The Global Initiative for Chronic Obstructive Lung Disease (GOLD) defines chronic obstructive pulmonary disease (COPD) as a "common, preventable and treatable disease that is characterized by persistent respiratory symptoms and airflow limitation that is due to airway and/or alveolar abnormalities usually caused by significant exposure to noxious particles or gases" (GOLD, 2017, p. x). Disease severity is influenced by exacerbations and comorbidities. COPD causes significant morbidity and mortality worldwide. Cigarette smoking is a well-known risk factor for development of COPD.

Background

It is estimated that more than 380 million people are living with COPD worldwide. COPD was responsible for 3 million deaths in 2012 and is projected to be the third leading cause of death by 2020 (GOLD, 2017). An estimated $52 billion is spent on care of the individual with COPD annually in the United States. In developing countries, the economic burden shifts from direct and indirect medical costs to lost workplace and home productivity. In addition, COPD contributes to significant disability worldwide.

Exposure to cigarette smoke is the most widely known cause of COPD. However, genetic factors, such as hereditary alpha-1 antitrypsin deficiency, predispose individuals to development of COPD. Additional risk factors include occupational exposure to chemicals, dust, fumes, and air pollution. Previously, men were more likely to be diagnosed with COPD than women. However, women are just as likely to develop COPD as males (GOLD, 2017). Individuals who experienced conditions that affected lung growth during gestation and childhood may be more likely to develop COPD than those who did not.

Inflammation of the lung and airways is a normal response when exposed to cigarette smoke or other noxious agents. Chronic inflammation may cause destruction of the lung tissue and disrupt the physiologic mechanisms that normally repair the lungs. These changes lead to reduced airway diameter and lung fibrosis. Airway changes lead to trapping of gas during expiration. Reduced expiratory volume is noted during spirometry. Patients with COPD have a reduction in forced expiratory volume (FEV) when expiration is measured over 1 second. This measurement is called FEV_1. In addition to airway changes, increased effort to breathe may lead to retention of carbon dioxide (GOLD, 2017).

COPD is a chronic, progressive disease that is characterized by periods of worsening symptoms, or exacerbations. Exacerbations may be triggered by infection, pollutants, or exposure to respiratory irritants. Patients experience more severe symptoms during an exacerbation and may require hospitalization.

All patients who complain of shortness of breath, chronic cough, or sputum production should be evaluated for COPD, regardless of risk factor exposure. A cough productive of sputum is seen in up to one third of patients (GOLD, 2017). The patient will undergo testing via spirometry to determine the extent of airflow limitation. Criteria for severity of airflow limitation in COPD may be classified as mild, moderate, severe, or very severe according to spirometry criteria defined by the GOLD (2017).

COPD often presents as one part of a complex patient health picture. Up to 40% of patients diagnosed with COPD may also be affected by heart disease (Grindrod, 2015). Other associated conditions include diabetes, hypertension, osteoporosis, and depression.

Medical management of COPD often involves the use of inhaled medications. A combination of long- and short-acting inhalers may be used to optimize therapy. Patients require significant instruction to ensure proper use of inhaled medications and individual administration technique should be assessed before changing medication or assuming a therapy is not effective (GOLD, 2017).

Clinical Aspects

ASSESSMENT

The nurse should suspect COPD in patients who present with complaints of progressive dyspnea, cough, and mucus production. Dyspnea is thought to be a better predictor of mortality than FEV and should be assessed during each encounter. It is recommended that facilities adopt a dyspnea or breathlessness rating scale to ensure consistency among assessments (Miller, Owens, & Silverman, 2015). Assess for risk factors, including cigarette smoking, exposure to secondhand cigarette smoke, or occupational exposure. Other diseases that mimic the symptoms of COPD include tuberculosis, asthma, congestive heart failure, and interstitial lung disease.

Physical assessment findings may include the following:

- Use of accessory muscles
- Changes in chest shape
- Cyanosis due to impaired arterial oxygenation
- Clubbing of the fingers
- Crackles or wheezes upon auscultation
- Cough productive of sputum
- Weight loss or signs of malnutrition

NURSING INTERVENTIONS, MANAGEMENT, AND IMPLICATIONS

Nursing management of the patient with COPD includes frequent observations of physiologic and mental status. Changes in respiratory function may be reflected via pulse oximetry, laboratory results (i.e., arterial blood gas), and mental status assessment. The nurse must recognize changes in status and consider indications of impending or actual respiratory failure or worsening disease.

Patients with COPD are likely to experience imbalanced nutrition due to high calorie expenditure caused by systemic inflammation and increased work of breathing (Hodson, 2016).

Nursing-related problems and the patient-specific plan of care should include consideration of oxygen imbalance, inadequate respiration, altered nutrition, activity intolerance, and risk for infection.

Nursing interventions include vital sign monitoring with frequent monitoring of oxygenation, administration of oxygen as ordered, assessment of dyspnea and signs of respiratory distress, medication management with oral or inhaled medications and oral or intravenous antibiotics, and education of the patient and significant other(s). Initiate appropriate nutritional screening and obtain consultation as indicated. Discharge planning includes anticipation of use of oxygen at home, need for assistive devices, and identification of challenges in obtaining or paying for medications.

OUTCOMES

Expected outcomes for any patient with COPD include activity tolerance, maintenance of adequate oxygenation, adequate nutrition, and adherence to prescribed medication regimen.

Following an exacerbation, expected outcomes include increased tolerance of activity, stable vital signs, absence of signs and symptoms of active infection, decreased sputum production, and a return to baseline oxygen requirements. Research has demonstrated that patients who receive the influenza vaccine experience a significant reduction in the number of COPD exacerbations when compared to those who do not receive the vaccine (GOLD, 2017). Evidence of the effectiveness of the pneumococcal vaccine is limited but it remains recommended for all patients aged 65 years and older (GOLD, 2017).

Summary

COPD is a preventable and treatable disease that often exists as a comorbidity with other diseases. Effective management of COPD includes medication, nutrition, preservation of physical function, and infection prevention. Assess for smoking during every patient encounter and encourage smoking cessation in those who actively smoke. Cessation of smoking is beneficial and may slow progression of the disease.

Global Initiative for Chronic Obstructive Lung Disease. (2017). Global initiative for chronic obstructive lung disease—Global strategy for the diagnosis, management and prevention of COPD. Retrieved from http://goldcopd.org/gold-2017-global-strategy-diagnosis-management-prevention-copd

Hodson, M. (2016). Integrating nutrition into pathways for patients with COPD. *British Journal of Community Nursing, 21*(11), 548–552. doi:10.12968/bjcn.2016.21.11.548

Miller, S., Owens, L., & Silverman, E. (2015). Physical examination of the adult patient with chronic respiratory disease. *MedSurg Nursing, 24*(3), 195–198.

■ COLORECTAL CANCER

Visnja Maria Masina
Crina V. Floruta

Overview

Colorectal cancer is the most common type of gastrointestinal cancer. Colorectal cancer is defined as the presence of a malignant mass of cells affecting the tissue of the large bowel (colon) or rectum. The etiology of colorectal cancer is multifactorial, involving genetic, environmental, and inflammatory factors that incite a sporadic genetic mutation in the gland cells of the epithelial lining of the affected tissue. These sporadic mutations of the colorectal tissue may result in dysregulated growth that can produce a malignant growth or tumor. Nurses play a key in role in helping patients understand their risk for colorectal cancer, strategies to minimize their risk and to detect early stages of the colorectal cancer, which is curable.

Background

Colorectal cancer is considered a disease of Western society; the incidence is relatively high in industrialized countries and low in less developed countries, such as those in Africa and Asia. In the United States, colorectal cancer is the third most common cause of cancer deaths following lung, prostate, and breast cancer in both men and women. The epidemiologic pattern of colorectal cancer suggests that diet and environmental factors play a major role in the pathogenesis of colorectal cancer (American Cancer Society [ACS], 2017).

Mortality rates have declined steadily in the past three decades, likely due to more effective screening programs and improvements in available treatment modalities. Trends in the declining incidence differ by age; however, for unknown reasons since 1992 there has been a 1.8% increase in the incidence of colorectal cancer in adults younger than age 50 years (ACS, 2017). In the United States, an estimated 95,520 new cases of colon cancer and 39,910 new cases of rectal cancer are expected to be diagnosed in 2017 (ACS, 2017).

The risk of colorectal cancer increases with age. Colorectal cancer occurs less frequently before age 40 years; 90% of cases occur after 50 years of age. The lifetime risk of developing colorectal cancer in the United States is approximately 5%. In addition to living in a Western society, risk factors for colorectal cancer include hereditary conditions such as familial adenomatous polyposis (FAP), inherited genetic conditions such as Lynch syndrome also known as *hereditary nonpolyposis colorectal cancer syndrome (HNPCC),* ulcerative colitis or Crohn's colitis (more than 10 years), personal or family history of colon polyps or cancer, and type 2 diabetes mellitus. Modifiable factors that increase risk for colorectal cancer include obesity, physical inactivity, long-term smoking, high consumption of red or processed meat, low calcium intake, moderate to heavy alcohol consumption, and very low intake of fruits and vegetables (ACS, 2017).

With early detection, colorectal cancer is a preventable and highly curable disease. Early-stage colorectal cancer is typically asymptomatic, making screening necessary to detect disease early. Whatever the causative factors, most colorectal cancers and adenocarcinomas in particular, thought to develop from adenomatous or serrated polyps. Although not all polyps progress to cancer, the evidence supports that most colorectal cancers arise from polyps. It is widely accepted that colorectal cancer-related morbidity and mortality can be reduced through early detection, removal of small polyps, and treatment of early-stage disease. National organizations, including the American Cancer Society (ACS), American Society for Gastrointestinal Endoscopy (ASGE), the National Comprehensive Cancer Network (NCCN), and American College of Gastroenterology (ACG) have established screening guidelines for average and increased-risk individuals. Routine screening for colorectal cancer and adenomatous polyps is recommended for asymptomatic adults aged 50 years and older. However, the individual's age and history should inform the frequency and mode of screening for colorectal cancer. Of all the screening methods for colorectal cancer, colonoscopy is considered the gold-standard screening modality.

Clinical Aspects

ASSESSMENT

Colon and rectal cancers are frequently conjoined but each tissue has distinct patterns of presentation, staging, and management of affected malignant tissue. Colon cancer can be categorized as right-sided or left-sided lesions. Abdominal pain, palpation of a mass on the right side, change in bowel habits, anemia, and weight loss are symptoms of ascending (right-sided) colon cancer. Pain, change in bowel habits, hematochezia, and bowel obstruction are symptoms characteristic to descending or left-sided colon cancer.

The evaluation of colon cancer includes complete history and physical examination; colonoscopy; laboratory studies, including complete blood count (CBC) to evaluate for anemia, basic metabolic panel (BMP) and liver function testing; and carcinoembryonic antigen (CEA), which has been found to provide some prognostic information and is used during surveillance. The tumor, node, and metastasis framework is used for staging colorectal cancer. Initial staging is done through radiographic imaging such as CT scans of chest, abdomen, and pelvis. MRI of the liver or PET scans are reserved for when metastatic lesions are suspected. Treatment options for colorectal cancer are dependent on the stage at diagnosis. Early-stage colorectal cancer is treated surgically; the majority of stage I and II cancers are curable by surgical resection. A combination of surgery, chemotherapy, and radiation are used to manage stage III and IV diseases. Patients are followed at regular intervals up to 5 years from the diagnosis to monitor recuperation and detect any evidence of recurrent disease.

Symptoms of rectal cancer include bright red blood mixed in stool, rectal bleeding, and change in bowel habits and or shape of stool, tenesmus, fatigue, anemia, and unintentional weight loss. Timely evaluation of symptoms is essential. In addition to the evaluation for colon cancer, patients with suspected rectal cancer undergo MRI of the pelvis for locoregional staging and a flexible or rigid proctoscopy to verify the location of the tumor in relation to the anal verge. Locally advanced rectal cancers (stage II and III) are treated through a multidisciplinary treatment approach consisting of neoadjuvant chemoradiation therapy, followed by surgical resection, and adjuvant chemotherapy.

OUTCOMES

Nurses play an important role in educating the public in recognizing early signs of colorectal cancer and following recommended screening guidelines. Nurses play an integral role in supporting and educating patients with colorectal cancer by being knowledgeable regarding risk factors, signs and symptoms, disease course, and current and emerging therapies. Timely patient–family education may minimize anxiety and promote compliance and self-management.

For patients undergoing surgical resection in whom formation of a stoma is possible, consultation with a wound ostomy and continence (WOC) nurse is beneficial. Choosing an appropriate stoma site, teaching stoma care, and counseling about living with a stoma makes the postoperative course smoother with less complications. Topics discussed at this initial visit include anatomy; stoma function and appearance; emptying and changing of the pouch system; obtaining supplies; and activities of daily living, including bathing/showering, diet, clothing, and sexuality (Mahoney, 2016).

Summary

Prevention and early detection are key to curing colorectal cancers. Nurses play a fundamental role in educating and supporting patients about a sensitive topic and helping individuals understand the importance of screening. If a diagnosis of cancer is made, the nurse plays a pivotal role in the patient's cancer treatment journey.

American Cancer Society. (2017). *Cancer facts and figures.* Atlanta, GA: Author.

Mahoney, M. (2016). Preoperative preparation of patients undergoing a fecal or urinary diversion. In J. Carmel, J. Colwell, & M. Goldberg (Eds.), *Wound, ostomy and continence nurses society core curriculum: Ostomy management* (pp. 99–112). Philadelphia, PA: Wolters Kluwer.

■ CORONARY ARTERY DISEASE IN ADULTS

Kate Cook
Mary T. Quinn Griffin

Overview

Coronary artery disease (CAD), defined clinically as a blockage or narrowing of the coronary vessels that impedes blood flow, is a common form of cardiovascular disease in adults. The disease continues to be a leading cause of death in the United States, claiming 385,000 lives annually (Ramos, 2014). CAD is the number one cause of death across ethnic groups in both developed and developing countries worldwide; thus it is considered a global crisis (Assimes & Roberts, 2016). There are a number of modifiable and nonmodifiable risk factors that identify patients at greatest risk for developing CAD. Initial nursing efforts must focus on accurate assessment of risk stratification and alteration of all modifiable risk factors identified. Patient management varies as a patient's disease progresses, and is depending on related clinical manifestations.

Background

The obstruction in blood flow associated with CAD is due to atherosclerosis, which occurs when fatty substances build up over time, forming a plaque that hardens the walls of the arterial blood vessels. Atherosclerosis begins when the innermost layer of the arterial vessels, the endothelium, is repeatedly subjected to injury. In response to this damage within the vessels, inflammatory processes occur, which, in turn, change the structure and biochemistry of the arterial walls. Macrophages are produced and transport lipids inside the walls of the arteries. Smooth muscle migrates into the areas of fatty accumulation, forming a plaque that may protrude into the vessel opening. Depending on the thickness of the plaque, this protrusion may be enough to restrict blood flow, causing ischemia. Plaques on the vessel walls are vulnerable to rupture, which can result in the sudden formation of a thrombus. A thrombus in a coronary vessel leads to obstruction of blood flow, and the potential for complications such as acute coronary syndrome or a myocardial infarction.

A variety of risk factors may, in combination, inflict the initial injury to the walls of the coronary vessels. Modifiable risk factors include elevated serum lipid levels, tobacco use, hypertension, diabetes mellitus, obesity, sedentary lifestyle, and stress. Nonmodifiable risks associated with CAD include age, family history of CAD, ethnicity, and gender. African Americans have a higher incidence of CAD than other racial groups. In terms of gender, males tend to have a higher likelihood of developing CAD at an earlier age when compared to females. Recent evidence suggests that the presence of high blood pressure, obesity, and high cholesterol have a similar effect on CAD-related outcomes in men and women. Prolonged tobacco use, however, is more hazardous to women. Women who have a history of specific pregnancy complications (such as preeclampsia or gestational diabetes), polycystic ovary disease, or early-onset menopause are at higher risk for morbidity and mortality related to CAD.

Patient teaching focuses on educating patients regarding prevention and management of modifiable risk factors. Collaborative management of patients with CAD varies greatly depending on physical manifestations and disease severity. Common interventions include pain management, pharmacological therapy, percutaneous coronary intervention (stenting), and coronary artery bypass graft.

Clinical Aspects

ASSESSMENT

In the absence of physical symptoms, such as angina pectoris, clinicians must rely on an accurate health history, risk assessment tools, and the observance of unexpected findings in the physical assessment to detect CAD. A three-generation family history and information related to age of onset of any known cases of CAD is useful in determining a patient's heritable risk (Assimes & Roberts, 2016). For patients who have not been diagnosed, risk factor assessment is a critical component of identifying patients at greatest risk. The American College of Cardiology and the American Heart Association recommend use of the Pooled Cohort Equations risk assessment scale to estimate the 10-year risk of atherosclerotic cardiovascular disease in patients (Goff et al., 2014). This scale uses an algorithm based on an individual's gender, age, race, total cholesterol laboratory values, along with history of hypertension, smoking, and diabetes to determine an individual's risk classification. The scale has been validated for use in both White and African American men and women.

A thorough physical assessment should be performed. Cardiovascular assessment related to decreased coronary perfusion, such as accurate blood pressure measurement in both arms, ankle–brachial index, heart rate, respiratory rate, pulse oximetry, capillary refill, and the quality and rhythm of bilateral pulses should be performed. Neck veins should be examined for distention, and the heart and lungs should be auscultated for adventitious sounds, indicative of fluid volume excess. The skin and mucous membranes should be assessed for color, temperature, and the presence of moisture.

Various laboratory tests are useful in determining a patient's risk for development of CAD. A fasting lipid profile (total cholesterol, low- and high-density lipoproteins, and triglycerides) is often performed to establish a baseline for patients. The information gained from this profile can be used to preventatively treat patients without CAD who are known to be at risk or to proactively treat patients diagnosed with CAD and reduce the chances of progression. C-reactive protein (CRP) is a measure of the level of inflammation in the body, and is considered a marker for cardiovascular risk. Elevated brain natriuretic peptide (BNP) and homocysteine levels are biomarkers associated with an increased risk for CAD and may be used as part of the diagnostic evaluation. Patients diagnosed with metabolic syndrome for diabetes are inherently at higher risk for cardiac disease. Therefore, fasting plasma glucose and hemoglobin A1c are also common diagnostic screenings.

There are several noninvasive imaging studies commonly associated with the detection of CAD. Exercise (for patients physically able to exercise) or pharmacological (if exercise is contraindicated) stress tests are often performed to determine the presence of ischemia (Ramos, 2014). If patients are asymptomatic but have a significant family history of CAD or a diagnosis of diabetes mellitus, a nuclear stress test may be useful in detecting disease. CT angiograms (CTAs) have the ability to visualize the coronary arteries and are a noninvasive method to detect the presence and severity of plaque in the vessel walls (Ramos, 2014).

NURSING INTERVENTIONS, MANAGEMENT, AND IMPLICATIONS

Nursing interventions, such as education, support, and behavioral counseling, have been proven effective in assisting patients diagnosed with or at risk for developing CAD. These interventions, however, can involve a costly and time-consuming process, and there is some debate regarding the proper methods for going about these interventions (Saffi, Polanczyk, & Rabelo-Silva, 2014). Behavioral counseling and education should be focused on modifiable risk factors that are placing patients at greater risk. Nurses can connect patients with community resources, such as weight management, exercise, and smoking cessation programs, which provide individuals with education, support, and accountability (Lachman et al., 2015).

Advances in treatment and cardioprotective medications have led to a recent decline in hospitalizations and mortality for patients with ischemic disease. Adherence to these medication regimens is critical for control of CAD-related symptoms; therefore, medication nonadherence could be considered a modifiable risk factor for complications (Lourenço et al., 2014). Nurse-conducted interventions for outpatients aimed at reinforcing the importance of prescribed treatments and identifying individual barriers to adherence to protocols appear to promote positive health behavior changes in clients.

OUTCOMES

Expected outcomes related to CAD vary depending on the clinical manifestations of the disease, as well as each patient's genetic risk and adherence to treatment protocols. Recent studies have shown that for patients at high genetic risk, management of modifiable risk factors is associated with a 50% lower risk of CAD (Khera et al., 2016). Therefore, nursing goals should focus on adherence to prescribed treatment and modification of risk factors in order to prevent disease progression and limit complications.

Summary

CAD is a broad term used to describe conditions that lead to blocked blood flow within the vessels that supply blood, oxygen, and nutrition to the heart. Patients diagnosed and treated for CAD are at high risk for reoccurrence and mortality. Genetic and modifiable lifestyle factors have long since been associated with susceptibility to this disease. Most recent, human genome studies based on an individual's genetic makeup have the potential ability to determine persons at highest risk for developing CAD as well as individuals who will best respond to therapy (Assimes & Roberts, 2016). Early identification and treatment of patients with CAD will lead to an increased quality of life for these patients coupled with decreased morbidity and mortality in this patient population.

Assimes, T. L., & Roberts, R. (2016). Genetics: Implications for prevention and management of coronary artery disease. *Journal of the American College of Cardiology, 68*(25), 2797–2818. doi:10.1016/j.jacc.2016.10.039

Goff, D. C., Jr., Lloyd-Jones, D. M., Bennett, G., Coady, S., D'Agostino, R. B., Gibbons, R., . . . Tomaselli, G. F. (2014). 2013 ACC/AHA guideline on the assessment of cardiovascular risk: A report of the American College of Cardiology/American Heart Association Task Force on Practice Guidelines [published correction appears in *Circulation, 129*(Suppl. 2), S74–S75]. *Circulation, 129*(Suppl. 2), S49–S73. doi:10.1161/01.cir.0000437741.48606.98

Khera, A. V., Emdin, C. A., Drake, I., Natarajan, P., Bick, A. G., Cook, N. R., . . . Kathiresan, S. (2016). Genetic risk, adherence to a healthy lifestyle, and coronary disease. *New England Journal of Medicine, 375*(24), 2349–2358. doi:10.1056/NEJMoa1605086

Lachman, S., Minneboo, M., Snaterse, M., Jorstad, H. T., Ter Reit, G., Scholte Op Reimer, W. J.; Response 2 Study Group. (2015). Community-based comprehensive lifestyle programs in patients with coronary artery disease: Objectives, design and expected results of Randomized Evaluation of Secondary Prevention by Outpatient Nurse Specialists 2 trial (RESPONSE 2). *American Heart Journal, 170*(2), 216–222. doi:10.1016/j.ahj.2015.05.010

Lourenço, L. B., Rodrigues, R. C., Ciol, M. A., São-João, T. M., Cornélio, M. E., Dantas, R. A., & Gallani, M. C. (2014). A randomized controlled trial of the effectiveness of planning strategies in the adherence to medication for coronary artery disease. *Journal of Advanced Nursing, 70*(7), 1616–1628. doi:10.1111/jan.12323

Ramos, L. M. (2014). Cardiac diagnostic testing: What bedside nurses need to know. *Critical Care Nurse, 34*(3), 16–27; quiz 28. doi:10.4037/ccn2014361

Saffi, M. A., Polanczyk, C. A., & Rabelo-Silva, E. R. (2014). Lifestyle interventions reduce cardiovascular risk in patients with coronary artery disease: A randomized clinical trial. *European Journal of Cardiovascular Nursing, 13*(5), 436–443. doi:10.1177/1474515113505396

■ CUSHING SYNDROME

Yolanda Flenoury
Jane F. Marek

Overview

The adrenal glands are an important part of the endocrine system and produce and secrete glucocorticoids, mineralocorticoids, and androgens. Cortisol, sometimes referred to as the stress hormone, is an adrenal glucocorticoid hormone regulated by the hypothalamus–pituitary–adrenal (HPA) axis. Cortisol is essential to homeostasis and regulates the body's physiologic response to stress, including maintaining blood glucose levels, immune response, blood pressure, and protein, carbohydrate, and fat metabolism. In 1912, Harvey W. Cushing identified the relationship between certain physical characteristics and a tumor in the pituitary gland, which became known as Cushing disease. Cushing syndrome, characterized by excess cortisol levels, refers to patients with the classic signs and symptoms described by Cushing, but the cause of the excess cortisol is not restricted to adrenocorticotropic hormone (ACTH)-secreting pituitary tumors.

Background

Cushing syndrome is estimated to affect 10 to 15 million people annually in the United States. The disease is more common in women than men and the median age at diagnosis is approximately 41 years (Lacroix, Feelders, Stratakis, & Nieman, 2015). Patients with active untreated Cushing syndrome have a mortality rate 1.7 to 4.8 times higher than the general population (Neiman et al., 2015). Most of the cases of Cushing syndrome are caused by the use of exogenous glucocorticoids, such as prednisone, used to treat other medical conditions. The majority of cases unrelated to steroid use are a result of ACTH-secreting pituitary adenomas. Less common causes of Cushing syndrome are adrenal tumors responsible for the excess release of cortisol, ectopic ACTH-secreting tumors associated with certain malignancies, and family history (Neiman et al., 2015).

Clinical manifestations of Cushing syndrome vary depending on the cause and duration of the excess cortisol levels. The typical manifestations of Cushing syndrome include central obesity with thin arms and legs, rounded or "moon" face, excess fat behind the neck and upper back, and weight gain (Quinn, 2016). Other manifestations include fatigue, mood swings, depression, increased thirst and urine output, amenorrhea, acanthosis on the neck, ruddy complexion, acne, thin skin that is easily bruised, hirsutism, and prominent purple striae on the abdomen, breasts, hips, and axilla (Urrets-Zavalía et al., 2016). On physical examination, patients with Cushing syndrome often have elevated blood pressure, muscle atrophy, and muscle weakness.

Diagnosis is based on the patient's history, presenting symptoms, laboratory tests, and imaging. No single laboratory test is specific for Cushing syndrome. The three laboratory tests recommended by the Endocrine Society are the 24-hour urine-free cortisol, late-night salivary cortisol, and the low-dose dexamethasone suppression test (Lacroix et al., 2016). The late-night salivary cortisol level is commonly used for initial screening and can be done at home by the patient at bedtime. Other tests to aid in diagnosis include midnight plasma cortisol levels, corticotropin-releasing hormone stimulation test, and a high-dose dexamethasone suppression test. Once the diagnosis of Cushing syndrome has been established, serum testing of morning ACTH levels is performed to differentiate between Cushing disease and ectopic ACTH syndrome. CT scans and/or MRI may be used to identify the location of the tumor causing the increased cortisol levels (Raff & Carroll, 2015).

Treatment for patients with Cushing syndrome depends on the etiology. Patients with Cushing syndrome related to steroid use who cannot be treated with other medications will generally have the dose reduced to diminish Cushing symptoms, but still treat their primary disease. There are several treatments for patients with ACTH-secreting pituitary tumors. The goal of surgical intervention for Cushing syndrome is removal of the tumor on the pituitary or adrenal gland. Endoscopic transsphenoidal surgery (microadenectomy or hypophysectomy) allows removal of the pituitary tumor without disrupting overall pituitary functioning (Neiman et al., 2015; Raff & Carroll, 2014). Many patients will eventually have normal HPA function, but pituitary function may be affected following extensive surgical resection. Patients who have had unsuccessful surgeries or who are not surgical candidates may be treated with radiation (Neiman et al., 2015). Pituitary radiation is effective for only approximately 40% to 50% of patients; unfortunately it may take months to years for patients to report an improvement in their symptoms. Medications can be used alone or in conjunction with surgery and/or radiation to treat Cushing syndrome. Adrenal enzyme inhibitors used to control excess cortisol production include ketoconazole (Nizoral), mitotane (Lysodren), amnioglutethimide (Cytadren), and metyrapone (Metopirone; Neiman et al., 2015).

Clinical Aspects

ASSESSMENT

Excess cortisol levels can cause a wide variety of psychosocial and physiologic alterations. Patients with Cushing syndrome may have body-image issues related to skin changes, hirsutism, and weight gain. The nurse should assess patients for body-image disturbances and be able to provide resources and support and help patients develop effective coping mechanisms. It is important for the nurse to monitor for other cortisol-related adverse effects, such as depression, mood swings, diabetes, hypertension, hypokalemia, deep vein thrombosis, infection, and osteoporosis. Patients with adverse effects should be provided with education regarding management and treatment options, as well as referred to appropriate providers (Neiman et al., 2015). Extremely elevated cortisol levels impair immunity and increase the risk for opportunistic infections and sepsis. The nurse should provide education related to age-appropriate vaccines (influenza, pneumococcal, and herpes zoster) and administer as appropriate (Neiman et al., 2015).

OUTCOMES

The primary treatment for Cushing syndrome is surgical intervention. Major surgical complications following pituitary surgery include diabetes insipidus, venous thromboembolic events (VTEs), and infection. Postoperatively, the nurse must monitor the patient for signs of diabetes insipidus, including polyuria, polydipsia, dehydration, tachycardia, hypotension, hypernatremia, elevated serum osmolality, and decreased urine osmolality. As patients with Cushing syndrome are at an increased risk of infection, postoperative care should include a thorough surgical site assessment and careful monitoring of temperature and laboratory values for changes related to infection. There is a normal and expected decrease in ACTH levels following adrenalectomy, which will result in cortisol levels dropping below normal. It is important to monitor patients for signs of adrenal insufficiency such as hypoglycemia, hyponatremia, hyperkalemia, and hypotension. Patients who have had an adrenalectomy will need to take cortisol replacement therapy for a period after surgery to allow for recovery of the HPA axis. The nurse should ensure that the patient has a proper understanding of why and when to take the cortisol replacement to mimic normal physiological secretion (Neiman et al., 2015; Raff & Carroll, 2104).

Cushing syndrome can cause alterations in coagulation factors, putting patients at risk for VTE. Nurses should carefully monitor and assess patients for signs of deep vein thrombosis (DVT) and pulmonary embolism (PE). The nurse should also collaborate with other members of the health care team to ensure that the patient has appropriate perioperative mechanical and/or pharmacological DVT prophylaxis. Patients who have had surgery to treat Cushing syndrome are still at risk for thrombosis up to a year postoperatively. Patients should have education regarding the symptoms of DVT and PE and the importance of seeking emergency care if they occur.

Summary

Most cases of Cushing syndrome are caused by the use of exogenous steroids. Whatever the cause, treatment goals include maintaining normal serum cortisol levels, minimizing adverse effects of steroid use, and avoiding signs of adrenal insufficiency. Steroid replacement therapy may be indicated following surgical treatment of Cushing syndrome or following long-term glucocorticoid treatment until the HPA axis returns to normal. If exogenous steroid treatment is necessary, the dose should be tapered to the lowest effective dose for the shortest duration to achieve desired outcomes. If possible, systemic therapy should be avoided. If the patient's medical condition makes treatment with corticosteroids unavoidable, the use of steroid-sparing immunosuppressive agents may be helpful in minimizing adverse effects. Patients at risk for osteoporosis being treated with long-term glucocorticoid therapy should be evaluated for treatment with bisphosphonates. Patients should be taught how to recognize signs of adverse effects associated with glucocorticoid therapy, including infection, VTE, osteoporosis, hyperglycemia, ulcers and gastrointestinal bleeding, and delayed wound healing.

Lacroix, A., Feelders, S., Stratakis, C. A., & Nieman, L. K. (2015). Cushing's syndrome. *Lancet, 386*(9996), 913–927. doi:10.1016/S0140-6736(14)61375-1

Neiman, L. S., Biller, B. M. K., Findling, J. W., Hassan Murad, M., Newell-Price, J., Savage, M. O., & Tabarin, A. (2015). Treatment of Cushing's syndrome: An Endocrine Society clinical practice guideline. *Journal of Clinical Endocrinology and Metabolism, 100*(8), 2807–2831. doi:10.1210/jc.2015-1818

Quinn, L. (2016). The endocrine system. In H. Craven (Ed.), *Core curriculum for medical-surgical nursing* (5th ed., pp. 311–328). Pitman, NJ: Academy of Medical–Surgical Nurses.

Raff, H., & Carroll, T. (2015). Cushing's syndrome: From physiological principles to diagnosis and clinical care. *Journal of Physiology, 593*(3), 493–506. doi:10.1113/jphysiol.2014.282871

Urrets-Zavalía, J. A., Espósito, E., Garay, I., Monti, R., Ruiz-Lascano, A., Correa, L., . . . Grzybowski, A. (2016). The eye and the skin in nonendocrine metabolic disorders. *Clinics in Dermatology, 34*(2), 166–182. doi:10.1016/j.clindermatol.2015.12.002

■ DEEP VEIN THROMBOSIS

Kelly K. McConnell

Overview

Deep vein thrombosis (DVT) or venous thrombosis in the leg, pelvis, or upper extremity may result in a venous thromboembolic event (VTE). A DVT occurs when a thrombus or clot is formed and there is dysregulation of the fibrinolytic system that prevents the breakdown or reabsorbtion of a thrombosis within the lumen of a venous blood vessel. Consequently, DVTs can cause an obstruction of blood flow preventing the delivery of oxygen and vital nutrients to tissues, and results in ischemic tissue injury or necrosis. Nursing care of the adult with a DVT is focused on early detection and the implementation of appropriate nursing interventions to optimize outcomes and decrease further morbidity or life-threatening complications.

Background

According to the Centers for Disease Control and Prevention (CDC), the exact number of people affected by VTE disease, including DVT, is unknown. As many as 900,000 Americans annually are likely to be affected by VTE disease; it is estimated that nearly two thirds of these adults have a detectable DVT (CDC, 2015). For adults who develop DVTs, the risk of recurrence is approximately 7% despite pharmacotherapy (McNamara, 2017). Venous thromboses are highly morbid, the 1-month mortality rate is as high as 6% for DVTs although postmortem studies suggest that this rate is likely to be significantly underestimated (Behravesh et al., 2017). In addition to the risk for acute mortality and, despite timely initiation of pharmacotherapy, DVT complications can lead to persistent chronic disease caused by impaired venous return, known as *post-thrombotic syndrome (PTS)*. Among those who have had a DVT, one half will have long-term complications, such as swelling, pain, discoloration, and scaling, in the affected limb after an acute DVT (CDC, 2015).

The Agency for Healthcare Research and Quality (AHRQ) suggests that DVT is one of the most common preventable causes of hospital deaths (AHRQ, 2016). The total estimated costs in the United States associated with VTE is between $13.5 and $69.5 billion, including an estimated cost of $10,000 to treat DVT plus any additional nonmedical expenses (AHRQ, 2016).

A DVT can occur when a vein's inner lining is damaged by physical, chemical, or biological factors. DVTs are primary located in the deep veins of the lower extremities but can also appear in the pelvis and upper extremities. Risk factors for DVT include a history of endothelial damage/dysfunction, venous stasis, and hypercoagulable states also known as *Virchow's triad*. Venous stasis can be caused by immobilization, including individuals on bedrest or who have recently been traveling for a long period of time or individuals with polycythemia, which can lead to endothelial injury. Endothelial damage/dysfunction causes include a history of smoking, hypertension, serious injuries or major trauma or surgery within the past 4 weeks, inflammation, and immune responses. Hypercoagulable causes of DVT include active malignancy (treatment within previous 6 months or palliative therapy), splenectomy, sickle cell disease, previous proven venous thromboembolism, reduced cardiac output (congestive heart failure), obesity, advanced age (older than 60 years old although DVTs can occur in any age), pregnancy and 6 weeks after childbirth, hormone replacement therapy and oral contraceptives, chronic obstructive pulmonary disease (COPD), chronic inflammatory disease of the digestive tract, varicose veins, and indwelling catheters and electrodes in great veins and right heart (CDC, 2015; National Institutes of Health [NIH], 2011). Approximately 5% to 8% of the U.S. population has one of several genetic risk factors, known as *inherited thrombophilias*, which increase the risk for thrombosis (CDC, 2015). Inherited diseases include factor V Leiden-acquired thrombotic disorder, antiphospholipid antibodies, heparin-induced thrombocytopenia, and thrombocytosis (NIH, 2011). There is also supporting evidence confirming that individuals with HIV have a higher incidence of clinically detected thromboembolic disease (NIH, 2011).

Clinical Aspects

ASSESSMENT

Nursing care of the patient with suspected DVT includes a review of the individual's history, physical assessment findings, laboratory and diagnostic findings. When obtaining a health history, risk factors leading to abnormal clotting should be identified and documented. When assessing an individual for DVT, it is important to understand that approximately only half of people show signs and symptoms. The signs and symptoms for DVT include unilateral pain or tenderness in the leg, which may be felt only when standing or walking, swelling to the extremity, warmth in the area that is swollen or painful, and redness or discoloration of the extremity (CDC, 2015). When symptoms develop slowly and without "classic" clinical symptoms for DVT, conducting a thorough physical assessment should be done in conjunction with laboratory and diagnostic tests to diagnose DVT in an effort to prescribe interventions that reduce the risk for VTE-associated morbidity and mortality.

In addition to physical assessment findings, there are several diagnostic and laboratory tests that can be used to confirm the diagnosis of DVT. The most common test for diagnosing DVT is ultrasound. If an ultrasound does not provide a clear diagnosis, a venography may be ordered. Other tests used to diagnose DVT include MRI and CT scanning. Laboratory tests may be recommended to help diagnose DVT. The D-dimer test measures a substance in the blood that is released when a blood clot dissolves. If there are high levels of the substance, a blot clot may be present but if the results are normal and there are few risk factors, DVT is unlikely (CDC, 2015). Additional blood tests may also be ordered for individuals at risk for an inherited blood clotting disorder, including those with reoccurring blood clots with unknown etiology or when blood clots are found in unusual locations (such as the liver, kidney, or brain) suggesting an inherited clotting disorder (NIH, 2011).

NURSING INTERVENTIONS, MANAGEMENT, AND IMPLICATIONS

DVT can be treated with systemic and endovascular approaches in an effort to improve the 5% all-cause mortality within 1 year attributed to VTE (Behravesh et al., 2017). Anticoagulants, including unfractionated heparin, low-molecular-weight heparin, and factor X_a inhibitors can be used to treat DVT. The duration of anticoagulant therapy is generally 6 months, but can vary depending on the individual patient.

Thrombin inhibitors may be used for patients unable to tolerate treatment with heparin. The use of thrombolytics is restricted to life-threatening or emergent situations due to their high risk for bleeding.

In addition to medications there are other treatments to prevent further complications from DVT, including a vena cava filter, thrombolysis, and compression stockings or intermittent pneumatic compression devices (IPCDs). A vena cava filter is inserted inside the vena cava and catches blood clots before they travel to the lungs, preventing a pulmonary embolism, but does not stop new blood clots from forming. Thrombolysis may be performed in severe cases of DVT when there is a risk for loss of limb. Compression stockings and IPCDs are used to reduce venous stasis and improve venous return from the lower extremities. Contraindications should be considered when implementing mechanical DVT interventions, including conditions that affect the lower extremities, conditions that compromise lower extremity blood flow, severe congestive heart failure, thigh circumference that exceeds the limit of the instructions, and sensitivity to latex (McNamara, 2017).

Nursing care of the patient with DVT should primarily focus on the prevention of worsening the condition and education related to controllable risk factors and prescribed pharmacotherapy management, including safe practices and the risk for bleeding.

Nursing interventions for individuals with DVT include minimizing positions that compromise blood flow; immobilizing limb and initiating bed rest to reduce risk of clot mobilization, elevating limb maintaining slight flexion while in bed; applying graduated compression stockings or IPCDs per protocol; assisting with progressive ambulation when allowed; applying a warm, moist compress as scheduled; assessing and reporting worsening signs or symptoms of DVT; administering analgesics as prescribed for pain and evaluating effectiveness; administering oxygen as ordered to maintain tissue perfusion; administering anticoagulants and thrombin inhibitors as ordered to reduce the risk of additional clotting; and monitoring laboratory values, including prothrombin time (PT)/international normalized ratio (INR) to assess warfarin (Coumadin) and activated partial thromboplastin time (aPTT) to assess heparin effectiveness and dosage.

Care of an individual with DVT includes checking for signs of complications, including pulmonary embolism, decreased tissue perfusion, and excessive bleeding, which can be life-threatening. Signs and symptoms of bleeding include obvious signs of bleeding (bruising, petechiae, petechial hemorrhaging in the sclera, hematuria, epitasis, blood in stool or oral cavity). Nurses should ensure good hydration to prevent increased blood viscosity; provide education pertinent to anticoagulation therapy, including dietary restrictions such as vitamin K-rich foods when taking warfarin (Coumadin) and there is risk for bleeding. For individuals of child-bearing age, the nurse should discuss contraception choices as oral contraceptive therapy can increase the risk for DVT.

OUTCOMES

Individual outcomes are dependent on the management of DVT. The goals for DVT therapy include stopping blood clots from enlarging, preventing blood clots from becoming an embolism to the lung, and reducing the recurrence of future blood clots. In addition to goals of therapy, individuals should be monitored for common side effects, such as bleeding, from pharmacotherapy to treat DVT. Individuals undergoing DVT treatment are usually initially hospitalized and then monitored closely at home by having regular blood tests measuring coagulability and effectiveness of pharmacotherapy.

Summary

DVT can lead to worsening morbidity and mortality rates in individuals who go untreated. Early detection and management are vital to the outcomes for individuals with DVT. Nurses play a pivotal role in assessing, monitoring, and providing care for patients with DVT. Implementing appropriate nursing interventions can reduce the additional risks associated with DVT. Utilizing evidence-based nursing practice standards and recommended pharmacologic and nonpharmacologic measures when caring for individuals with DVT can promote better outcomes and decrease worsening morbidity and mortality rates.

Agency for Healthcare Research and Quality. (2016). *Executive summary: Preventing hospital acquired venous thromboembolism: A guide for effective quality improvement*. Rockville, MD: Author. Retrieved from https://www.ahrq.gov/professionals/quality-patient-safety/patient-safety-resources/resources/vtguide/vtguidesum.html

Behravesh, S., Hoang, P., Nanda, A., Wallace, A., Sheth, R. A., Deipolyi, A. R., . . . Oklu, R. (2017). Pathogenesis of thromboembolism and endovascular management. *Thrombosis, 3039713*, 1–13. doi:10.1155/2017/3039713

Centers for Disease Control and Prevention. (2015). Venous thromboembolism (blood clots). Retrieved from https://www.cdc.gov/ncbddd/dvt/data.html

McNamara, S. A. (2014). Patient safety first: Prevention of venous thromboembolism. *AORN Journal, 99*(5), 642–647. doi:10.1016/j.aorn.2014.02.001

National Institutes of Health. (2011). What is deep vein thrombosis? Retrieved from https://www.nhlbi.nih.gov/health/health-topics/topics/dvt

■ DIABETES INSIPIDUS

Danielle M. Diemer

Overview

Diabetes insipidus (DI), not to be mistaken with diabetes mellitus, is a rare disorder that can be debilitating. A hormone called *antidiuretic hormone (ADH)*, also referred to as *vasopressin*, helps regulate the kidneys' fluid balance of water and sodium. In DI, there is a deficiency, or lack of ADH. Large amounts of diluted and odorless urine are excreted and patients experience increased thirst (National Institute of Diabetes and Digestive and Kidney Disease [NIDDK], 2015). Nursing care for individuals with DI focuses on early recognition of intake and output to deliver appropriate nursing care and education to both the patients and their families.

Background

In the United States, three in 100,000 individuals are affected by DI. Most of the cases of DI develop in childhood or early adulthood (Cumulative Index to Nursing and Allied Health Literature [CINAHL], 2016).

There are four different types of DI. Neurogenic and nephrogenic are the most common types. Neurogenic DI (also known as *central DI*) is caused by a lack of ADH. This occurs when there is damage to the hypothalamus or pituitary gland or in some cases an inherited defected gene. Nephrogenic DI is caused by the kidneys' inability to respond to ADH. Certain medications, chronic kidney disease, or inherited gene changes can cause this type of DI (National Institute of Health [NIH], 2016). The other two less common forms of DI are dipsogenic and gestational. In dipsogenic DI (also known as *primary polydipsia*), individuals experience excess thirst resulting in increased fluid intake from a problem with the thirst mechanism. This form of DI is often associated with psychiatric disorders (Sanjay et al., 2016). Gestational DI can occur during pregnancy, usually in the third trimester. The abnormality is that the placenta prohibits the mother's ADH from working properly (Tritos, 2013).

There are several factors that contribute to an individual's risk for developing DI. Medications that interfere with the kidneys' reabsorption of water can place an individual at risk. Also adrenal insufficiency, sickle cell anemia, Langerhans cell histiocytosis, genetic problems, polycystic kidney disease, and increased levels of calcium in the blood place individuals at risk for DI (CINAHL Information Systems, 2016).

The most significant complication of DI is dehydration. If the DI is not treated and becomes severe, seizures, permanent brain damage, or death can occur (NIDDK, 2015). Other complications include mental status changes, fatigue, lethargy, tachycardia, hypotension, fever, headaches, decreased body temperature, hypernatremia, and hypokalemia (CINAHL Information Systems,

2016). Immediate medical attention is needed in individuals experiencing dizziness, confusion, or sluggishness (NIDDK, 2015).

Treatment is aimed at determining the underlying cause or the type of DI. This initial treatment and management may require hospitalization. Once treated, there are usually no severe problems or issues with early death (NIH, 2016).

Clinical Aspects

ASSESSMENT

It is important for nurses to obtain a thorough medical and family history. The documentation of the individual's physical assessment and laboratory data are also important. During the history, it is important for the nurse to ask what home medications the patient is taking. Lithium is an example of a medication to be aware of that can cause DI. Other questions to ask the individuals are whether they are experiencing symptoms of polydipsia, polyuria, or nocturia. Inquiring about a family history of DI is also an important question for the nurse to ask (NIH, 2016).

During the physical assessment, the nurse should focus on looking for signs of dehydration (NIDDK, 2015). Other assessment findings of DI include increased urine output (regardless of intake), water cravings, and possibly fevers (CINAHL Information Systems, 2016). Laboratory tests that can be ordered include urinalysis; 24-hour urine, serum and urine osmolality/osmolality; and fluid deprivation test. A CT scan or MRI could also be ordered (CINAHL Information Systems, 2016).

NURSING INTERVENTIONS, MANAGEMENT, AND IMPLICATIONS

Nursing care of an individual with DI should focus on preventing severe hydration. Some nursing-related problems include fluid volume deficit, sleep disturbances, activity intolerance/fatigue, anxiety, and patient/family knowledge deficit (Vera, 2012).

OUTCOMES

The expected outcomes of evidence-based nursing care focus on keeping the symptoms under control and preventing dehydration from progressing to severe dehydration. Nursing monitoring of intake/output is a key element to determine the reduction of progression of the disorder during treatment.

Summary

Individuals diagnosed with DI may initially need to be hospitalized. A thorough medical/family history and assessment can help with the early diagnosis of DI. Once the type of DI is determined, then treatment will help with preventing any long-term complications.

CINAHL Information Systems. (2016). *Quick lessons: Diabetes insipidus*. Glendale, CA: Author.

National Institute of Diabetes and Digestive and Kidney Disease. (2015). *Diabetes insipidus*. Washington DC: U.S. Department of Health and Human Services. Retrieved from http://www.niddk.nih.gov/health-information/health -topics/kidney-disease/diabetes-insipidus/pages/facts.aspx

National Institutes of Health. (2016). Diabetes insipidus. Retrieved from https://medline plus.gov/ency/article/000377.htm

Sanjay, K., Abdual Hamid, Z., Sunil, M. J., Bipid, S., Subhanker, C., Awadhesh Kumar, S., . . . Harshad, M. (2016). Diabetes insipidus. *Indian Journal of Endocrinology and Metabolism, 20*(1), 9–21. doi:10.4103/2230-8210.172273

Tritos, N. (2013, July). Diabetes insipidus. In A. Klibanski & J. Schlechte (Eds.), *Fact sheet: Diabetes insipidus* (pp. 1–2). Retrieved from http://www.hormone.org/ questions-and-answers/2013/diabetes-insipidus

Vera, M. (2012). 3 Diabetes insipidus nursing care plans. Retrieved from http:// nurselabs.com/diabetes-insipidus-nursing-care-plans

■ DIABETES MELLITUS

Mary Beth Modic

Overview

Diabetes mellitus (DM) is a serious, complex, and progressive disease. DM refers to a group of metabolic diseases in which the pancreas does not produce insulin or the body cannot effectively use the insulin that is made. This results in high blood glucose levels that are strongly associated with macrovascular complications (e.g., coronary heart disease, peripheral vascular disease, cerebrovascular) and microvascular complications (e.g., retinopathy, nephropathy, and neuropathy).

There are several different types of DM, most notably type 1, type 2, and gestational (American Diabetes Association, 2016a). Type 1 DM (T1DM) occurs when the beta cells of the pancreas are compromised by autoimmune insults. Individuals with T1DM do not have functional beta cells that produce insulin, resulting in their need for exogenous replacement of insulin. Type 2 DM (T2DM) occurs when the body becomes resistant to insulin due to the metabolic alterations that occur with obesity. Similar to individuals with T1DM, the beta cells of individuals with T2DM or heightened states of insulin, resistance eventually lose their secretory function, and exogenous insulin supplementation is required. By the time a person is diagnosed with T2DM, it is estimated that there is a 50% decline in beta cell function (Petznick, 2011). There are other types of DM that occur as a result of pregnancy, malnutrition, genetic disorders, surgery, and medications. However, these other subtypes of DM occur in 1% to 5% of the population.

Therefore, this entry focuses on the nursing care for individuals with T1DM and T2DM. Although all DM care should be customized to the individual and context, nursing care for patients with DM is typically directed at normalizing blood glucose, promoting effective self-management practices, and assisting them to live a normal life (Schreiner, 2016).

Background

DM affects 23.6 million Americans and 422 million people worldwide, with 5% of those diagnosed with T1DM and 90% with T2DM (Centers for Disease Control and Prevention [CDC], 2014). The cost of diabetes in the United States is estimated at $245 billion—$176 billion attributed to medical expenditures and $69 billion to lost work and wages (CDC, 2014). African Americans, Hispanics, and Native Americans are at greater risk of developing T2DM than Caucasians. Complications of diabetes include heart disease, dyslipidemia, stroke, renal failure, blindness, and amputations. Diabetes is the seventh leading cause of death but is often underreported on death certificates (CDC, 2014). Diabetes is a significant public health concern as Americans grow older, consume more calorically dense foods, become more sedentary, and obese.

There are three laboratory studies that are used to diagnose diabetes. A fasting blood glucose of 126 mg/dL (7 mmol/L) or greater on two separate occasions constitutes a diagnosis of diabetes, blood glucose values between 100 and 125 mg/dL identify a person with prediabetes, and a test result less than 100 mg/dL is normal. A second diagnostic test is an oral glucose tolerance test (OGTT) that requires the individual to fast for 8 hours and drink 75 g of glucose. The individual's blood is drawn at 1 hour and 2 hours postingestion of the glucose. A glucose value of 200 mg/dL or greater at the 2-hour interval results in a diagnosis of diabetes. A glycated hemoglobin test also known as *A1c* measures the average glucose value in the blood for the previous 2 to 3 months. A test result of greater than 6.5%, which is equivalent to a glucose value of 140 mg/dL, also provides a diagnosis of diabetes (American Diabetes Association, 2016b).

Clinical Aspects

ASSESSMENT

A diagnosis of DM may be acute, in the case of T1DM, when a child is brought to the health care provider because of polyuria (excessive urination), polydipsia (excessive thirst), polyphagia (excessive hunger), and weight loss. Parents or caregivers have noted very wet diapers, excessive trips to the bathroom as well as extreme thirst, hunger and weight loss in their child. In the case of T2DM, many of the complications associated with diabetes are already present when a diagnosis of diabetes is rendered.

In addition to gathering an accurate past medical history of the person's type and duration of DM and performing a physical assessment, it is essential that the individual's perception of success in performing daily diabetes self-care activities be explored. Physical activity, dietary practices, frequency of blood glucose monitoring, medication adherence, presence and degree of stress, and sleep patterns should be examined (Meece, 2015). Frequency and severity of hypoglycemic events, if the individual is prescribed insulin, should be reviewed as persons with T1DM typically experience two symptomatic hypoglycemic events a week and one severe episode per year (Hanefield, Duetting, & Bramlage, 2013).

NURSING INTERVENTIONS, MANAGEMENT, AND IMPLICATIONS

Nursing care of the adult with DM is directed at normalizing blood glucose levels, preventing hypoglycemia and hyperglycemia crises, and assessing the individual's ability to safely manage his or her diabetes.

Individuals with DM may present to the emergency department in hyperglycemic crisis. There are two conditions that warrant hospitalization: Diabetic ketoacidosis (DKA) and hyperglycemic hyperosmolar syndrome (HHS). DKA is most common in individuals with T1DM and is a state of absolute insulin deficiency. Dehydration, accumulation of ketone bodies, and metabolic abnormalities are also present in DKA. When the body does not have enough insulin to get glucose into the cells, the cells use fat to provide fuel. The breakdown of fat produces fatty acids and ketones that build up in the bloodstream. The individual will present with complaints of nausea, polyuria, polydipsia, weakness, and fatigue. The kidneys work to get rid of the ketones and the glucose, which leads to ketonuria (ketone bodies in the urine) and glycosuria (glucose in the urine). Laboratory results that indicate severe DKA include glucose (greater than 250 mg/dL), pH (greater than 7.00), bicarbonate (greater than 18 mEq/L), anion gap (greater than 12), and presence of serum and urine ketones. The anion gap is a calculated laboratory value that identifies the cause of metabolic acidosis. Treatment for DKA includes fluid resuscitation, insulin therapy, correction of other metabolic derangements, and investigation of the precipitating cause.

HHS is a condition in which a person, often elderly with T2DM, presents with significant hyperglycemia, hyperosmolality, and dehydration. (Pasquel & Umpierrez, 2014). Laboratory results that indicate HHS include glucose (greater than 600 mg/dL), serum osmolality (320 mOsm/kg), pH (greater than 7.30), bicarbonate (greater than 15 mEq/L), anion gap (variable), and small amounts of serum and urine ketones. Treatment is focused on fluid replacement, and normalizing glucose, osmolality, and electrolytes. Underlying infections are the primary precipitators of HHS with 40% to 60% being caused by pneumonia and 5% to 16% produced by urinary tract infections (Pasquel & Umpierrez, 2014).

Hypoglycemia can be a life-threatening event. It results from too little food, too much exercise, alcohol consumption, an unusual eating pattern, or too much insulin. The glucose threshold alert value for hypoglycemia is 70 mg/dL and a clinically significant hypoglycemic event is defined at 54 mg/dL (American Diabetes Association, 2016b). The severity of the event is not determined by the glucose value, but rather by the severity of the symptoms. As the glucose begins to drop, individuals begin to feel anxious, irritable, and tachycardiac. In response to hypoglycemia, glucagon, a counter-regulatory hormone is released. If the hypoglycemic event is not attended too quickly, the glucose will continue to drop and the individual can lose consciousness, seize, become comatose, and die as a result of glucose deprivation to the brain.

Depression is a common comorbid condition in individuals with diabetes, affecting 15% to 20% of people with diabetes overall (Friis, Consedine & Johnson, 2015). Individuals who suffer with depression have greater difficulty in following their prescribed medical regimen. Feelings of fatigue, lack of appetite, and feelings of hopelessness can impede a person's ability to perform the requisite self-management practices that must be performed daily to achieve metabolic control.

Priority nursing interventions for the patient with diabetes include monitoring of blood glucose, preventing glucose excursions (hyper and hypoglycemia), coordinating insulin administration with blood glucose monitoring and meal consumption, trending and interpreting glucose results, and supporting the individual in successful diabetes self-care practices.

OUTCOMES

The expected outcomes of evidence-based nursing care are directed at optimizing glucose control. Effective diabetes management requires that the individual living with diabetes is recognized as the expert on his or her life. Nurses and other health care team members need to be vigilant to the daily obstacles that can impede a person's ability to eat healthfully, be physically active, take diabetes medication as prescribed, monitor blood glucose correctly, interpret glucose results accurately, and seek out medical attention appropriately. Referrals to outpatient diabetes self-management education (DSME) programs, medical nutrition therapy, social work, and case management are warranted when a person with diabetes is noted to be struggling to follow the self-care practices that have been recommended and prescribed.

Summary

A diagnosis of DM is life-altering. The self-management of DM requires vigilance and significant behavioral self-regulation to follow the prescribed regimen. Nurses have an integral role in educating, supporting, and affirming these individuals to prevent complications and assist them to flourish in living with diabetes.

American Diabetes Association. (2016a). Classification and diagnosis of diabetes: Section 2. *Diabetes Care, 40*(Suppl. 1), S11–S24. doi:10.2337/dc17-S005

American Diabetes Association. (2016b). Classification and diagnosis of diabetes: Section 6. *Diabetes Care, 40*(Suppl. 1), S48–S56. doi:10.2337/dc17-S009

Centers for Disease Control and Prevention. (2014). *National diabetes statistics report: Estimates of diabetes and its burden in the United States*. Atlanta, GA: U.S. Department of Health and Human Services. Retrieved from https://stacks.cdc.gov/view/cdc/23442

Friis, A., Consedine, N., & Johnson, M. (2015). Does kindness matter? Diabetes, depression, and self-compassion: A selective review and research agenda. *Diabetes Spectrum, 29*(4), 252–257. doi:10:1111/codi.12781

Hanefield, M., Duetting, E., & Bramlage, P. (2013). Cardiac implications of hypoglycemia in patients with diabetes—A systematic review. *Cardiovascular Diabetology, 135*(12), 1–11. doi:10.1186/1475-2480-12-135

Meece, J. (2015). Improving adherence through better conversation. *AADE in Practice, 3*(4), 52–57. doi:10.1177/2325160316639021

Pasquel, F., & Umpierrez, G. (2014). Hyperosmolar hyperglycemic state: A historic review of the clinical presentation, diagnosis and treatment. *Diabetes Care, 37*(11), 3124–3131. doi:10.2337/dc14-0984

Petznick, A. (2011). Insulin management of type 2 diabetes mellitus. *American Family Physician, 84*(2), 183–190.

Schreiner, B. (2016). Teaching across the life span. *AADE in Practice, 2*(4), 28–31. doi.10.1177/2325160315624888

■ DIVERTICULAR DISEASE

Rhoda Redulla

Overview

Diverticular disease is a very common gastrointestinal (GI) disorder that can lead to hospitalization; diverticular bleeding is the most common cause of GI bleeding (Mosadeghi, Bhuket, & Stollman, 2016). Diverticular disease is also the most common finding during colonoscopy (Mosadeghi et al., 2016). Diverticular disease includes diverticulosis and diverticulitis. Diverticula are outpouchings or herniations of the mucosa in the wall of the large intestine. Diverticulitis is inflammation of diverticula and diverticulosis is the presence of noninflamed diverticula. The clinical course of diverticular disease is varied. Many patients have asymptomatic diverticular disease, others may experience acute complications, such as GI bleeding, fistulae formation, or perforation, whereas others may have chronic diverticular disease.

Background

Diverticular disease is a common and increasing problem in developed countries such as the United States, Australia, United Kingdom, and France. Age is a strong risk factor; the prevalence increases with age. Over 50% of adults older than 70 years have diverticula and 80% remain asymptomatic; an estimated 20% of patients with diverticulosis will eventually develop diverticulitis (Strate, 2014). Men and women are equally affected. Diverticular disease accounts for approximately 814,000 hospitalizations per year in the United States and an estimated 2.7 million outpatient visits (Feuerstein & Falchuk, 2016).

Lifestyle factors have long been associated with diverticular disease. Diets low in fiber and lack of fecal bulk were thought to be major contributing factors to the disease, especially in Western countries. However, there is conflicting evidence that a high-fiber diet and frequent bowel movements result in a higher incidence of diverticular disease (Mosadeghi et al., 2016). Low dietary fiber is thought to increase colonic transit time and decrease the volume of stool, which in turn increases intraluminal pressure in the colon. Other theories attribute the formation of diverticula to changes in collagen synthesis in the bowel wall, abnormal colonic motility, and dysfunction of colonic neurotransmitters (Mosadeghi et al., 2015). Alterations in connective tissue, known as *collaginosis* or *herniosos*, are thought to be responsible for Saint's triad, which includes hiatal hernia, diverticulosis, and cholelithiasis. Chronic, low-grade inflammation is thought to play a role in patients with mild symptoms (symptomatic uncomplicated diverticular disease [SUDD]; Mosadeghi et al., 2016). Other factors contributing to diverticular disease include lack or decrease in physical activity, genetics, poor bowel habits (ignoring or suppressing the urge to have a bowel movement), obesity, aspirin, use nonsteroidal anti-inflammatory drug (NSAID) use, steroid use, alcohol consumption, diets high in red meat, and the effects of aging (Feuerstein & Falchuk, 2016; Mosadeghi et al., 2016).

Diverticula form when increased pressure within the lumen of the large intestine causes bowel mucosa to form pouches through defects in the colon wall. Meckel's diverticulum or true diverticula penetrate through all layers of the bowel wall, in contrast, pseudodiverticula only involve the mucosa and submucosal layers. The circular and longitudinal muscles often thicken or hypertrophy in the area affected by diverticula. This narrows the bowel lumen, increasing intraluminal pressure. Contraction of the muscles in response to normal stimuli, such as meals, may occlude the narrowed lumen, further increasing intraluminal pressure. Although diverticula can occur anywhere in the GI tract, they are commonly found in the sigmoid colon, which has the highest intraluminal pressure in the bowel (Morris, Regenbogen, Hardiman, & Hendren, 2014). The high pressure causes mucosa to herniate through the muscle wall, forming a diverticulum. Areas where nutrient blood vessels penetrate the circular muscle layer are the most common sites for diverticula formation. Bleeding can occur from a rupture in any of the vessels lining a diverticulum. The severity of bleeding ranges from mild rectal bleeding to hemorrhage, hypotension, and impending shock. Most episodes of bleeding are self-limiting but endoscopic evaluation may be warranted for evaluation and treatment (Strate, 2016).

The etiology of diverticulitis is not completely understood. Feces or undigested food may collect in the outpouchings causing obstruction, distention, and decreased blood supply. An overgrowth of colonic bacteria may result in inflammation, localized necrosis of the bowel wall, and microperforation. Diverticulitis can range from mild to severe; larger perforations may lead to abscess or fistula formation and peritonitis.

Clinical Aspects

ASSESSMENT

More than two thirds of patients with diverticular disease are asymptomatic. Symptoms depend on the location, severity of disease, and presence of inflammation and complications. The most common clinical finding is cramping left lower quadrant abdominal pain; other symptoms include constipation, diarrhea, bloating, and painless rectal bleeding (Thompson, 2016). Weakness and fatigue may also develop as the disease progresses. The clinical presentation of diverticulitis ranges from no signs of infection to acute peritonitis. Depending on the location and severity of the inflammation, other symptoms, such as nausea, vomiting, and a low-grade fever, may occur. The abdomen should be inspected for masses, distention, and tenderness. The older adult may only report vague abdominal pain. Diagnosis is made by history and physical examination. Diagnostic testing includes hemoglobin and hematocrit, white blood cell count, stool for occult blood, and abdominal x-rays to identify perforation. Upper GI series or barium enema can be used to locate diverticula, but should not be performed during periods of acute inflammation.

During assessment, the nurse obtains a health history focusing on the onset and duration of pain, dietary habits, bowel patterns, presence of rectal bleeding, usual activity level, and presence of other risk factors. For recurrent episodes, the diagnosis is usually determined with a focused history and physical examination by the health care provider (Strate, Peery, & Neumann, 2015).

NURSING INTERVENTIONS, MANAGEMENT, AND IMPLICATIONS

Applicable nursing diagnoses for the patient with diverticulitis include acute pain, altered bowel elimination pattern, and deficient knowledge. Nursing interventions are specific to presenting symptoms and decrease the risk of the potential complications of perforation, bleeding, and peritonitis. Interventions for pain management include administration of opioid analgesics to manage severe pain. The nurse should monitor the patient for signs of infection, including assessing the temperature every 4 hours; fever more than 38.3°C (101°F) may indicate increased inflammation or spread of inflammation. The older adult may present with only a slight temperature elevation or change in mental status. The nurse also monitors the patient's vital signs, observing for signs of bleeding and fluid volume deficit. Monitoring the patient's fluid volume status is particularly important for patients presenting with diarrhea. Bowel rest is usually indicated, especially for the patient with acute diverticulitis. The patient should be monitored for fluid and electrolyte imbalances; IV fluid and electrolyte replacement may be indicated. Other nursing interventions include performing a complete abdominal assessment, monitoring for distention and tenderness every 4 to 8 hours or more often as indicated. Significant changes, based on an ongoing assessment, should be promptly reported to the provider.

Evidence on dietary modification, particularly a high-fiber diet to reduce the risk of complications, remains undefined (Stollman, Smalley, & Hirano, 2015). Known benefits have been inconsistent. A stool softener may be prescribed but laxatives are not indicated for the patient with diverticular disease. During acute exacerbations, laxatives and enemas are contraindicated due to their effects on intestinal motility.

OUTCOMES

A priority nursing intervention is to provide patient education on the disease process, prevention of complications, dietary modifications, and treatment regimen. The expected outcome for the patient with acute diverticulitis is to remain free from complications, including abscess formation, fistula, bowel perforation, peritonitis, and hemorrhage. The patient should also be able to verbalize knowledge of strategies to prevent further episodes of acute disease and complications.

Individuals who are overweight or obese are at increased risk for developing diverticular disease. Smoking may also increase the risk of developing the condition. Patient education therefore includes the importance of maintaining a normal weight and avoidance or cessation of smoking (Strate et al., 2015).

No evidence exists to support avoiding intake of nuts and seeds to reduce the risk for diverticulitis in patients with known diverticulosis. Intake of nuts, corn, popcorn, and berries is not associated with increased risk for diverticular disease. Risk reduction strategies include limiting intake of red meat, maintaining a regular exercise pattern, avoiding the use of NSAIDs, and avoiding activities that increase intra-abdominal pressure (Strate et al., 2015).

Patients with mild symptoms are usually managed on an ambulatory basis. Medical treatment for acute diverticulitis includes oral (metronidazole and ciprofloxacin or trimethoprim-sulfamethoxazole) or intravenous antibiotics and diet modification. Indications for hospitalization include the presence of complications (bleeding, fistula formation, peritonitis, dehydration), the inability to tolerate oral fluids, fever, persistent abdominal pain, the presence of significant comorbidities, or lack of adequate support at home. Management strategies include pain management and bowel rest. Intravenous antibiotics have routinely been administered to patients admitted with acute uncomplicated diverticulitis. The most recent guidelines recommend the selective, rather than routine use of IV antibiotics (Peery & Stollman, 2015; Stollman et al., 2015). This recommended change in practice is based on results indicating no significant difference in the time to resolution of symptoms, complications, duration of hospital stay, and risk of recurrence between patients treated with intravenous (IV) antibiotics versus those treated with IV fluids alone (Peery & Stollman, 2015). There is growing inclination to withhold antibiotics when there is no risk for complicated disease (Johnson, 2016; Peery & Stollman, 2015; Stollman et al., 2015).

Surgical resection of the diseased segment of colon is often indicated if there is no clinical improvement within 48 hours despite supportive therapy. Emergency surgery may be indicated for patients with bowel obstruction, perforation, fistula, abscess, or peritonitis. A colon resection is the most commonly performed procedure; a temporary or permanent colostomy may be necessary (Peery & Neumann, 2015). An evolving discussion related to surgical approach in recurrent diverticulitis is elective surgery. However, there is insufficient evidence to support the benefits of elective surgery as a treatment for diverticular disease (Stollman et al., 2015). If creation of an ostomy is a possibility, a consult with a wound, ostomy, and continence (WOCN) nurse should be initiated.

Summary

Diverticular disease has become increasingly common in recent years. Etiologic theories and the approach to treatment has also significantly evolved (Regenbogen, Hardiman, Hendren, & Morris, 2014).

Emerging evidence does not support the theory of a low-fiber diet as a major causative factor in the etiology of diverticular disease. A high-fiber diet has recently been linked to an increased risk of diverticulitis. More research is indicated before a change in practice occurs. Because of the evidence supporting the role of chronic low-grade inflammation in the etiology of diverticular disease, more research is needed to evaluate the effectiveness of mesalamine for symptom relief and prevention of diverticulitis (Mosadeghi et al., 2015). The benefit of probiotics has not been demonstrated, but they may be prescribed (Feuerstein & Falchuk, 2016). Nursing management includes supportive measures based on presenting symptoms and patient education to prevent recurrent episodes. Some cases of uncomplicated diverticulitis may not require antibiotics. However, in severe diverticulitis, hospitalization is required. Recurrent disease may also prompt the need for surgery.

Feuerstein, J. D., & Falchuk, K. R. (2016). Diverticulosis and diverticulitis. *Mayo Clinic Proceedings, 91*(8), 1094–1104. doi:10.1016/j.mayocp.2016.03.012

Johnson, D. (2016). New guidelines on acute diverticulitis: How will they change clinical practice? *Medscape*. Retrieved from http://www.medscape.com/viewarticle/857275

Morris, A. M., Regenbogen, S. E., Hardiman, K. M., & Hendren, S. (2014). Sigmoid diverticulitis: A systematic review. *Journal of the American Medical Association, 311*(3), 287–297. doi:10.1001/jama.2013.282025

Mosadeghi, S., Bhuket, T., & Stollman, N. (2015). Diverticular disease: Evolving concepts in classification, presentation, and management. *Current Opinion in Gastroenterology, 31*(1), 50–55. doi:10.1097/MOG.0000000000000145

Peery, A. F., & Stollman, N. (2015). Antibiotics for acute uncomplicated diverticulitis: Time for a paradigm change? *Gastroenterology, 149*(7), 1650–1651. doi:10.1053/j.gastro.2015.10.022

Regenbogen, S. E., Hardiman, K. M., Hendren, S., & Morris, A. M. (2014). Surgery for diverticulitis in the 21st century: A systematic review. *JAMA Surgery, 149*(3), 292–303. doi:10.1001/jamasurg.2013.5477

Stollman, N., Smalley, W., & Hirano, I. (2015). American gastroenterological association institute guideline on the management of acute diverticulitis. *Gastroenterology, 149*(7), 1944–1949. doi:10.1053/j.gastro.2015.10.003

Strate, L. L. (2014). Diverticular disease. National Institute of Diabetes and Digestive and Kidney Diseases. Retrieved from https://www.niddk.nih.gov/health-information/digestive-diseases/diverticulosis-diverticulitis

Strate, L. L., Peery, A. F., & Neumann, I. (2015). American Gastroenterological Association Institute technical review on the management of acute diverticulitis. *Gastroenterology, 149*(7), 1950–1976. doi:10.1053/j.gastro.2015.10.001

Thompson, A. E. (2016). Diverticulosis and diverticulitis. *Journal of the American Medical Association, 316*(10), 1124. doi:10.1001/jama.2016.3592

■ ENDOCARDITIS

Courtney G. Donahue
Celeste M. Alfes

Overview

Infective endocarditis (IE) is an inflammation of the endocardium, the endothelial membrane that lines the heart chambers and valves. IE is a potentially lethal disease that occurs when bacteria or fungi invade the bloodstream and the endocardial tissue. The epidemiology of IE has become more complex with the multitude of health care-associated factors that predispose the patient to infection (Baddour et al., 2015).

Background

IE is an uncommon infectious disease seen in approximately three to seven cases per 100,000 persons per year and deaths related to endocarditis are estimated to be one per 100,000 cases per year (Baddour et al., 2015). Although this disease is relatively rare, IE continues to have increased morbidity and mortality. IE is now the third or fourth most common life-threatening infection syndrome. Although the major risk factor for IE, rheumatic fever, has decreased significantly, the incidence of IE remains high. IE has changed from a disease primarily of the young, to one of the elderly, related to the fact that individuals are living longer with chronic heart disease and are having more invasive medical procedures (Josephson, 2014).

Patients most susceptible to acquiring IE include people who have congenital heart defects, damaged or artificial heart valves, or implanted medical devices in the heart or blood vessels. Other risk factors include poor dental hygiene and intravenous drug users. Furthermore, those undergoing invasive procedures and surgeries are at higher risk for bloodstream infections that can result in endocarditis (Josephson, 2014). The most common bacteria associated with IE are *Staphylococcus aureus, Enterococci, and Streptococci* organisms. The incidence of IE caused by *S. aureus* has increased and is now the most common causative organism in the industrialized world (Baddour et al., 2015).

Nosocomial infections acquired during a hospital stay contribute to the incidence of endocarditis. Nosocomial infections are acquired secondary to procedures, such as a pacemaker implantation, or various catheter insertions. These infections are more prevalent in men than in women with a ratio of 2:1 (Baddour et al., 2015). Signs and symptoms of IE include but are not limited to fever, malaise, and fatigue. A heart murmur, weight loss, and coughing are present in 35% of cases and small, painful petechiae (Osler's nodes) under the fingernails or toenails can also be present as well as small dark painless flat spots on the palms of the hands or soles of the feet (Janeway lesions).

Clinical Aspects

ASSESSMENT

IE is a relatively uncommon condition that presents with a multitude of non-cardiac symptoms, making diagnosis of IE challenging (Josephson, 2014). The single most definitive test result is a positive blood culture. Current practice guidelines recommend at least three blood cultures from three different venipuncture sites to confirm diagnosis (Nishimura et al., 2014). The cultures enable the health care professional to determine which bacteria is the infective agent in the bloodstream. Treatment with antibiotics can then be determined regarding resistance and sensitivity.

Echocardiography is another common diagnostic marker used to diagnose IE using sound waves to create pictures of the heart, which may show damage. A transthoracic echo (TTE), which allows the health care professional to look at images of the patient's heart and determine whether there is vegetation on its structures may be ordered. If suspicion remains likely for diagnosis of IE, then a transesophageal echocardiogram (TEE) will also be ordered to provide additional information to support the diagnosis. An EKG may also be ordered as a supplement to determine whether there are any arrhythmias present (Nishimura et al., 2014).

NURSING INTERVENTIONS, MANAGEMENT, AND IMPLICATIONS

Nurses play a vital role in the care and detection of endocarditis. A thorough physical assessment can help detect the signs and symptoms of endocarditis. It is important to note that a complete and thorough medical and surgical history is crucial to knowing whether the patient has had a valve replacement, intravenous drug abuse, or cardiac history that would preclude the patient to IE.

Nurses also have a very important role in preventing IE. Sterile dressing changes of peripherally inserted central catheter (PICC) lines, intravenous lines, and arterial–venous fistulas are vital to preventing IE associated with central line bloodstream infections. Furthermore, providing comprehensive education on dental hygiene to both the patient and family can help prevent IE. Oftentimes, patients are not aware of how important their dental hygiene and dental prophylaxis are to their overall health and that poor dental hygiene is a precursor to acquiring IE. Daily adherence to a strict oral hygiene regimen along with routine visits to one's dentist who is aware of the patient's IE history is vital.

The two approaches to treating IE are the use of intravenous antibiotics for 2 to 6 weeks and cardiac surgery (Josephson, 2014). Infectious disease physicians collaborate with the primary care physician in determining the best choice of antibiotic. In some cases, the damage from the infection requires surgery to remove or repair a heart valve. Surgery is implicated in patients who have a vegetation of more than 10 mm in diameter. This is often seen in IE caused by fungi as this can become harder to treat. The proportion of patients undergoing surgery has increased to approximately 50% of those affected. Mortality from endocarditis usually occurs from congestive heart failure.

Endocarditis can continue to affect the patient after antibiotic therapy is initiated. The risk of embolization occurs in 22% to 50% of IE cases (Nishimura et al., 2014). Recent research has shown that the rate of embolic events dramatically decreases during and after the first 3 weeks of antibiotic therapy. Up to 65% of embolic events involve the central nervous system with more than 90% of these emboli lodged in the middle cerebral artery with the potential to cause a cerebrovascular accident, one of the many possible neurologic complications (Thuny et al., 2005). Despite the risk of emboli, anticoagulation therapy is controversial in patients post-IE. Some authorities recommend continuing anticoagulation therapy in patients with mechanical valve IE (Nishimura et al., 2014). However, most research concludes that it should be discontinued in all forms for at least 2 weeks in patients who have had an embolic event (Thuny et al., 2005).

OUTCOMES

Although IE is rare, it is a very serious disease. After antibiotic therapy, thorough follow-up is important to prevent a recurrence of endocarditis. Teaching the patient signs and symptoms to look for in endocarditis, including fever, malaise, and fatigue, is beneficial to preventing recurrence. A repeat echocardiogram is recommended to obtain a new baseline after treatment of the infection. A thorough dental evaluation is recommended to rule out all active sources of oral infection. All indwelling intravenous catheters used to infuse antibiotics should be removed immediately upon cessation of antibiotics. Developing heart failure is commonly seen in patients who experience IE. Follow-up for patients includes a thorough workup to determine whether any heart failure is present.

Summary

IE is a complex disease generally requiring management by a team of physicians and allied health care providers. Nurses are key members of the health care team and can greatly influence the outcome of the patient with endocarditis. It is important for nurses to closely assess their patients and identify those at increased risk for developing IE. Monitoring vital signs closely, drawing blood cultures regularly, and assessing the skin for peripheral embolization are key to patient outcomes. Nurses can also convey their knowledge of endocarditis to the patients and their families to assist them in understanding the disease process, management, and long-term care for this disease. With proper nursing and medical care, patients can return to their lives after IE, rejoining the community stronger than before.

Baddour, L. M., Wilson, W. R., Bayer, A. S., Fowler, V. G., Tleyjeh, I. M., Rybak, M. J., . . . Taubert, K. A. (2015). Infective endocarditis in adults: Diagnosis, antimicrobial therapy, and management of complications: A scientific statement for healthcare professionals from the American Heart Association. *Circulation, 132*(15), 1435–1486. doi:10.1161/CIR.0000000000000296

Josephson, L. (2014). Infective endocarditis: A review for nurses. *Dimensions of Critical Care Nursing, 33*(6), 327–340. doi:10.1097/DCC.0000000000000081

Nishimura, R. A., Otto, C. M., Bonow, R. O., Carabello, B. A., Erwin, J. P., Guyton, R. A., . . . Thomas, J. D. (2014). 2014 AHA/ACC guideline for the management of patients with valvular heart disease. *Journal of the American College of Cardiology*, 1–185. doi:10.1016/j.jacc.2014.02.536

Thuny, F., Di Salvo, G., Disalvo, G., Belliard, O., Avierinos, J. F., Pergola, V., . . . Habib, G. (2005). Risk of embolism and death in infective endocarditis: Prognostic value of echocardiography: A prospective multicenter study. *Circulation, 112*(1), 69–75. doi:10.1161/CIRCULATIONAHA.104.493155

■ FRACTURES

Joseph D. Perazzo

Overview

Fractures are a form of skeletal trauma in which the continuity of bone tissue is lost, often referred to as a "break." Fractures occur when the force exerted on a bone exceeds the pressure the bone can withstand, and can be the result of force as seen in traumatic injuries or the result of a weakened bone matrix as seen in osteoporosis. Fractures can occur in any bone and, depending on location and severity, can lead to chronic pain, deformity, and even permanent disability (American Academy of Orthopedic Surgeons [AAOS], 2017). Nursing care for people who experience fractures is focused on safety, preventing further injury, alleviating pain, assisting with self-care, education, and promoting rehabilitative efforts to regain mobility and function (Hinkle & Cheever, 2014).

Background

Fractures can affect individuals across the life span, but are most commonly seen in young males between 15 and 24 years of age and in adults aged 65 years and older (Huether & McCance, 2016). The causes and specific sites of fractures differ across the life span, with traumatic fractures (e.g., tibial, clavical, humeral) affecting younger persons, and fragility fractures (e.g., wrist, hip, ribs, and spine) having a higher incidence in older adults as the result of pathological bone loss (e.g., age, osteoporosis; Huether & McCance, 2016). Other fractures, such as those to the skull, hands, and feet, are also related to traumatic injury, including workplace accidents (AAOS, 2017). According to the Global Alliance of Musculoskeletal Health (Watkins-Castillo, Yelin, & Weinstein, 2017), health care providers treat more than 18 million fractures annually, a figure expected to increase substantially as the population of older Americans increases. Perhaps the most damaging aspect of fractures is the potential for long-term physical and psychosocial complications, including chronic pain and disability (Watkins-Castillo et al., 2017). Fractures, along with other musculoskeletal injuries, cost Americans more than $200 billion annually in direct health care costs, and more than $70 billion in indirect costs due to disability and lost productivity (Watkins-Castillo et al., 2017).

There are many different categorizations and classifications of fractures, many outside the scope of this entry. Common fractures include:

- *Oblique*: Angular fracture (diagonal) caused by direct or indirect injury to bone
- *Transverse*: Horizontal fracture across the bone, direct or indirect injury to bone
- *Comminuted*: Multiple-segment fracture "shatter," caused by direct injury to bone
- *Linear*: Fracture along the vertical axis of the bone, caused by overuse

■ *Depressed*: Fracture driven inward, seen in skull and facial fractures
■ *Spiral*: Fracture twists around bone shaft, caused by rotating force (e.g., athletics)
■ *Stress*: Bone matrix breaks in response to repeated loading and unloading (e.g., running)
■ *Closed*: Fracture does not break the skin, caused by direct or indirect injury to bone
■ *Open*: Fracture breaks through skin, caused by moderate to severe trauma
■ *Pathologic*: Fracture at site of weakened bone matrix, caused by low bone mineral density (Hinkle & Cheever, 2014; Huether & McCance, 2016)

Although fractures can affect people of any age, certain groups have an elevated risk for fractures, including young people at high risk for trauma and overuse (e.g., athletes), as well as postmenopausal women and individuals with chronic diseases that decrease bone mineral density (e.g., cancer, HIV). Other risk factors for fractures include malnutrition, decreased physical function (fall risk), low body mass index (BMI), alcohol use, smoking, and taking medications known to weaken bone (e.g., glucocorticoids; Huether & McCance, 2016). A key difference between traumatic and nontraumatic fractures is the level of force, energy, or activity that resulted in fracture; stress fractures occur through repetitive force, traumatic fractures are caused by significant (moderate to severe) force, and fragility fractures can occur regardless of force because of weak bone, sometimes during normal daily activities (Hinkle & Cheever, 2014; Huether & McCance, 2016).

The pathophysiology of fractures is defined by the specific causes of the fracture, as well as the ability of the bone to regain integrity during the healing process. Fracture healing occurs in three phases: (a) the inflammatory phase (immediate: 4 weeks), (b) the repair phase (1–2 months), and (c) the remodeling phase (up to 6 months; Huether & McCance, 2016; Kalfas, 2001). In the inflammatory phase, a hematoma forms at the site of the injured bone, leading to infiltration of inflammatory cells and fibroblasts, leading to formation of granulation and vascular tissue that allows the process of repairing to begin. Mesenchymal cells that differentiate into bone-forming cells (osteoblasts) migrate to the area and new blood vessels are formed to deliver oxygen and nutrients (Huether & McCance, 2016; Kalfas, 2001). Soft new bone tissue (osteoid) and cartilage are woven to create a bridge between the fracture fragments, creating a soft, fragile "callus" that is mineralized and hardened in a process known as *ossification*. Immobilization is particularly important during this phase. In the remodeling phase, osteoblasts and bone resorption cells (osteoclasts) work together to repair the physical structure of the bone and provide tissue to strengthen the new bone (Hinkle & Cheever, 2014; Huether & McCance, 2016; Kalfas, 2001). Remodeling is promoted by mechanical forces (e.g., weight bearing), and continues over time to continually strengthen the new bone and remove bone tissue where necessary, resulting in healed bone with appropriate anatomical structure. From first response to postdischarge rehabilitation, clinical interventions drive this process through efforts to stabilize, align, immobilize, and eventually stimulate bones to promote optimal healing (Hinkle & Cheever, 2014; Huether & McCance, 2016; Kalfas, 2001).

Clinical Aspects

ASSESSMENT

Fractures are diagnosed and monitored using x-ray imaging that allows clinicians to determine the site and severity of a fracture and to determine a course of action that will promote optimal healing. Clinical fracture interventions vary depending on the type of fracture, but share the goal of accomplishing reduction, immobilization, and restoration of function (Hinkle & Cheever, 2014).

NURSING INTERVENTIONS, MANAGEMENT, AND IMPLICATIONS

Reduction refers to the process of placing bones in their appropriate anatomical alignment. In a closed reduction, bones are manually manipulated into alignment and held in place using casts, splints, or percutaneous pinning. In an open reduction, a surgical approach is used in which fracture fragments are aligned and held in place with the use of internal fixation devices (e.g., pins, screws, plates, nails; Hinkle & Cheever, 2014).

Immobilization refers to interventions designed to keep bones in appropriate anatomical position that will lead to proper healing. Specific immobilization interventions are chosen based on the site and severity of a fracture, and include casts, bandages, and splints, which are used for simpler fractures often for long bones. *Fixation* refers to external and internal fixators used to maintain alignment, often used with more severe or more complex fractures. Traction involves the use of pulling force to promote bone alignment and is especially important in maintaining overall anatomical alignment of the injured body part; this includes skin traction (e.g., Buck's extension traction) and skeletal traction (Brunner et al., 2014). Finally, functional restoration includes all efforts to help individuals regain use of the injured body part and includes all matter of physical rehabilitative efforts, ranging from gradual range of motion to vigorous physical activity (Hinkle & Cheever, 2014).

Immediately following injury, particularly in the case of open fractures, individuals can have significant bleeding caused by injuries directly and indirectly associated with the broken bones. One of the most serious complications occurs with open femoral fractures in which the femoral artery can be torn causing acute hemorrhage, and is treated by fracture stabilization and blood volume restoration. Another potential (though rarely fatal) complication associated with fractures are fat emboli that can gain access to the vascular compartment, leading to occlusion of blood vessels that supply vital organs. Compartment syndrome is a complication that occurs when one of the body's 46 anatomic compartments, such as those in the extremities, loses blood flow, potentially leading to necrotic tissue loss. Finally, during healing, the complication of nonunion can occur when bones are not properly aligned and can lead to loss of function, chronic pain, deformity, and crepitus (AAOS, 2017; Hinkle & Cheever, 2014; Huether & McCance, 2016).

Nursing care of adults who experience fractures is focused on promoting patient safety, preventing further complication to fractures, and promoting optimal healing. Priority nursing diagnoses include careful assessment of fracture sites and sites of fixation for swelling and signs of infection, assessing and managing pain, careful asepsis and proper positioning of fixation and traction devices, ensuring immobilization, promoting early mobility when appropriate, and providing emotional support and patient education regarding expectations related to prognosis, hospitalization, surgical interventions, and future limitations (Hinkle & Cheever, 2014; Huether & McCance, 2016).

Outcomes

The outcomes of priority nursing interventions are directly associated with promoting optimal fracture healing. Swelling and drainage at the fracture site can alert nurses to malalignment, further complication of injuries, or infections at fixation or surgical sites (Hinkle & Cheever, 2014; Huether & McCance, 2016). Pain, often quite significant, is common in the early stages of fracture healing, but should improve with time. Sudden onset of increased pain (not associated with movement) can be a sign of complicated healing or compartment syndrome. Patients should maintain immobilization until clinical assessments indicate that movement would not jeopardize healing or patient safety (Hinkle & Cheever, 2014). Nurses should ensure that the patient completes required range of motion and mobilization to prevent bone loss and promote bone remodeling. Finally, patients should understand timelines related to healing, mobility restrictions, and be educated about healing following clinical encounters, potential physical limitations they may encounter, and ways to promote bone remodeling, particularly those related to diet and physical activity (AAOS, 2017; Hinkle & Cheever, 2014; Huether & McCance, 2016).

Summary

Fractures are a significant injury that can affect people of all ages and affect many different parts of the body. Optimal healing of fractures requires timely intervention and careful assessment of injuries. Nurses play a vital role in helping patients to tolerate, maintain, and understand the phases of fracture healing, both in and out of the clinical environment, which help patients to regain as much function as possible following injury.

American Academy of Orthopedic Surgeons. (2017). Fractures (broken bones). Retrieved from http://orthoinfo.aaos.org/topic.cfm?topic=a00139

Hinkle, J., & Cheever, K. H. (2014). *Brunner & Suddarth's textbook of medical–surgical nursing*. Philadelphia, PA: Wolters Kluwer Health.

Huether, S. E., & McCance, K. L. (2016). *Understanding pathophysiology (5th ed.)*. St. Louis, MO: Elsevier Health Sciences.

Kalfas, I. H. (2001). Principles of bone healing. *Neurosurgical Focus, 10*(4), E1. doi:10.3171/foc.2001.10.4.2

Watkins-Castillo, S. I., Yelin, E., & Weinstein, S. (2017). The burden of musculoskeletal diseases in the United States: Facts in brief. Retrieved from http://www.boneandjoint burden.org/facts-brief

■ GALLBLADDER AND BILIARY TRACT DISEASE

Andrea Marie Herr

Overview

The main function of the gallbladder is storage and release of bile. Most gallbladder disease is a result of inflammation of the gallbladder or obstruction of the biliary tree, usually by stones, causing biliary stasis. Common gallbladder problems are cholecystitis and cholelithiasis. Cholelithiasis, or gallstones, are crystallized deposits containing cholesterol and/or bilirubin (Tiderington, Lee, & Ko, 2016). Surgical management of gallstones is considered to be the gold standard and is safe and effective; more than 750,000 cholecystectomies are performed annually (Pak & Lindseth, 2016). Other less common conditions include gallbladder polyps and benign or malignant tumors. Disorders of the biliary tract include choledocholithiasis, primary sclerosing cholangitis, and cholangiocarcinoma.

Background

GALLBLADDER DISEASE

Gallbladder disease is the second most common gastrointestinal discharge diagnosis in U.S. hospitalizations (Pak & Lindseth, 2016). Gallstones affect 10% and 20% of the adult population; gallbladder disease is more prevalent in women (Pak & Lindseth, 2016). There are two main types of gallstones; the majority of stones are made up of cholesterol and are yellow-green-colored and pigment stones, which are brown or black and contain bilirubin. Inflammation of the gallbladder, or cholecystitis, can be acute or chronic and commonly occurs as a result of gallstones, but can occur without stones (acalculous cholecystitis). Acalculous cholecystitis is associated with a higher morbidity and mortality rate than calculous cholecystitis. Acalculous cholecystitis is associated with critically ill patients with sepsis, burns, or who are on mechanical ventilation.

Most patients with cholethiliasis are asymptomatic. When gallstones are acutely symptomatic, they commonly cause biliary colic, a result of transient blockage of a bile duct, which is characterized by right-upper-quadrant pain, often radiating to the back or right shoulder and lasting longer than 30 minutes and nausea and vomiting (Pak & Lindseth, 2016). Other more chronic symptoms include a dull ache, intolerance of fatty foods, dyspepsia, and increase in flatulence. The treatment and management of acute and chronic cholecystitis is laparoscopic cholecystectomy. Medical treatment includes shock-wave lithotripsy and medical dissolution therapy. Dissolution therapy, primarily with bile acids, has largely been replaced with cholecystectomy, but may be indicated for some patients. There is a high rate of stone recurrence following treatment (Tiderington et al., 2016).

Both malignant and benign tumors can be found in the gallbladder. Benign tumors that are found in the gallbladder are papillomas, adenomyomas, or cholesterol polyps. Malignant tumors of the gallbladder, primarily adenocarcinomas, are relatively rare, but are the most common and aggressive cancer of the biliary tract (Kanthan, Senger, Ahmed, & Kanthan, 2015). Risk factors for gallbladder cancer include chronic inflammation, gallstones, gallbladder polyps, age, female gender, obesity, genetics, and ethnicity (Kanthan et al., 2015). Abdominal ultrasound, CT, or MRI can identify the tumor location. An endoscopic ultrasound (EUS) with biopsy or endoscopic retrograde cholangiopancreatography (ERCP) with tissue sampling can be used for diagnosis. Treatment modalities include surgery, radiation, and chemotherapy, alone or in combination, depending on tumor staging and grading.

Surgery is the only curative approach to gallbladder cancer. However, only about 20% of tumors are diagnosed early enough for a surgical cure. Most patients with gallbladder cancer are asymptomatic, making early diagnosis difficult. Most gallbladder cancers are discovered incidentally or diagnosed at an advanced stage (Kanthan et al., 2015).

BILIARY TRACT DISEASE

Choledocholithiasis is a gallstone in the common bile duct and can cause biliary obstruction, biliary colic pain, elevated liver function tests, cholangitis, and gallstone pancreatitis. About 11% to 21% of patients with gallstones also have common bile duct stones (Costi, Gnocchi, Di Mario, & Sarli, 2014). Intraoperative cholangiography can identify stones in the biliary tree; ERCP can be performed for stone removal. Lithotripsy may be used to break up a very large stone for easier removal (Costi et al., 2014).

Primary sclerolsing cholangitis (PSC) is a chronic, idiopathic inflammatory disease of the bile ducts. The disease is characterized by fibrosis of the bile duct and ultimately leads to end-stage liver disease (Hirschfield, Karlsen, Lindor, & Adams, 2013). PSC is linked to inflammatory bowel disease (IBD); approximately 60% to 80% of patients with PSC also have IBD. PSC results in biliary strictures, recurrent cholangitis, and biliary cirrhosis; approximately 50% of patients eventually need a liver transplant (Hirschfield et al., 2013).

Cholangiocarcinoma is a rare cancer of the bile duct, and is classified as intra- or extrahepatic based on the location of the tumor. Risk factors include PSC and ulcerative colitis. Symptoms include signs of biliary obstruction, weight loss, and abdominal pain. Five-year survival rates vary from 15% to 30% for localized cancers to 2% for stage 4 malignancies (American Cancer Society [ACS], 2017). Most tumors are unable to be surgically removed. Treatment options include surgical resection, radiation/chemotherapy, and palliative therapy with biliary stenting to maintain biliary drainage.

Clinical Aspects

ASSESSMENT

An understanding of the risk factors associated with gallbladder disease is useful in helping nurses identify patients at risk, provide information regarding preventive strategies, and to provide education and resources for disease management (Pak & Lindseth, 2016). Patients at risk for cholelithiasis include females older than 40 years, Native American or Mexican American ethnicity, and obesity (Pak & Lindseth, 2016). Other risk factors include sedentary lifestyle, dyslipidemia, rapid weight loss, treatment with estrogen therapy, type 2 diabetes, and family history. Nursing interventions and management include healthy dietary and lifestyle changes, weight loss, nutrition guidance, education on signs/symptoms of gallstone disease, and strategies to reduce modifiable risk factors. Choledocholithiasis is usually discovered at either the time of gallbladder surgery or when a patient presents with symptoms of biliary duct obstruction.

Diagnostic studies include complete blood count, liver function tests, and serum amylase and lipase to differentiate among types of gallbladder disorders and complications of gallbladder disease. Abdominal ultrasound and cholescintigraphy (hepatobiliary iminodiacetic acid [HIDA] scan) are commonly used to diagnose cholelithiasis and cholecystitis. Magnetic resonance cholangiopancreatography (MRCP) and ERCP are indicated if choledocholithiasis is suspected; ERCP can be used diagnostically or therapeutically to remove stones or place stents.

OUTCOMES

Patients may be hospitalized for acute cholecsytitis. Treatment consists of bowel rest, intravenous (IV) fluids, and IV antibiotics. Complications of cholecystitis include gangrenous gallbladder, perforation, and peritonitis. Surgical options include laparoscopic, percutaneous, and open cholecystectomy. Perioperative nursing care consists of pain management, prevention of postoperative complications, and discharge education. The nursing care for patients with gallbladder cancer is focused on perioperative care if the tumor is resectable and oncology care for a patient who may undergo chemotherapy and/or radiation as treatment.

Summary

Gallbladder disease is found in 10% to 20% of the adult population and is a frequent cause for hospitalization (Shabanzadeh, Sørensen, & Jørgensen, 2016). Gallstones are common in the population, but only a small percentage of patients with gallstones are symptomatic (Tiderington et al., 2016). A better understanding of the risk factors for gallbladder and biliary tract disease is beneficial for nurses to better provide education about reducing the risk of disease and preventing complications for those already diagnosed (Pak & Lindseth, 2016).

American Cancer Society. (2017). Survival statistics for bile duct cancers. Retrieved from https://www.cancer.org/cancer/bile-duct-cancer/detection-diagnosis-staging/survival-by-stage.html

Costi, R., Gnocchi, A., Di Mario, F., & Sarli, L. (2014). Diagnosis and management of choledocholithiasis in the golden age of imaging, endoscopy and laparoscopy. *World Journal of Gastroenterology, 20*(37), 13382–13401. doi:10.3748/wjg.v20.i37.13382

Hirschfield, G. M., Karlsen, T. H., Lindor, K. D., & Adams, D. H. (2013). Primary sclerosing cholangitis. *Lancet, 382*(9904), 1587–1599. doi:10.1016/S0140-6736(13)60096-3

Kanthan, R., Senger, J.-L., Ahmed, S., & Kanthan, S. C. (2015). Gallbladder cancer in the 21st century. *Journal of Oncology, 2015,* 967472. doi:10.1155/2015/967472

Pak, M., & Lindseth, G. (2016). Risk factors for cholelithiasis. *Gastroenterology Nursing, 39*(4), 297–309. doi:10.1097/SGA.0000000000000235

Shabanzadeh, D. M., Sørensen, T. L., & Jørgensen, T. (2016). Abdominal symptoms and incident gallstones in a population unaware of gallstone status. *Canadian Journal of Gastroenterology and Hepatology, 2016,* 9730687. doi:10.1155/2016/9730687

Tiderington, E., Lee, S. P., & Ko, C. W. (2016). Gallstones: New insights into an old story. *F1000Research, 5,* 1817. doi:10.12688/f1000research.8874.1

■ GASTRIC CANCER

Una Hopkins
Jane F. Marek

Overview

Cancer of the stomach is the third leading cause of cancer deaths globally, with an estimated 700,000 deaths occurring annually. Once the leading cause of cancer-related deaths in the United States, gastric cancer is now the 15th most common cancer. The decline in the incidence of stomach cancer in the United States is thought to be a result of recognition of risk factors, including *Helicobacter pylori* infection, poor refrigeration, and an increase in consumption of fresh foods and vegetables. Despite the declining incidence in the United States, the prognosis remains poor, because most patients are diagnosed with advanced stage disease and few, if any, curative options. This is clearly reflected when comparing the 5-year survival rates for stage 1 cancer (57%–71%) compared with stage 3 (9%–20%) and stage 4 (4%; American Cancer Society [ACS], 2017). The disease is more prevalent in Central and Eastern Europe, Central and South America, and Asia; more than 70% of gastric cancer is found in developing countries. The highest rate of gastric cancer is in Korea, followed by Mongolia and Japan (World Cancer Research Fund International [WCRFI], 2015). The ACS estimates 28,000 new cases of gastric cancer and 10,960 deaths for 2017 (ACS, 2017). In the United States, the incidence of gastric cancer is higher among Asian Americans, Pacific Islanders, Hispanics, Native Americans, and African Americans, and least common among Whites.

Background

There are two types of gastric cancer: intestinal and diffuse. Most cases of gastric cancer are adenocarcinomas and histologically resemble cancers arising from the intestinal tract. Other types of gastric cancer include lymphomas, gastrointestinal stromal tumors, carcinoids, and squamous cell. Adenocarcinomas originate in the mucosal layer of the stomach and then spread outward. The liver is the most common site of metastasis (48%), followed by the peritoneum (32%), lung (15%), and bone (12%); the site of metastasis varies on location of the gastric lesion (Riihimäki et al., 2016).

Dietary and lifestyle factors impact the risk of gastric cancer. A diet high in salt; processed meat; fish, fried, pickled, and smoked foods; and low in fiber and fresh fruits and vegetables increase an individual's risk for gastric cancer. Obesity, smoking, and a family history of gastric cancer are also risk factors. Other contributing factors include *H. pylori* and Epstein–Barr infection, chronic atrophic gastritis, gastric ulcers, pernicious anemia, intestinal metaplasia, familial adenomatous polyposis, and hereditary nonpolyposis colorectal cancer (Lynch syndrome; Ajani et al., 2016).

Gastric cancer is generally asymptomatic until late stages when it has progressed through the muscularis and serosa layers of the stomach. Clinical manifestations include indigestion, dysphagia, loss of appetite, bloating, nausea, weight loss, melena, hematemesis, and pain in the upper abdomen. Gastric outlet obstruction, small bowel obstruction, pleural effusion, and jaundice may occur with advanced metastatic disease.

There are no routine screening guidelines for gastric cancer. Diagnostic tests include esophagogastroduodenscopy (EGD), endoscopic ultrasound, and upper gastrointestinal series and barium swallow. Chest x-ray, CT, and positron emission tomography may be indicated to evaluate for metastases. Tumor markers, such as carcinoembryonic antigen (CEA) and carbohydrate antigen (CA19-9), may be used to evaluate the effectiveness of treatment.

Once a diagnosis of gastric cancer has been made through biopsy, the tissue should be tested for human epidermal growth factor receptor 2 (HER-2/neu or HER-2) levels. This molecular marker was originally discovered in breast cancer and is associated with other malignancies, including gastric and gastroesophageal cancer. HER-2 overexpression in gastric cancer varies from 4.4% to 53.4% (Abrahao-Machado & Scapulatempo-Neto, 2016). Trastuzumab (Herceptin), a monoclonal antibody that targets HER-2, is approved for gastric cancer. Testing for HER-2 must be done to identify patients who might benefit from this treatment and other molecular HER-2 agents being evaluated for treatment of gastric cancer (Abrahao-Machado & Scapulatempo-Neto, 2016). Treatment for gastric cancer depends on the location, size, and staging of the tumor.

A multidisciplinary team consisting of surgeons, radiation oncologists, gastroenterologists, dieticians, and nurses offers the best approach to care. According to National Comprehensive Cancer Network guidelines, early-stage cancers are treated with endoscopic mucosal resection or partial or total gastrectomy (Ajani et al., 2016). Chemotherapy can be used preoperatively or postoperatively in addition to radiation depending on the tumor stage. Chemotherapy and radiation may be indicated for unresectable tumors and palliation.

Clinical Aspects

ASSESSMENT

Nurses play a significant role in teaching and supporting the patients and their families throughout the cancer continuum. From providing support as patients cope with a new diagnosis of gastric cancer, teaching about the expected outcomes following surgery, chemotherapy, or radiation, to advocating for patients and their families at the end of life, nurses are the primary caregivers.

When caring for patients who have undergone surgical treatment of gastric cancer, nurses can implement evidence-based interventions to improve patient outcomes. These interventions include an interactive education program about gastric cancer, treatment, and symptom management; the Modified Hospital Elder Life Program (HELP) consists of early mobilization, nutritional assistance, and therapeutic cognitive activities, and perioperative interventions, including self-management of pain, management of enteral and abdominal drains, and dietary education. These interventions resulted in a decrease in delirium and improvement in functional and nutritional status, improvement in patients' knowledge about the disease process and treatments, improvement in coping skills and quality of life, and reduced postoperative complications and improvement in quality of life (Gomes et al., 2016).

OUTCOMES

The goal of surgical treatment is to improve survival, reduce symptoms, and maintain quality of life with the minimal amount of adverse effects. Five-year survival rates following surgical treatment of gastric cancer have improved and have been reported to be as high as 33% to 50% (Shan, Shan, Morris, Golani, & Saxena, 2015). A systematic review of patients' health-related quality of life (HRQOL) scores following partial and total gastrectomy demonstrated that HQOL was negatively impacted 1-month postsurgery but returned to preoperative levels or better 1 year after surgery. Patients continued to have gastrointestinal symptoms 6 months after surgery. Patients who underwent partial gastrectomy had better HQOL scores in the physical, emotional, and functional status domains and returned to preoperative levels faster than patients who underwent total gastrectomy (Shan et al., 2015). Nurses can apply these findings by ensuring that the patients undergoing partial and total gastrectomy are prepared to experience a decline in overall health and functional status in the first few months following surgery and understand this will most likely improve with time.

Monitoring the patient's nutritional status following gastric resection or gastrectomy is a priority. If patients are unable to tolerate oral feedings, parenteral nutrition may be indicated until the patient is able to tolerate enteral feeding. Most patients experience dumping syndrome following gastric resection. The nurse can reassure the patient that these symptoms usually lessen or resolve after several months and teach the patient dietary modifications to reduce their occurrence. A nutritional consult should be initiated to plan strategies to best meet the patient's nutritional needs while in the hospital and after discharge. Most patients experience a 20% weight loss over the first 3 to 6 months after surgery. Following gastrectomy, the patients require lifelong injections of vitamin B_{12} due to the loss of parietal cells and intrinsic factor necessary for absorption of vitamin B_{12} in the ileum.

Summary

Gastric cancer continues to be a leading cause of cancer deaths worldwide and a global health concern, despite declining rates in the United States. Gastric cancer is difficult to diagnose early due to its nonspecific symptoms in early stages, which contribute to the poor prognosis associated with this disease. Screening for gastric cancer is controversial and varies by geographic region. Screening programs have been implemented in Korea, Japan, and other countries with a high incidence of gastric cancer, but there are no evidence-based recommendations for the United States. Infection with *H. pylori* is a known risk factor for gastric cancer, and testing and treating *H. pylori* is relatively easy and inexpensive. More research is needed to examine the effectiveness of screening for *H. pylori* infection as a method of reducing the incidence of gastric cancer, especially in countries where the disease is prevalent (Herrero, Parsonnet, & Greenberg, 2014). The World Health Organization identified evaluating the effectiveness of screening and treating *H. pylori* infection as a method to reduce the incidence of gastric cancer as a global priority (Wald, 2014). Clinical trials are underway in several countries. Nurses can play a role in prevention by health-promotion teaching and risk reduction strategies.

Management of the patient with gastric cancer depends on the health of the individual, stage of disease, and treatment modality. Maintaining quality of life, managing symptoms, and promoting optimal nutrition are priorities of care for patients with any stage of gastric cancer. Nurses can provide information regarding resources and psychosocial support for patients with unresectable disease as they face end-of-life decisions. A multidisciplinary approach and supportive care are essential components of care for the patients and their families throughout the disease process.

Abrahao-Machado, L. F., & Scapulatempo-Neto, C. (2016). HER2 testing in gastric cancer: An update. *World Journal of Gastroenterology, 22*(19), 4619–4625. doi:10.3748/wjg.v22.i19.4619

Ajani, J. A., D'Amico, T. A., Almhanna, K., Bentrem, D. J., Chao, J., Das, P., . . . Sundar, H. (2016). Gastric cancer, version 3.2016, NCCN clinical practice guidelines in oncology. *Journal of the National Comprehensive Cancer Network, 14*(10), 1286–1312.

American Cancer Society. (2017). What are the key statistics about stomach cancer? Retrieved from https://www.cancer.org/cancer/stomach-cancer/about/key-statistics.html

Gomes, N. C. R. P., Vilaca de Brito Santos, C. S., Rodrigues Bettencourt de Jesus, M. M. G., & da Silva Henriques, M. A. (2016). Effectiveness of nursing interventions in the postoperative recover of gastric cancer patients: A systematic literature review. *Journal of Nursing Referencia, 4*(11), 111–119. doi:10.12707/RIV16050

Herrero, R., Parsonnet, J., & Greenberg, E. R. (2014). Prevention of gastric cancer. *Journal of the American Medical Association, 312*(12), 1197–1198. doi:10.1001/jama.2014.10498

Riihimäki, M., Hemminki, A., Sundquist, K., Sundquist, J., & Hemminki, K. (2016). Metastatic spread in patients with gastric cancer. *Oncotarget, 7*(32), 52307–52316. doi:10.18632/oncotarget.10740

Shan, B., Shan, L., Morris, D., Golani, S., & Saxena, A. (2015). Systematic review on quality of life outcomes after gastrectomy for gastric carcinoma. *Journal of Gastrointestinal Oncology, 6*(5), 544–560. doi:10.3978/j.issn.2078-6891.2015.046

Wald, N. J. (2014). The treatment of *Helicobacter pylori* infection of the stomach in relation to the possible prevention of gastric cancer. In IARC *Helicobacter pylori* Working Group (Ed.), *Helicobacter pylori eradication as a strategy for preventing gastric cancer* (pp. 174–180). Lyon, France: International Agency for Research on Cancer. Retrieved from http://www.iarc.fr/en/publications/pdfs-online/wrk/wrk8/index.php

World Cancer Research Fund International. (2015). Stomach cancer statistics. Retrieved from http://www.wcrf.org/int/cancer-facts-figures/data-specific-cancers/stomach-cancer-statistics

■ GASTRITIS

Maria G. Smisek

Overview

Gastritis is inflammation or swelling of the mucosal lining in the stomach (Cohen & Hull, 2015; Porth, 2015). Gastritis can be acute or chronic in nature and is considered one of the most common problems affecting the stomach. The National Institute of Diabetes and Digestive and Kidney Disease (NIDDK) estimates 60 to 70 million people in the United States have some form of a digestive disease resulting in 36.6 million office visits, 21.7 million hospitalizations, 245,921 deaths, and a total cost of $141.8 billion in direct and indirect care (NIDDK, 2014b).

Background

Gastritis is a disorder affecting the mucosa of the stomach. The epithelial lining of the stomach is usually impermeable to the gastric secretions produced, creating a mucosal barrier. In gastritis, the mucosa undergoes inflammatory changes that can lead to ulceration or bleeding. Common threats affecting the integrity of the mucosal lining are irritation, infections (predominately *Helicobacter pylori*), injury to the stomach lining due to trauma or surgery or an autoimmune response (NIDDK, 2014c). Contributing factors include excessive alcohol intake, ingesting food contaminated with bacteria, gastroesophageal reflux, chemicals, infection, and surgical procedures or trauma. Severe gastritis can erode the mucosa, forming a peptic ulcer in the membrane of the esophagus, stomach, or duodenum (Cohen & Hull, 2015, NIDDK, 2014a).

Gastritis may be acute or chronic and presents as erosive or nonerosive. Erosive gastritis occurs when the stomach lining begins to wear down, exhibiting ulcerations and erosions. Nonerosive gastritis causes inflammation to the stomach lining without subsequent ulceration or erosion. Approximately 30% to 40% of the population of the United States develops an *H. pylori* infection, lying dormant for years before exhibiting signs and symptoms (Kulnigg-Dabsch, 2016; NIDDK, 2014b).

Acute gastritis is an acute episode of inflammation of the stomach mucosa, which is typically a self-limiting condition that resolves in several days postremoval of the aggravating agent. Damage to the stomach lining from inflammation can be a result of exposure to nonsteroidal anti-inflammatory drugs (NSAIDs); foods or liquids that have low acidity or high alkalinity, such as alcohol, coffee, and spicy foods, chemical agents, or radiation. A reduction in mucus production and/or an increase in acidity lead to tissue damage. Progression from acute to chronic disease depends on the affected location in the stomach. Extreme physiologic stress related to serious medical or surgical intervention weakens the mucosa making it susceptible to an acute hemorrhage gastritis (Porth, 2015).

Chronic gastritis is an absence of grossly visible erosion and chronic inflammatory changes to the epithelium that persists for more than 3 months (Cohen & Hull, 2015, NIDDK, 2014c). Without treatment, chronic gastritis may persist for years leading to atrophy of the glandular epithelium and serious complications. Chronic gastritis has three major types: *H. pylori* gastritis, chronic autoimmune gastritis, and chemical gastropathy (Porth, 2015). *H. pylori* gastritis is the result of *H. pylori* bacteria causing a chronic inflammation of the antrum and body of the stomach. Possible modes of transmission are fecal–oral, oral–oral, and environmental (Porth, 2015). The *H. pylori* bacteria interferes with the mucosal barrier of the stomach and damages its lining. Prevent infection by following good hygiene: eat only food washed and cooked properly, wash with soap and water after using the restroom and before eating. Damage to the stomach lining related to NSAIDs use, alcohol consumption, exposure to chemicals or trauma can progress from an acute phase to chronic if untreated.

Autoimmune gastritis is chronic inflammation that eventually results in mucosal atrophy. The immune system attacks healthy parietal cells in the lining of the stomach affecting iron and B_{12} absorption and consequently causing pernicious anemia (Kulnigg-Dabsch, 2016). Pernicious anemia is a decrease in red blood cells due to inability to absorb B_{12}. Chemical gastritis is the result of exposure to bilious, pancreatic, or duodenal secretions. This form is seen typically in clients with abdominal surgery such as gastroduodenostomy or gastrojejunostomy (Porth, 2015).

Clinical Aspects

ASSESSMENT

A detailed history, including prescription and over-the-counter medications used, past illnesses along with the onset, duration, relieving, and aggravating factors related to signs and symptoms of acute or chronic exposure, should be taken. Findings may include long-term use of known irritants: aspirin, other NSAIDs, or chemotherapy. Dietary history may identify poor nutritional habits, allergies, alcohol, coffee, and tobacco use. Travel history, especially to developing countries, can indicate exposure to *H. pylori* or other bacteria. Complaints of dizziness, fatigue, pallor, shortness of breath may indicate anemia secondary to gastrointestinal (GI) bleeding (NIDDK, 2014c; Porth, 2015; Sipponen, 2015). Epigastric pain, anorexia, nausea, and vomiting may reveal abdominal distension, bloating and tenderness on physical exam. It is important to recognize any episode of dark stools, blood in emesis or coffee grounds indicates bleeding (Cohen & Hull, 2015; NIDDK, 2014c; Porth, 2015).

Diagnostic studies can be invasive or noninvasive based on history and physical findings. A blood test identifies anemia and stool for occult blood indicates GI bleeding. A noninvasive urea breath test can identify *H. pylori*, whereas an upper endoscopy visualizes the anatomy of the stomach and duodenum. Signs of irritation or ulceration indicate active gastritis. A small biopsy taken during the procedure rules out *H. pylori* and direct treatment.

Following diagnosis, a plan of care is developed between the physician and the client. Successful treatment is indicated when the symptoms are resolved and, in the case of *H. pylori*, the bacteria is eliminated (Porth, 2015).

Nursing-related problems include pain (acute or chronic) related to disruption of mucosal lining of the stomach as evidenced by use of irritants (NSAIDs, smoking, extreme stress), infection (*H. pylori*), trauma or surgery and infection related to ulceration of duodenum as evidenced by *H. pylori* bacteria (via biopsy), burning pain in abdomen, anorexia, and weight loss.

NURSING INTERVENTIONS, MANAGEMENT, AND IMPLICATIONS

Nursing interventions include assessing the client's past and present pain level (using a 1 to 10 scale), assessing for signs of infection, administering pain medication and antibiotics as ordered, and educating the client on the effect irritants, such as NSAIDs, alcohol, coffee, and smoking, have on stomach mucosa. Teaching should include alternative treatment for discomfort, setting treatment goals, implications for revision of intervention depending on client response, and identifying patient understanding through verbalization and return demonstration. The nurse should also supply the patients and their families with a list of community resources to assist compliance.

OUTCOMES

Although some people with gastritis have no pain or discomfort, others have been living with pain and discomfort. Inflammation and swelling can cause destruction of the epithelial lining of the stomach. Left untreated, gastritis can lead to peptic ulcers, anemia, erosion, and hemorrhage. Complaints of epigastric pain or other GI symptoms and a history of exposure to GI irritants suggests gastritis. Management of gastritis is done by treating the underlying cause and reducing the amount of acid in the stomach. Repeated use of irritants and medications can exacerbate the condition leading to hospitalization and long-term treatment.

Summary

Patient education is a key element in the treatment of patients with gastritis. Education regarding *H. pylori* and the suspected mode of transmission can assist in preventing exposure (NIDDK, 2014c; Porth, 2015). Early diagnosis of gastritis and its causitive agent can facilitate a speedy recovery. Identifying client concerns regarding treatment plan, cost, and access to that treatment are an essential nursing responsibility.

Cohen, B. J., & Hull, K. L. (2015). *Memmlers's the human body in health and disease* (13th ed., pp. 432–458). Philadelphia, PA: Wolters Kluwer.

Kulnigg-Dabsch, S. (2016). Autoimmune gastritis. *Wiener Medizinische Wochenschrift, 166*(13), 424–430. doi:10.1007/s10354-016-0515-55

National Institute of Diabetes and Digestive and Kidney Disease. (2014a). Definition & facts for peptic ulcers (stomach ulcers). Retrieved from https://www.niddk.nih.gov/health-information/digestive-diseases/peptic-ulcers-stomach-ulcers/definition-facts

National Institute of Diabetes and Digestive and Kidney Disease. (2014b). Digestive diseases statistics for the United States. Retrieved from https://www.niddk.nih.gov/health-information/health-statistics/Pages/digestive-diseases-statistics-for-the-united-states.aspx

National Institute of Diabetes and Digestive and Kidney Disease. (2014c). Gastritis. Retrieved from https://www.niddk.nih.gov/health-information/digestive-diseases/gastritis

Porth, C. M. (2015). Disorders of gastrointestinal function. In C. M. Porth (Ed.), *Essentials of pathophysiology* (4th ed., pp. 696–723). Philadelphia, PA: Wolters Kluwer.

Sipponen, P. M. H.-I. (2015, June 3). Chronic gastritis. *Scandinavian Journal of Gastroenterology, 50*(6), 657–667. doi:10.3109/00365521.2015.1019918

■ GASTROESOPHAGEAL REFLUX DISEASE

Kelly Ann Lynn

Overview

Gastroesophageal reflux is a normal process that occurs in healthy adults and children when stomach contents briefly back up or "reflux" into the esophagus. Gastroesophageal reflux disease (GERD) is a consensus diagnosis that refers to the bothersome symptoms or complications that occur as a result of gastroesophageal reflux (Vakil, van Zanten, Kahrilas, Dent, Jones, & Global Consensus Group, 2006). Patients with GERD may be at increased risk of developing esophageal stricture, Barrett's esophagus, and esophageal cancer (Francis et al., 2013; Katz, Gerson, & Vela, 2013). GERD has been indicated in increased morbidity related to aspiration, particularly with intubated patients and exacerbation of symptoms for patients with asthma. Nursing care of patients with GERD focuses on prevention of complications, education, and management of symptoms and medications.

Background

Incidence of GERD is fairly common and is reported to affect 20% to 30% of the U.S. population (Katz et al., 2013; Kleiman et al., 2013). GERD may affect up to 40% of the U.S. population (Francis et al., 2013; Vaezi et al., 2016). Although there is no significant demographic predisposition to GERD, incidence is lower in Eastern Asia as compared to Western Europe and North America (Lightdale & Gremse, 2013). GERD is present in both adult and pediatric populations.

The costs associated with GERD are astounding. Kleiman et al. (2013) reported 5.5 million U.S. outpatient visits in 2002 and 76,000 inpatient admissions in 2005 for GERD-related care, and over $10 billion spent on acid-reducing medications in 2004. Likewise, Francis et al. (2013) note national expenditures ranging from $9.3 billion to $12.1 billion for GERD-related care.

GERD is associated with weakness or malfunction of the lower esophageal sphincter (LES), which connects the esophagus to the stomach. GERD affects the LES, a muscle connecting the esophagus and stomach. Gastric contents back up, or reflux, into the esophagus due to changes in LES muscle tone or increased pressure below the sphincter. Other factors contributing to the pathophysiology of GERD include decreased esophageal motility, which may be related to underlying diseases like achalasia or possibly the result of allergies or other inflammatory reactions. Pregnancy, obesity, and hiatal hernias also increase the incidence of GERD.

Patients with GERD typically present with complaints of heartburn, regurgitation, and sour taste in the mouth. These are also called *esophageal symptoms*. Atypical presentation (extraesophageal symptoms) include chronic cough, hoarseness, sore throat, worsening oral health, recurrent earache and ear infections, and nocturnal asthma (Katz et al., 2013; Lightdale & Gremse, 2013). More bothersome symptoms include vomiting, pain, and difficulty swallowing.

Clinical Aspects

ASSESSMENT

A thorough nursing assessment is essential for patients with GERD. This includes a comprehensive patient history with targeted questions related to eating habits and symptom triggers and remedies. Physical assessment should include accurate measurement of the patient's height and weight. Swallowing ability and gag reflex must be assessed to determine risk for aspiration. Patients presenting with pain (chest pain radiating to neck, jaw, and arm) need immediate evaluation to rule out myocardial infarction (MI) and angina as GERD symptoms can mimic these life-threatening conditions.

Review of essential laboratory values includes cardiac enzymes to rule out MI for patients presenting with chest pain, complete blood count (CBC) to assess for anemia, serum chemistry to assess for electrolyte imbalances and malnutrition, and serum iron studies (transferrin, total iron binding capacity, transferring saturation, or ferritin) are collected to help differentiate if an anemia is related to an iron-deficiency or chronic inflammation.

Review of medications is an essential part of the nursing assessment. Anticholinergic medications may delay gastric emptying and should be used cautiously in patients with GERD. Some pain medications (i.e., nonsteroidal anti-inflammatory drugs [NSAIDs] and aspirin) may cause gastritis and GI bleeding and should therefore be avoided.

Older children and adult patients may be prescribed an 8-week course of a proton pump inhibitor (PPI) to alleviate symptoms of GERD as a first-line therapy. PPIs should be taken 30 to 60 minutes before the first meal of the day for maximum efficacy. It is essential to review the prescribed schedule for PPI administration as studies have shown up to 70% of primary care practitioners in the United States advised patients to take the PPI at bedtime (Katz et al., 2013). Nurses should counsel patients on the appropriate dose and timing of PPIs.

NURSING INTERVENTIONS, MANAGEMENT, AND IMPLICATIONS

Nursing care of patients with GERD should be tailored to the patients' symptoms and clinical status. The focus of care should be prevention of the serious consequences related to GERD. Optimizing compliance with medication, diet, and lifestyle modifications will reduce symptoms of GERD and promote quality of life.

It is important that the nurses involved in the care of patients with GERD educate patients on all aspects of treatment and management. All medications should be reviewed for potential adverse interactions and side effects. Patients should be educated on proper administration of medications to maximize the effective relief of symptoms.

Knowledge of simple lifestyle modifications and medication therapy may be the only measures needed to reach treatment goals. Patients who are unresponsive to medical management and who are experiencing considerable distress from symptoms may be referred for esophageal testing (endoscopy, esophageal pH study, manometry) and/or surgical intervention. These patients need education about the planned interventions and specific issues related to various surgical options (fundoplication, myotomy). Symptoms can be alleviated by educating patients and their families about dietary recommendations and lifestyle modifications. Some eating habits can help manage symptoms of heartburn and reflux. Patients should be advised to practice mindful eating in a calm and relaxed environment, chew thoroughly, and avoid eating while standing. Remind patients to eat small meals and snacks to avoid overeating and abdominal distention. Dinner should be a lighter meal and patients should wait 2 to 3 hours after eating before they lie down.

Some foods and beverages cause the LES to relax and thus increase gastric secretions and acid level in the stomach subsequently causing "heartburn" and reflux symptoms. Patients should be educated to stay away from foods that are known to exacerbate symptoms. These include fruits and vegetables like bell peppers, tomatoes, and tomato sauce; citrus fruits and juices; beans; and cabbages. Heavy, high-fat, and fried foods should be avoided as well as spicy food, mints, and chocolate. Caffeine, carbonated beverages, and alcohol, especially red wine, should be avoided.

Patients should be encouraged to consume a healthy diet of lean protein, low-fat dairy products, heart-healthy fats, and whole grains. Some dietary additions that may alleviate symptoms include ginger, Chamomile tea, and fermented foods (i.e., kimchee, sauerkraut, kefir, tempeh, miso, plain yogurt, or kombucha). Keeping a food journal may help patients identify foods that trigger symptoms. Once a patient has achieved thorough and complete remission of symptoms through medication and lifestyle modifications, he or she may slowly reintroduce foods one at a time to ensure that they do not exacerbate symptoms.

Patients with GERD are encouraged to adopt healthy lifestyle habits. Weight loss, avoiding alcohol and smoking, and incorporating stress-reducing behaviors (exercise, yoga, meditation) all correlate with symptom relief. Patients should avoid tight clothing as this can increase pressure on the LES and exacerbate symptoms. Likewise, lying flat can promote reflux so patients are encouraged to sleep on several pillows.

Management of GERD symptoms centers around lifestyle and diet modification. Adherence to these modifications may cause stress for patients and their families. Parents of children and babies with GERD may become hypervigilant about the child's appetite, nutrition intake, and eating behaviors. This may lead to increased anxiety and tension around meals. Nurses must offer patients and their families support and encouragement as they manage their symptoms.

OUTCOMES

The expected outcomes of evidence-based nursing care for patients with GERD are effective management of symptoms and medications prescribed to treat them, increased quality of life, decreased incidence of serious consequences of GERD like aspiration pneumonia and exacerbation of asthma, and reduced sequelae of disease (i.e., Barrett's esophagus, esophageal adenocarcinoma).

Summary

GERD is a complicated health issue that can affect people of all demographics. The symptoms of GERD can adversely affect quality of life. Diagnosis can be elusive and effective management may rely on trial and error. Nursing care is essential to supporting patients through this process while promoting compliance with care plans and minimizing unnecessary distress and morbidity.

Francis, D. O., Rymer, J. A., Slaughter, J. C., Choksi, Y., Jiramongkolchai, P., Ogbeide, E., . . . Vaezi, M. F. (2013). High economic burden of caring for patients with suspected extraesophageal reflux. *American Journal of Gastroenterology, 108*(6), 905–911. doi:10.1038/ajg.2013.69

Katz, P. O., Gerson, L. B., & Vela, M. F. (2013). Guidelines for the diagnosis and management of gastroesophageal reflux disease. *American Journal of Gastroenterology, 108*(3), 308–328; quiz 329. doi:10.1038/ajg.2012.444

Kleiman, D. A., Sporn, M. J., Beninato, T., Metz, Y., Crawford, C., Fahey, T. J., & Zarnegar, R. (2013). Early referral for 24-hour esophageal pH monitoring may prevent unnecessary treatment with acid-reducing medications. *Surgical Endoscopy, 27*(4), 1302–1309. doi:10.1007/s00464-012-2602-z

Lightdale, J. R., & Gremse, D. A.; Section on Gastroenterology, Hepatology, and Nutrition. (2013). Gastroesophageal reflux: Management guidance for the pediatrician. *Pediatrics, 131*(5), e1684–e1695. doi:10.1542/peds.2013-0421

Vaezi, M. F., Brill, J. V., Mills, M. R., Bernstein, B. B., Ness, R. M., Richards, W. O., . . . Patel, K. (2016). An episode payment framework for gastroesophageal reflux disease. *Gastroenterology, 150*(4), 1019–1025. doi:10.1053/j.gastro.2016.02.037

Vakil, N., van Zanten, S. V., Kahrilas, P., Dent, J., & Jones, R.; Global Consensus Group. (2006). The Montreal definition and classification of gastroesophageal reflux disease: A global evidence-based consensus. *American Journal of Gastroenterology, 101*(8), 1900–1920; quiz 1943. doi:10.1111/j.1572-0241.2006.00630.x

■ GOUT

Maria A. Mendoza

Overview

Gout is a hereditary disease caused by deposits of uric acid crystals (monoso-dium urate) in the peripheral joints leading to inflammation. The most common site of inflammation is usually in the metatarsophalangeal joint of the great toe. Gout is also known as *gouty arthritis* and is the most common form of inflammatory arthritis. From 2007 to 2008, the National Health and Nutrition Survey (NHANES) found that 3.9% (8.3 million) of adults (20 years and more) self-reported a diagnosis of gout, a 1.2% increase over the past decade (Centers for Disease Control and Prevention [CDC], 2016). Men are afflicted more often (5.9%) than women (2.0%) with Black men affected about twice as often as White men (10.9% vs. 5.8%) (CDC, 2016). Data from the Health Professionals Follow-up Study showed an increased risk of all-cause mortality and cardiovas-cular disease mortality in men with gout (CDC, 2016). A diagnosis of gout has been associated with a poor quality of life (CDC, 2016). The major challenge to nurses caring for patients with gout is managing pain during acute episodes as well as preventing recurrent attacks.

Background

Gout can become a chronic disease with long remissions followed by acute exac-erbations. Acute attacks are caused by excessive intake of rich food and alcohol, particularly beer. Gout is a complex disorder with both genetic and environmen-tal risk factors, including increased age, hyperuricemia, dietary habits (intake of alcohol, sweetened beverages, fructose, seafood, meat, dairy product, coffee, and vitamin C), diuretic use, obesity, insulin resistance and metabolic syndrome, and impaired kidney function (Fuerst, 2015; Hainer, Matheson, & Wilkes, 2014; Harding, 2016).

Urates, a form of uric acid, are by-products of purine metabolism, a sub-stance present in all body tissues and foods. Urates are excreted through the kidneys to maintain a serum uric acid level between 4 and 6.8 mg/dL. Increased production coupled with decreased excretion of urates results in hyperuricemia (serum level greater than 6.8 mg/dL). It is interesting to note that hyperuricemia does not always progress to gout unless there is crystallization of urates, result-ing in inflammation.

The clinical presentation of gout includes extremely painful, inflamed, tender joints. It can involve any joint in the body but the metatarsophalangeal joint of the great toe is a common site because of the increased pressure on this joint during walking. Patients also report weakness, nausea, chills, and frequent uri-nation. Untreated gout can lead to serious injury. Urate crystals can accumulate in the kidneys, leading to stone formation, and in the joints (tophi). Tophi are found in the fingers and in cartilage, such as the ears, and can lead to inflammation, scarring, and deformity. Appearance of tophi is commonly referred as *tophaceous gout*. A definitive diagnosis of gout is made through synovial fluid analysis for urate crystals in the affected joint. However, in primary care, a diagnosis of gout may be made through the patient's history and clinical presentation, including a rapid acute onset of symptoms, unilateral metatarsophalangeal joint involvement, and prior episodes (Harding, 2016). The uric acid level is not diagnostic as half of the patients with acute gout have normal levels; obtaining a baseline value is recommended to monitor the effectiveness of therapy (Harding, 2016; Qaseem, Harris, & Forciea, 2016).

Clinical Aspects

ASSESSMENT

The nurse should perform a comprehensive history to determine the presence of the aforementioned risk factors. Physical assessment includes vital signs, height and weight, body mass index (BMI), examination of the involved joint, signs of insulin resistance markers such as acanthosis nigricans, and assessment for tophi in joints and ears. Laboratory screening for uric acid may be ordered as well as examination of the synovial fluid from joint aspirate to look for urate crystals.

NURSING INTERVENTIONS, MANAGEMENT, AND IMPLICATIONS

Applicable nursing diagnoses for the patient with gout include pain, acute or chronic; deficient knowledge; and impaired physical mobility.

The following interventions are primarily based on the American College of Physician's guidelines for managing the patient with gout (Qaseem et al., 2017).

Medication and dietary adherence is of primary importance during prophylactic treatment. The nurse is responsible for teaching the patient about the actions, side/adverse effects, and proper administration of prescribed medications. Acute attacks of gout are managed with pharmacologic treatment. Numerous randomized controlled trials (RCTs) show that colchicine and non-steroidal anti-inflammatory drugs (NSAIDs), such as naproxen, indomethacin, and sulindac, are effective in controlling pain in acute gout. Gastrointestinal adverse effects are common and these medications should be taken with food. Corticosteroids are used in acute exacerbations and their inflammatory effect is equivalent to NSAIDs. Patients should be taught signs of adverse effects of NSAIDs and steroids. Patients should be taught to avoid aspirin and niacin, which can precipitate acute episodes by raising uric acid levels.

To prevent flares, patients should observe some dietary restrictions. Foods high in purine, such as organ meats, beef, lamb, pork, and seafood, are to be avoided. Other food restrictions include sugar-sweetened drinks and fruit juices containing high-fructose corn syrup, vegetables and fruits high in vitamin C, nuts, whole grains, and legumes. The patient should be encouraged to drink at least eight glasses of fluids daily to prevent uric-related urolithiasis. Excessive emotional and physical stress, surgery, and acute illness can also cause a flare. The evidence on dietary counseling showed mixed results. A randomized controlled study by Holland and McGill (2014) demonstrated that diet education resulted in significant improvement in knowledge of the intervention group but had no effect on serum urate level at 6 months.

Urate-lowering therapy is considered in patients with tophi, a history of two or more acute episodes of inflammation per year, stage 2 or higher chronic kidney disease (CKD), or a history of urolithiasis. RCTs show that the use of low-dose colchicine and NSAID or NSAID alone is effective in reducing the risk of acute attacks in patients initiating urate-lowering therapy. Allopurinol is the first line of treatment, gradually titrated every 2 to 5 weeks to reach desired serum uric acid level. Lower doses are used in patients with significant CKD. A more expensive medication, febuxostat, does not require dose adjustment in CKD. Probenecid is prescribed for patients with contraindications to either allopurinol or febuxostat with no history of urolithiasis and creatinine clearance above 50 mL/min. The nurse should inform the patient not to take aspirin, which would cancel the effects of the drug. Prophylaxis may continue for 3 months in persons without tophi and up to 6 months if tophi are present.

Nonpharmacological pain management, such as topical ice application on the affected joints 30 minutes four times a day, nonweight bearing on affected joints, and bedrest, are recommended during severe attacks.

The nurse plays a supportive role during acute episodes that affect the functional and mobility status of the patient. The environment has to be assessed to ensure patient safety. Provisions of safety and mobility aids may be necessary. Emotional support should be provided as needed.

Summary

Gout is an inflammatory disease of the peripheral joints caused by accumulation of urate crystals with both genetic and environmental risk factors. Typical presentation is an acute onset of unilateral joint redness, swelling, and pain. Analysis of synovial fluid from the involved joint for presence of urate crystals is the gold standard for diagnosing gout, but diagnosis is usually made from history and clinical presentation in primary care. Gout is managed by pharmacologic treatment during acute episode and as prophylaxis. The nurse's responsibility is supporting the patient in managing symptoms, reducing flares, and monitoring effects of therapy. Patient education related to diet counseling, medication teaching, and lifestyle modification is an important part of nursing care.

Centers for Disease Control and Prevention. (2016). Arthritis. Retrieved from https://www.cdc.gov/arthritis/basics/gout.html

Fuerst, M. L. (2015). How common is gout in the United States, really? *Rheumatology Network, 11*(11), 649–662.

Hainer, B. L., Matheson, E., & Wilkes, R. T. (2014). Diagnosis, treatment, and prevention of gout. *American Family Physician, 90*(12), 831–836.

Harding, M. (2016). An update on gout for primary care providers. *Nurse Practitioner, 41*(4), 14–21; quiz 21. doi:10.1097/01.NPR.0000481510.32360.fa

Holland, R., & McGill, N. W. (2015). Comprehensive dietary education in treated gout patients does not further improve serum urate. *Internal Medicine Journal, 45*(2), 189–194. doi:10.1111/imj.12661

Qaseem, A., Harris, R. P., & Forciea, M. A.; Clinical Guidelines Committee of the American College of Physicians. (2017). Management of acute and recurrent gout: A clinical practice guideline from the American College of Physicians. *Annals of Internal Medicine, 166*(1), 58–68. doi:10.7326/M16-0570

■ GUILLAIN–BARRÉ SYNDROME

Kathleen Marsala-Cervasio

Overview

Guillain–Barré syndrome (GBS) is the most common acute inflammatory poly-neuropathy characterized by rapid, progressive, and symmetrical neuromuscular paralysis (Willison, Jacobs, & van Doorn, 2016). The annual incidence in the United States is 0.6 to 1.9 per 100,000 persons per year with 0.6 per 100,000 cases in children, and 2 to 7 per 100,000 persons per year in the elderly (Willison et al., 2016). It is believed that this disease is an autoimmune disorder triggered by infections, surgery, or vaccinations (Walling & Dickson, 2013). A severe man-ifestation of the disease triggers respiratory failure in approximately 25% of all cases and is fatal in 5% to 10% of cases worldwide (Walling & Dickson, 2013). GBS requires intensive nursing care to identify rapid progression and interven-tion as well as specific teaching and rehabilitation. Early detection of GBS is crucial to management of the syndrome.

Background

GBS is a fulminant polyradiculoneuropathy, characterized by progressive weak-ness and diminished to absent myotatic reflexes (Willison et al., 2016). First reported in the literature in 1834, this syndrome is believed to be triggered by infection stimulating an antiganglioside antibody production (Rajabally & Uncini, 2012). In approximately 70% of cases of GBS, symptoms occurs 1 to 3 weeks after an acute infectious process (Rajabally & Uncini, 2012). The organ-isms most commonly involved are *Campylobacter jejuni*, *Mycoplasma pneumo-nia*, *Haemophilus influenza*, cytomegalovirus, Epstein–Barr virus, and influenza (Willison et al., 2016). According to Rajabally and Uncini (2016), the adminis-tration of antirabies, influenza, and swine flu vaccines were all associated with an increase in the incidence of GBS.

Clinical Aspects

Clinical features of GBS include areflexia, progressive limb weakness initially in the legs, and uncommon sensory loss to the bulbar, facial, and respiratory func-tion within 2 to 4 weeks after onset, the time of maximum severity of symptoms (Willison et al., 2016). Typically, after a month of symptom onset, remyelination occurs and the recovery process begins, lasting from weeks to years, often with residual effects.

Additional GBS symptoms include autonomic dysfunction and pain. Pain is the first reported symptom accompanied with numbness and tingling in the hands and feet bilaterally (Willison et al., 2016). Progressive symmetrical weak-ness occurs from the distal to proximal extremities with diminished reflexes, proprioception, and vibratory sensation (Moore & Shepard, 2014). Autonomic dysfunction may be characterized by arrhythmias, blood pressure instability, respiratory dysfunction, dysphagia, dysarthria, and facial paralysis. Children initially present with the inability to walk in over 50% of GBS cases; rarely is the syndrome seen in infants (Willison et al., 2016). Recently, Zika virus and dengue fever have been responsible for reported cases of GBS outside the United States (van den Berg et al., 2014).

ASSESSMENT

Assessment for GBS begins with a history, specifically asking about either viral gastrointestinal or respiratory infections in the 2 weeks prior to symptom onset. Physical findings may include difficulty in walking, numbness in the hands and feet, body weakness, and functional decline in the prior few days. As GBS progresses, there is fever and bladder and bowel dysfunction (van den Berg et al., 2014). Laboratory tests may include a cytological examination of cerebral spinal fluid, which usually reveals an increased level of protein. Immunoglobulins and serum protein electrophoresis may have decreased levels of immunoglobulin (IgA). Blood tests may reveal cytomegalovirus or Epstein–Barr virus, and stool cultures may identify *C. jejuni*. Other diagnostic studies may include nerve conduction velocity studies, electromyography, electrocardiogram, and pulmonary function tests. Plasma exchange therapy and intravenous immune globulin therapy have been shown to haste recovery (Rosen, 2012).

NURSING INTERVENTIONS, MANAGEMENT, AND IMPLICATIONS

Initial nursing assessment consists of a history, complete physical, and psychosocial evaluation of potential signs or symptoms of GBS. Documentation must include recent travel as well as recent viral illnesses, vaccinations, and surgeries. Recent and current medications should be reviewed with the medical team. A neurological assessment should include the Glasgow Coma Scale, particular evaluation of muscle strength in all extremities, and questions for the presence of numbness and tingling of extremities, particularly the lower extremities. Filaments may be used for extremity sensory assessment. A complete set of vital signs should include oxygen saturation and a pain assessment. The respiratory system is thoroughly evaluated. If the patient is in a monitored environment, all vital signs should be continuously monitored with alarm settings on to identify any deviations quickly. As the nurse proceeds to continue assessing the patient, specific questions about bladder and bowel incontinence will be evaluated.

Safety is a priority and nurses should include a fall-prevention protocol that includes three rails up, call bell in reach, and frequent checks for activities of daily living. Weakness can also lead to other injuries like burns from hot drinks. Skin breakdown may occur and therefore prevention is key and implementation of skin care protocols a priority. Constant observation for incontinence is necessary to prevent skin breakdown. Patients with GBS should be on aspiration precautions with oxygen and suction at the bedside and the head of the bed up.

Venous thrombosis prevention by passive or active range of motion, intermittent pneumatic compression devices, or anticoagulant prophylaxis may be indicated. Referral to physical therapy, plus occupational and speech therapy for swallowing assessment may be indicated. The nurse should ensure communication, assess coping mechanisms, screen for depression, and plan for rehabilitation with the patients and their families.

OUTCOMES

The administration of corticosteroids has not demonstrated any benefit to prognosis. Supportive therapy includes pain management, monitoring vital signs, frequent respiratory assessments, and a focus on preventing complications while hospitalized. Neurological problems will persist in up to 20% of patients with GBS, and one half of these patients will be severely disabled (van den Berg et al., 2014).

Summary

GBS is potentially life-threatening; no cure is known. A history and physical findings with specific questions by the registered nurse (RN) can identify early symptoms and intervention. GBS requires an interdisciplinary approach to care, recovery, and long-term rehabilitation. Increased awareness of GBS screening is vital in a time of identification of new organisms, that is, Zika, increased use of vaccinations, and increased surgical interventions.

Moore, A. S., & Shepard, L. H. (2014). Myasthenia gravis vs. Guillain–Barré syndrome—What's the difference? *Nursing Made Incredibly Easy, 12*(4), 20–30.

Rajabally, Y. A., & Uncini, A. (2012). Outcome and its predictors in Guillain–Barre syndrome. *Journal of Neurology, Neurosurgery, and Psychiatry, 83*(7), 711–718. doi:10.1136/jnnp-2011-301882

Rosen, B. A. (2012). Guillain–Barré syndrome. *Pediatrics in Review, 33*(4), 164–70; quiz 170. doi:10.1542/pir.33-4-164

van den Berg, V., Walgaard, C., Drenthen, J., Fokke, C., Jacobs, B., & van Doorn, P. (2014). Guillain–Barré syndrome: Pathogenesis, diagnosis, treatment, and prognosis. *Neurology,* (10), 469–482.

Walling, A. D., & Dickson, G. (2013). Guillain–Barré syndrome. *American Family Physician, 87*(3), 191–197.

Willison, H. J., Jacobs, B. C., & van Doorn, P. A. (2016). Guillain–Barré syndrome. *Lancet, 388*(10045), 717–727. doi:10.1016/S0140-6736(16) 00339-1

■ HEART FAILURE

Arlene Travis

Overview

Heart failure (HF) is a common condition associated with significant mortality, morbidity, reduction in quality of life, and health care costs. Nurses play an important role in the care of patients with HF. Well-informed nurses, skilled in the care of patients with HF, make significant contributions to the health and well-being of these patients.

HF is a syndrome characterized by the inability of the heart to supply the body with sufficient blood and oxygen to meet its metabolic needs. HF is a chronic condition, with no cure, characterized by flares in disease severity, requiring life-long management to control symptoms and maintain optimal cardiac function. Patients with HF are subject to episodes of rapid worsening of symptoms, at which point chronic HF becomes acute HF (also known as *acute decompensated HF*), which usually requires hospitalization.

HF is a major public health problem and a global epidemic, affecting approximately 25 million people worldwide and 5.8 million in the United States (Ambrosy et al., 2014; Roger, 2013). The incidence of HF increases sharply with age (Go et al., 2012) and the number of people with HF is expected to rise dramatically due to the aging of the world's population. The number of Americans with HF is projected to increase from 5.8 million in 2012 to 8.5 million by 2030. One of five Americans will develop HF in their lifetime, and about 50% of patients with HF die within 5 years of diagnosis (Centers for Disease Control and Prevention [CDC], 2015). HF is one of the leading causes of hospitalizations in the United States and is responsible for 1 million hospitalizations every year (Pfuntner, Wier, & Stocks, 2013). Costs associated with HF place a significant economic burden on the health care system. In 2012, the cost of HF care in the United States was about $32 billion, and is anticipated to soar to $70 billion by 2030 (Heidenreich et al., 2013.) Hospitalizations account for the majority of the costs of caring for HF patients.

Background

HF begins when an event or insult to the heart impairs its ability to function, causing a reduction in cardiac output (CO). HF can be classified as ischemic or nonischemic depending on the underlying cause. The majority of patients (65%) have ischemic HF. In ischemic HF, decreased oxygenation of the myocardium, usually caused by coronary artery disease, results in decreased CO. In nonischemic HF, factors, such as hypertension or valve disease, cause the decrease in CO.

HF is categorized as systolic or diastolic. This distinction is based on the ejection fraction (EF), a measure of left ventricular (LV) function. EF is measured as the percentage of blood (which has filled the LV in diastole) that is pumped out during systole. In systolic HF (also known as *HF with reduced EF*), the EF is below normal. In diastolic HF (also known as *HF with preserved EF*), the EF remains normal or even high. Diastolic HF is caused by impaired ventricular filling during diastole, resulting in insufficient volume available to be pumped from the LV, whereas systolic HF is caused by impaired pumping action of the LV during systole.

CO (the volume of blood pumped by the heart in 1 minute) is determined by heart rate (HR) and stroke volume (SV), the volume of blood that is pumped from the LV in one myocardial contraction (systole). SV is determined by the interaction of three factors: *preload, afterload,* and *contractility. Preload* refers to volume of blood that fills the heart, *contractility* refers to the force with which the ventricle contracts, and *afterload* refers to the resistance the heart must overcome for blood to exit the ventricle (Butler, 2012).

When CO is reduced, the body attempts to compensate by activating mechanisms that affect both SV and HR (Rogers & Bush, 2015). HR is controlled by the sinoatrial node (SA), which is influenced by the sympathetic nervous system (SNS). Sympathetic activation is one of the key pathophysiologic mechanisms underlying HF; when the CO drops, the SNS is stimulated and HR increases.

Another underlying pathophysiologic process of HF is activation of the renin–angiotensin–aldosterone system (RAAS). As a result of decreased CO, renal perfusion is decreased. As a compensatory mechanism, the RAAS is activated causing the release of angiotensin II and aldosterone. Angiotensin II raises blood pressure (BP), increases afterload, and stimulates aldosterone production, which then leads to sodium and fluid retention and increased preload.

Initially, compensatory mechanisms are successful in restoring CO; however, this is short lived. In fact, these compensatory mechanisms have unintended consequences that actually cause the syndrome of HF. Activation of the SNS increases HR, temporarily restoring CO, but also places additional stress on an already struggling heart, which tires, and CO falls. Activation of the RAAS increases preload and afterload, which initially raise CO; however, additional strain is placed on the heart, and CO decreases even more. Compensatory mechanisms are reactivated over and over in response to successive reductions in CO, and a self-perpetuating cycle of unintended consequences (reduced CO and fluid and sodium retention) is established, which causes HF.

Clinical Aspects

The clinical presentation of HF is directly related to unintended effects of compensatory mechanisms. Reduced CO causes reduced oxygen delivery to the body tissues, causing symptoms of fatigue, activity intolerance, and alterations in mental status. Sodium and fluid retention cause edema, orthopnea, weight gain, pulmonary congestion, dyspnea, and pulmonary edema.

ASSESSMENT

Understanding the pathophysiology of HF is crucial in guiding patient assessment. Patients with HF should be assessed for orientation, cognition, mood, energy level, and activity tolerance, as these reflect CO and tissue oxygenation. Lungs should be auscultated for crackles, which result from volume overload and impaired cardiac function. The heart should be auscultated for rate and rhythm, and for the S3 heart sound, which indicates increased intravascular volume. Cardiac murmurs may reflect valve disease and a displaced apical impulse suggests cardiac enlargement.

Patients should be assessed for indications of fluid retention, such as peripheral edema, anasarca, jugular venous distinction, and abdominal distention. Patients with chronic HF may have reduced appetite and nutritional deficiencies. Body weight and changes in weight are critical assessments for HF patients. Increasing weight is a sign of worsening HF, and a weight gain of more than 2 pounds in 1 day or 5 pounds in a week is a red flag and should be reported to the provider.

Vital signs are critical assessments for HF patients. An elevated BP increases afterload, reducing CO. Low blood pressure may reflect insufficient CO, which can compromise tissue oxygenation. Increased HR, especially at rest, is an indicator of cardiac dysfunction. Arrhythmias interfere with cardiac function and should be addressed. Respiratory rate and shortness of breath increase with worsening HF.

Laboratory tests include a metabolic panel and brain natriuretic peptide (BNP). Hyponatremia is associated with poor outcomes in HF patients, as is renal dysfunction. BNP is a hormone produced by the ventricles in response to volume overload and is elevated in persons with HF. BNP levels less than 100 pg/mL indicate no HF, if greater than 400 pg/mL HF is likely; clinical judgment should be used for findings within those ranges. As HF severity increases, BNP levels also increase; with effective treatment of HF, BNP levels should decrease. Patients hospitalized for acute HF should have BNP measured upon admission and in preparation for discharge. Chest x-rays shows size and position of the heart as well as pulmonary congestion. Echocardiography is done to evaluate LV function and determine the EF.

In addition to physical assessment, nurses should assess patients' knowledge and understanding of HF and their role in disease management. HF requires a significant amount of self-management and patients who understand the disease process and management strategies have better outcomes (Yancy et al., 2013). These assessments allow the nurse to plan appropriate patient education. Health literacy should also be assessed and patient teaching should be tailored to the patient's health literacy level.

NURSING INTERVENTIONS, MANAGEMENT, AND IMPLICATIONS

Pharmacologic therapy and lifestyle modification are the cornerstones of HF management. Medications used to treat HF block or reduce the effects of compensatory mechanisms. Beta-adrenergic antagonists (beta blockers) and angiotensin-converting-enzyme-inhibitors (ACEI) and angiotensin II receptor blockers (ARB) are mainstays of pharmacologic therapy for HF. Beta blockers act by reducing the negative effects of catecholamine stimulation on the myocardium by inhibiting SNS activity. ACEI, ARB, and aldosterone antagonists all block the effects of RAAS activation.

Diuretics, especially the loop diuretics furosemide and bumetanide, are almost always used in the treatment of HF, as they mobilize and eliminate fluid, reduce shortness of breath, and reduce the demand on the heart due to fluid overload. Devices, such as implantable cardiac defibrillators (ICD), may be used to decrease risk of sudden cardiac death. Biventricular pacemakers for "cardiac resynchronization therapy" may be used to optimize synchronous operation of all four chambers of the heart. Newer medications for HF include ivabradine, which directly reduces HR and valsartan-sacubitril, a potent inhibitor of the RAAS (Yancy et al., 2013.) Nursing interventions include patient education on therapeutic effects and side effects and on the importance of adherence to a medication regimen.

Lifestyle modifications for HF patients usually include some fluid and sodium restriction; however, these should be individualized for each patient. Patients with HF should be taught the benefits of smoking cessation and advised to remain physically active and exercise as tolerated to prevent deconditioning. Essential self-management activities include taking medications as directed, adhering to dietary recommendations, attending follow-up appointments, remaining active, understanding the signs and symptoms of worsening failure, and monitoring daily weight (Yancy et al., 2013). Nursing interventions to support lifestyle modification include counseling and teaching patients about risk factor reduction, disease and symptom management, diet, activity, and self-management strategies. Nurses play a key role in patient education and motivation and are often the primary educators for the patients and their families.

OUTCOMES

The desired outcomes of treatment for patients with HF are preventing mortality due to HF, preventing progression of disease, optimizing quality of life, and preventing hospitalizations. Adherence to medical and lifestyle recommendations supports these goals. Patients with HF have the highest rates of unplanned (within 30 days) readmission of all discharge diagnoses. In 2015, 22% of Medicare HF patients had unplanned readmissions (Medicare.gov, 2016). The Centers for Medicare & Medicaid Services (CMS) can impose financial penalties on hospitals with excessive readmissions. In 2016, an estimated 75% of U.S. hospitals were subject to financial penalties for readmissions (Rice, 2015), representing millions of dollars of lost revenue.

Nurses can play a key role in reducing avoidable readmissions as they have primary responsibility for patient education and discharge preparation. Nurses are ideally positioned to evaluate patient readiness for discharge in areas such as (a) knowledge of disease process, (b) physical and functional status, and (c) anticipated support at home, and can intervene if necessary. Patients evaluated by nurses as having low readiness for discharge have higher risk for readmission. Lack of social support is related to poor outcomes in patients with HF (Weiss, Costa, Yakusheva, & Bobay, 2013), and nurses may intervene by involving social services or case management to obtain needed assistance. HF may also cause cognitive impairment and depression, which increase readmission risk. Nurses can assess patients for these problems and mobilize the health care team for management strategies if indicated.

Managing HF can be challenging and demoralizing to patients, and nurses can provide much-needed counseling, emotional support, and encouragement.

Summary

HF is a complex problem with significant mortality and impact on patient quality of life that is influenced by medical, individual, social, and health care delivery system factors. Incidence and prevalence increase dramatically with an aging population. Management by multidisciplinary teams that include nurses is associated with better patient outcomes. Nurses will be called on to practice to the full extent of their scope to meet the health care needs of millions of HF patients, and are ideally positioned to use their knowledge and skills to improve outcomes and prevent readmissions in this growing patient population.

Ambrosy, A., Fonarow, G., Butler, J., Chioncel, O., Greene, S., Vaduganathan, M., . . . Gheorghiade, M. (2014). The global health and economic burden of hospitalizations for heart failure. *Journal of the American College of Cardiology, 63*(12), 1123–1133. doi:10.1016/j.jacc.2013.11.053

Butler, J. (2012). An overview of chronic heart failure management. *Nursing Times, 108*(14/15), 16–20. Retrieved from http://www.nursingtimes.net/clinical-archive/cardiology/an-overview-of-chronic-heart-failure-management/5043315.fullarticle

Centers for Disease Control and Prevention. (2015). Heart failure fact sheet. Retrieved from http://www.cdc.gov/dhdsp/data_statistics/fact_sheets/docs/fs_heart_failure.pdf

Go, A., Mozaffarian, D., Roger, V., Benjamin, E., Berry, J., Borden, W., . . . Turner, M. (2012). Heart disease and stroke statistic—2013 update: A report from the American Heart Association. *Circulation, 127*(1), e6–e245. doi:10.1161/cir.0b013e31828124ad

Heidenreich, P., Albert, N., Allen, L., Bluemke, D., Butler, J., Fonarow, G., . . . Trogdon, J. G. (2013). Forecasting the impact of heart failure in the United States: A policy statement from the American Heart Association. *Circulation: Heart Failure, 6*(3), 606–619. doi:10.1161/hhf.0b013e318291329a

Medicare.gov. (2016). Medicare hospital comparison of care. Retrieved from https://www.medicare.gov/hospitalcompare/search.html

Pfuntner, A., Wier, L., & Stocks, C. (2013). Statistical brief #162: Most frequent conditions in U.S. hospitals, 2011. Healthcare Cost and Utilization Project, Agency for Healthcare Quality and Research. Retrieved from http://www.hcupus.ahrq.gov/reports/statbr

Rice, S. (2015). Most hospitals face 30-day readmissions penalty in fiscal 2016. Modern Healthcare. Retrieved from http://www.modernhealthcare.com/article/20150803/NEWS/150809981

Roger, V. (2013). Epidemiology of heart failure. *Circulation Research, 113*(6), 646–659. doi:10.1161/circresaha.113.300268

Rogers, C., & Bush, N. (2015). Heart failure. *Nursing Clinics of North America, 50*(4), 787–799. doi:10.1016/j.cnur.2015.07.012

Weiss, M., Costa, L., Yakusheva, O., & Bobay, K. (2014). Validation of patient and nurse short forms of the readiness for hospital discharge scale and their relationship to return to the hospital. *Health Services Research, 49*(1), 304–317. doi:10.1111/1475-6773.12092

Yancy, C. W., Jessup, M., Bozkurt, B., Butler, J., Casey, D., & Drazner, M., . . . Wilkoff, B. L. (2013). 2013 ACCF/AHA guideline for the management of heart failure: A report of the American College of Cardiology Foundation/American Heart Association task force on practice guidelines. *Circulation, 128*(16), e240–327. doi:10.1161/cir.0b013e31829e8776

■ HEMOLYTIC ANEMIA

Rebecca M. Lutz
Charrita Ernewein

Overview

Hemolytic anemia (HA) is the expression of an underlying disease process. Hemolysis of the red blood cell (RBC) is a form of anemia resulting from the decrease in circulating RBCs (Barcellini & Fettizzo, 2015; Manchanda, 2015). HA may be acute or chronic, mild to severe, intravascular or extravascular, inherited or acquired (Bunn, 2017; Doig, 2015; Manchanda, 2015). An in-depth patient history, with the benefit of laboratory testing, aids diagnosis. Treatment is based on the differentiation of the underlying pathology (Cornett, 2017).

Background

Anemia is a general term indicating a decrease in circulating RBCs caused by a disease or deficiency and characterized by a decrease in the hemoglobin or hematocrit levels (Manchanda, 2015). Anemia results from a decrease in RBC production, an increase in RBC destruction, with an inability of the bone marrow to sufficiently compensate for the hemolysis, or a decrease in total blood volume (Barcellini & Fettizzo, 2015; Doig, 2015; Manchanda, 2015). The World Health Organization (WHO) estimated that 1.62 billion persons (24.8%) worldwide are affected by some form of anemia (WHO, 2008). The impact of HA on morbidity and mortality, quality of life, and levels of disability is linked to the severity of the underlying disorder and available treatment.

The RBC is produced by the bone marrow through the process of erythropoiesis. With a life span of 120 days, the primary function of the RBC is the exchange of gases within the body. Hemoglobin, a protein within the RBC, binds to oxygen in the lungs for transport to the tissues. In the event of hemolysis, decreasing levels of circulating oxygen stimulate the release of erythropoietin from the kidneys. Erythropoietin stimulates bone marrow to increase RBC production. Increased RBC production allows the body to compensate for hemolysis (Bunn, 2017; Doig, 2015; Manchanda, 2015).

Inherited hemolytic disorders result from intracellular (intrinsic) defects of the cell, enzyme deficiencies resulting in altered cell metabolism, or hemoglobin disorders (Bunn, 2017; Doig, 2015; Manchanda, 2015). Hereditary disorders include spherocytosis, elliptocytosis, xerocytosis, and stomatocytosis. The most common form, hereditary spherocytosis, is an autosomal dominant mutation. Glucose-6-phosphate dehydrogenase (G6PD) deficiency, an enzymatic disorder, is the most common X-linked chromosomal disorder. Inherited hemoglobin disorders, such as sickle cell (autosomal recessive) and thalassemia (autosomal dominant), result in acute, chronic, or episodic HA.

Acquired hemolytic disorders result from extracellular (extrinsic) factors such as infections, trauma, chemical exposures, or immunological disorders

(Bunn, 2017; Doig, 2015; Manchanda, 2015). Acquired hemolytic disorders result from an array of causes: bacterial or protozoal infections, mechanical heart valves or dialysis, chemical exposure to toxins such as drugs or venoms, or autoimmune or alloimmune responses. Autoimmune hemolytic anemia (AIHA) results from the production of antibodies: immunoglobulin G (IgG; warm agglutinin syndrome) or immunoglobulin M (IgM; cold agglutinin syndrome).

Clinical Aspects

ASSESSMENT

Clinical manifestations of HAs are dependent on the type and severity of the anemia (Barcellini & Fettizzo, 2015; Cornett, 2017). The most direct indicators of the clinical severity of HAs are the hemoglobin level and the level of hemolysis. Hemoglobin values at diagnosis are also important predictors of patient outcomes, correlating with the risk of death and multiple therapy lines (Barcellini & Fettizzo, 2015). Clinical presentation of patients with HA is influenced by the onset of the anemia, focusing on whether the onset was abrupt or gradual. Close monitoring of hemoglobin levels is a critical component in disease management and treatment response evaluation (Barcellini & Fettizzo, 2015).

Signs and symptoms of HA vary based on the type and severity of the disease and directly arise from hemolysis. Mild cases of HA may present without signs and symptoms. The most common symptom of all types of anemia is fatigue (Cornett, 2017). Clinically, the main signs of HA include jaundice, splenomegaly, and dark urine. Patients may also present with fatigue, pallor, dizziness, hypotension, shortness of breath, and tachycardia (Cornett, 2017; Doig, 2015).

Laboratory features of HA specifically relate to the hemolysis and erythropoietic response of the bone marrow (Cornett, 2017). Diagnostic testing initially includes a complete blood count (CBC), peripheral smear, reticulocyte count, serum bilirubin, lactate dehydrogenase (LDH), haptoglobin alanine aminotransferase (ALT), and a Coombs test (Capriotti & Frizzell, 2016). If HA is suspected, specific testing would be required for a definitive diagnosis of a specific type of HA.

Nursing assessment and interventions for patients with potential anemia involve the collection of subjective and objective data. The nurse should collect a detailed review of patients' medical history, medications, and their family medical history. Frequent monitoring of vital signs and oxygen saturation is also indicated. The nurse should be proficient in understanding laboratory values. Appropriate nursing diagnoses applicable to patients with HA include hypoxemia, activity intolerance based on fatigue, risk for injury, and deficient knowledge. Specific nursing interventions are dependent on the etiology of the HA. Interventions should be directed at establishing balance in daily activities while safely integrating rest and exercise. Patient education, monitoring, and follow-up are significant in relation to promoting positive patient outcomes (Cornett, 2017).

Treatment of HA varies based on the type, cause, and severity of the disease. Age, family medical history, and overall health are other factors that affect treatment. Management also includes blood transfusions, medications, surgery, plasmapheresis, blood and bone marrow transplants, and lifestyle changes (Bass, Tuscano, & Tuscano, 2014). Blood transfusions are required to treat severe or life-threatening HA. Medicines, primarily glucocorticoids, are the mainstay in treating some types of HA, especially AIHA. Plasmapheresis, a process that removes antibodies from the blood, can be used to treat immune HA after other treatments have failed. Splenectomy can stop or reduce high rates of RBC destruction (Bass et al., 2014). The goals of treatment include reducing or stopping RBC destruction, increasing RBC count to therapeutic levels, and treatment of the underlying cause of the condition.

OUTCOMES

There are many causes of HA and positive outcomes depend on the cause and severity (Cornett, 2017). Mild HA may require no treatment; yet severe HA requires prompt treatment to avoid mortality. Some causes of acquired HA can be prevented. Avoidance of triggers is effective in certain types of HA. Acquired forms of HA may resolve if the cause is identified and treated (Bass et al., 2014). Ongoing treatment may be required for inherited HA (Cornett, 2017).

Summary

HAs are a group of heterogeneous diseases, inherited or acquired, causing challenges in diagnosis and treatment (Barcellini & Fettizzo, 2015). With over 1.62 billion persons affected by anemia, the impact of HA is based on the underlying disorder and available treatment options. Signs and symptoms of HA vary based on the type and severity of the disease, yet clinically, the main signs of HA include jaundice, splenomegaly, and dark urine (Cornett, 2017). Although diagnostic testing, medical management, and nursing interventions vary based on the type, cause, and severity of the disease, the goals of treatment remain consistent to improve long-term patient outcomes.

Barcellini, W., & Fettizzo, B. (2015). Clinical application of hemolytic markers in the differential diagnosis and management of hemolytic anemia. *Disease Markers, 2015,* 635670. doi:10.1155/2015/635670

Bass, G., Tuscano, E., & Tuscano, J. (2014). Diagnosis and classification of autoimmune hemolytic anemia. *Autoimmune Reviews, 13,* 560–564. doi:10.1016/j.autrev.2013.11.010

Bunn, H. F. (2017). Overview of the anemias. In J. C. Aster & H. F. Bunn (Eds.), *Pathophysiology of blood disorders* (2nd ed., pp. 32–46). New York, NY: McGraw-Hill. Retrieved from http://accessmedicine.mhmedical.com.ezproxy.hsc.usf.edu/book.aspx?bookid=1900

Cornett, P. (2017). Hemolytic anemia. In E. Bope & R. Kellerman (Eds.), *Conn's current therapy* (pp. 371–376). Philadelphia, PA: Elsevier.

Doig, K. (2015). Introduction to increased destruction of erythrocytes. In E. Keohane, L. Smith, & J. Walenga (Eds.), *Rodak's hematology: Clinical principles and applications* (5th ed., pp. 348–356). St. Louis, MO: Elsevier. Retrieved from http://site.ebrary.com/lib/univsouthfl/reader.action?docID=11073954

Manchanda, N. (2015). Anemias: Red blood cell morphology and approach to diagnosis. In E. Keohane, L. Smith, & J. Walenga (Eds.), *Rodak's hematology: Clinical principles and applications* (5th ed., pp. 284–296). St. Louis, MO: Elsevier. Retrieved from http://site.ebrary.com/lib/univsouthfl/reader.action?docID=11073954

World Health Organization. (2008). Worldwide prevalence of anemia 1993–2005. Retrieved from http://apps.who.int/iris/bitstream/10665/43894/1/9789241596657_eng.pdf

■ HEPARIN-INDUCED THROMBOCYTOPENIA

Bette K. Idemoto
Jane F. Marek

Overview

Heparin-induced thrombocytopenia (HIT) is an abnormal clotting response to heparin and a complication of heparin therapy in susceptible patients. Heparin is an anticoagulant that has been used for more than 90 years as prophylaxis and treatment of venous or arterial clots in a variety of conditions, including venous thromboembolic disease (deep vein thrombosis [DVT] and pulmonary embolus [PE]), acute coronary syndrome, atrial fibrillation, and cerebrovascular accident. Heparin is also used during transfusions, dialysis, and to maintain patency of some venous access devices. A normal platelet count ranges from 150,000 to 450,000 platelets per microliter of blood. Thrombocytopenia or low platelet count can range from mild to severe and places the patient at an increased risk for bleeding. Unfortunately, patients treated with heparin for anticoagulation may experience a paradoxical clotting response thought to be related to an antibody-mediated cascade. Diligent monitoring of the platelet count after exposure to heparin is important for early detection of this abnormal response, known as HIT.

Background

The clotting mechanism involves a complex reaction of cell activation, adhesion, and platelet aggregation. This reaction can be lifesaving by stopping bleeding; however, overactivation may result in the formation of blood clots or thrombi. Blood clots within vessels and organs can lead to skin necrosis, limb ischemia and possible amputation, end-organ damage, and death.

Over 30 years ago, clinicians began to report case studies with thrombocytopenia in patients who had been exposed to heparin. These patients presented with an abrupt decline in platelet count and paradoxical platelet aggregation. Central features of the HIT syndrome include thrombocytopenia and increased platelet aggregation. HIT may develop within hours or up to 14 days after initiation of heparin therapy. Type 1 HIT is a nonimmunologic response that occurs within hours of exposure to heparin and results in a mild transient thrombocytopenia. Type 1 HIT is usually self-limiting and heparin therapy may be continued with close monitoring to detect possible clotting. In contrast, type 2 HIT typically occurs 5 to 10 days after exposure to heparin and is a potentially life-threatening clotting response that activates an immune response resulting in clotting complications (Greinacher, 2015).

It is believed that HIT is caused by the development of antibodies that stimulate platelets after administration of heparin. Heparin and platelet factor 4 (PF4) bind to form an antigen (immunoglobulin [IgG]) in susceptible patients, depending on the particular type of heparin administered, unfractionated heparin (UFH), or low-molecular weight heparin (LMWH). An altered immune response leads to the formation of HIT antibodies (heparin-PF4 antibodies), which in turn, activate the prothrombotic microparticles leading to thrombocytopenia and thrombosis. This thrombosis has occasionally been called *white clot syndrome*.

Although all patients treated with heparin are at risk for developing HIT antibodies, most persons will not develop type 2 HIT. It is estimated that 1% to 8% of patients treated with heparin may develop antibodies, but only half of those develop arterial or venous thrombosis. Patients at increased risk include those with extended periods of prophylactic anticoagulation such as following orthopedic or cardiopulmonary bypass surgery. A higher incidence of type 2 HIT is seen in postoperative patients treated with UFH than patients treated with LMWH (Junqueira, Zorzela, & Perini, 2017). Type 2 HIT risk factors include Caucasian race, female, and age more than 66 years. Contributing factors include previous exposure to heparin, with or without HIT or heparin-induced thrombocytopenia and thrombosis (HITT).

Clinical Aspects

ASSESSMENT

The clinical signs of type 2 HIT include ecchymosis at the heparin injection site and pain, weakness, numbness, and redness or swelling of the extremity. Limb ischemia is seen with DVT; thrombus can cause pulmonary emboli, stroke, acute myocardial infarction, all of which would require anticoagulation. Systemic reactions include chills, fever, dyspnea, and chest pain. Unlike most heparin reactions that result in active bleeding, HIT usually does not cause bleeding, rather patients will develop venous thromboembolism or HITT.

Diagnosis of HIT can be challenging; failure to recognize HIT may result in thrombosis, amputation, or death. Inaccurate diagnosis may result in thrombosis or hemorrhage. Other causes of thrombocytopenia include sepsis with disseminated intravascular coagulation, liver disease, immune thrombocytopenia, and medications (Warkentin, 2016). Many clinicians use the 4-T score to differentiate HIT from other causes of thrombocytopenia (Crowther et al., 2014). Each criterion has a maximum point value of 2; a total score of 0–3 indicates low probability of HIT, 4–5 intermediate probability, and 6–8 high probability. The 4 scoring criteria (4-Ts) are *thrombocytopenia* severity (platelet count greater than 50% and platelet nadir greater than or equal to 20), *timing* of platelet count fall (clear onset between days 5 and 14 or less than or equal to 1 day prior heparin exposure within 30 days), *thrombosis* or other sequelae, and the likelihood of *other* causes of thrombocytopenia. Obesity is associated with increased rates of HIT in patients in critical care units and patient "thickness" could be considered the 5th T in the 4-T scoring system (Bloom et al., 2016). The 4-T score is used in conjunction with other patient assessment data to determine the diagnosis of HIT. The patient with HIT may present with multiple symptoms, including signs of DVT, PE, or stroke and other symptoms, including flushing, chills, fever, dyspnea, and chest pain. Laboratory assessment includes platelet count less than 50,000/mm³ or sudden drop of 30% to 50% from baseline; heparin-induced platelet aggregation (HIPA) assay, serotonin release assay (SRA) to identify the HIT antigen, and enzyme-linked immunosorbent assay (ELISA) used to detect the HIT antigen, although false positives and lack of specificity limit the usefulness of the test (Nagler, Bachmann, ten Cate, & ten Cate-Hoek, 2016).

NURSING INTERVENTIONS, MANAGEMENT, AND IMPLICATIONS

Management includes recognition of patients at risk for HIT and assessing the patient for other possible causes of thrombocytopenia. Judicious use of heparin according to clinical practice guidelines can reduce unnecessary or prolonged treatment with heparin, thus reducing the risk of HIT. Early mobilization, exercise, and prevention of dehydration may all decrease the need for prophylactic subcutaneous heparin therapy, thus decreasing exposure to heparin and ultimately the risk of HIT. Discharge teaching should include education about HIT, risk factors, and signs and symptoms of HIT that may occur after discharge and before follow-up medical appointments. Patients should be taught to report unusual bruising and signs and symptoms of DVT and PE immediately to the provider.

Early recognition and diagnosis results in improved patient outcomes (Al-Eidan, 2015). All nurses should be aware of the potential for HIT. Strict guidelines and evidence-based interventions regarding maintenance of central venous access devices, implanted ports, and hemodialysis catheters should be followed to avoid unnecessary exposure to heparin. Ongoing physical assessment is important for early recognition and prevention of complications of HIT. Medication teaching should include a clear communication about exposure to heparin and delayed side effects of heparin after discharge.

OUTCOMES

The current standard for anticoagulation and heparin therapy is to obtain both baseline and ongoing laboratory values to monitor the platelet count, the major indicator of HIT. Evidence-based guidelines from the American College of Chest Physicians (ACCP; Garcia, Baglin, Weitz, & Samama, 2012) provide the standard of care for anticoagulation practices. The expertise of hematologists and vascular medicine specialists is an integral part of the interdisciplinary team's plan to manage patients with this complex phenomenon.

General principles of care of patients with HIT include immediate cessation of all heparin (including flushes, coated catheters, dialysate), laboratory testing to confirm the presence of the HIT antigen, alternative anticoagulation measures until the risk of thrombosis is satisfactorily eliminated, careful monitoring of the platelet count, and ongoing assessment for new thrombotic events (McGowan et al., 2016). Administering platelets is not recommended because they may exacerbate the hypercoagulable state.

The ACCP (Garcia et al., 2012) recommends limiting platelet transfusions to patients with severe thrombocytopenia and bleeding or those undergoing an invasive procedure with an increased risk of bleeding. Warfarin is not recommended as it can make the thrombosis worse in HIT; warfarin therapy should not be initiated until the platelet count has recovered to a minimum of 150 × 10^9/L. Patients should be treated with alternative anticoagulation; bivalirudin (Angiomax) and argatroban (Acova) are direct thrombin inhibitors currently approved for intravenous use in the United States (Garcia et al., 2012). Nursing care should follow the evidence-based guidelines, which have been specified for interdisciplinary teams (Vaughn et al., 2014).

Summary

Although the occurrence of HIT is infrequent, HIT can have devastating outcomes, such as DVT, PE, limb amputation, and death. It is imperative that nurses and all members of the health care team understand the devastating effects of unrecognized and untreated type 2 HIT. Efforts to limit unnecessary exposure to heparin are crucial. Patients receiving heparin must be carefully monitored with routine assessment of the platelet count. Discharge education regarding activity and recognizing the signs and symptoms of HIT is essential for prevention and early detection of HIT or HITT. Future trends include the development of selective anticoagulants with decreased side effects and sensitive diagnostic laboratory tests to adequately detect HIT and alternatives for anticoagulation.

Al-Eidan, F. A. (2015). Pharmacotherapy of heparin-induced thrombocytopenia: Therapeutic options and challenges in the clinical practices. *Journal of Vascular Nursing, 33*(1), 10–20. doi:10.1016/j.jvn.2014.07.001

Bloom, M. B., Zaw, A. A., Hoang, D. M., Mason, R., Alban, R. F., Chung, R., . . . Margulies, D. R. (2016). Body mass index strongly impacts the diagnosis and incidence of heparin-induced thrombocytopenia in the surgical intensive care unit. *Journal of Trauma and Acute Care Surgery, 80*(3), 398–403; discussion 403. doi:10.1097/TA.0000000000000952

Crowther, M., Cook, D., Guyatt, G., Zytaruk, N., McDonald, E., Williamson, D., . . . Warkentin, T. E. (2014). Heparin-induced thrombocytopenia in the critically ill: Interpreting the 4Ts test in a randomized trial. *Journal of Critical Care, 29*(3), 470.7–470.15. doi:10.1016/j.jcrc.2014.02.004

Garcia, D. A., Baglin, T. P., Weitz, J. I., & Samama, M. M. (2012). Parenteral anticoagulants: Antithrombotic therapy and prevention of thrombosis, 9th ed: American College of Chest Physicians evidence-based clinical practice guidelines. *Chest, 141*(2 Suppl.), e24S–e43S. doi:10.1378/chest.11-2291

Greinacher, A. (2015). Heparin-induced thrombocytopenia. *New England Journal of Medicine, 373*(19), 1883–1884. doi:10.1056/NEJMc1510993

Junqueira, D. R., Zorzela, L. M., & Perini, E. (2017). Unfractionated heparin versus low molecular weight heparins for avoiding heparin-induced thrombocytopenia in postoperative patients. *Cochrane Database of Systematic Reviews, 2017*(4), CD007557. doi:10.1002/14651858.CD007557.pub3

McGowan, K. E., Makari, J., Diamantouros, A., Bucci, C., Rempel, P., Selby, R., & Geerts, W. (2016). Reducing the hospital burden of heparin-induced thrombocytopenia: Impact of an avoid-heparin program. *Blood, 127*(16), 1954–1959. doi:10.1182/blood-2015-07-660001

Nagler, M., Bachmann, L. M., ten Cate, H., & ten Cate-Hoek, A. (2016). Diagnostic value of immunoassays for heparin-induced thrombocytopenia: A systematic review and meta-analysis. *Blood, 127*(5), 546–557. doi:10.1182/blood-2015-07-661215

Vaughn, D. M., Mazur, J., Foster, J., Lazarchick, J., Boylan, A., & Greenberg, C. S. (2014). Implementation of a heparin-induced thrombocytopenia management program reduces the cost of diagnostic testing and pharmacologic treatment in an academic medical center. *Blood, 124*(21), 4848.

Warkentin, T. E. (2015). Heparin-induced thrombocytopenia in critically ill patients. *Seminars in Thrombosis and Hemostasis, 41*(1), 49–60. doi:10.1055/s-0034-1398381

■ HIATAL HERNIA

Maricar P. Gomez

Overview

Hiatal hernia is a condition in which abdominal contents, most commonly of the stomach, protrude through the esophageal hiatus in the diaphragm, and into the thoracic cavity. Hiatal hernias are common in Western countries, specifically in the adult population, affecting more women than men (Qureshi, 2016). Nursing care of patients with hiatal hernia is often directed at assessment of symptoms and education to minimize symptoms and severity of herniation.

Background

Hiatal hernias are classified as either sliding or paraesophageal. Sliding, or type I, hiatal hernias constitute about 90% of hiatal hernia cases and occur when the gastroesophageal junction (GEJ) slides freely in and out of the thorax during changes in position or intra-abdominal pressure. Paraesophageal hernias (PEH) are further categorized by extent of herniation (types II, III, or IV). In type II hernias, the gastric fundus migrates above the diaphragm while the GEJ remains in the native subdiaphragmatic position. Type III is a combination of both types I and II, whereas the GEJ and gastric fundus protrude into the thorax through a pathologically widened esophageal hiatus. Finally, type IV refers to the presence of other abdominal visceral contents within the hernia sac such as omentum, spleen, pancreas, colon, or small bowel (Kohn et al., 2013).

Most adults with hiatal hernias are asymptomatic. Symptoms caused by hiatal hernias are a result of intermittent obstruction of the gastrointestinal tract and a lax or unsupported lower esophageal sphincter allowing reflux. Obstruction is a result of a herniated intrathoracic stomach compressing the adjacent esophagus along with angulation of the GEJ when stomach becomes progressively displaced into the chest. Rarely, patients develop acutely severe chest or epigastric pain and/or severe vomiting due to complications of volvulus or strangulation. Volvulus occurs when the intrathoracic stomach twists and subsequently obstructs the gastrointestinal tract. Strangulation of the stomach is a consequence of acute gastric volvulus. The blood supply to the stomach is interrupted and, if emergent surgery is not performed, gastric ischemia, necrosis, and even perforation of the stomach can ensue (Cohn & Soper, 2017).

The true incidence is difficult to approximate given that many people with hiatal hernias are asymptomatic and never diagnosed. Certain chronic conditions increase the propensity of developing hiatal hernia, including obesity, pregnancy, and abdominal ascites. These conditions promote herniation of organs from the positive pressure environment within the abdomen to a negative pressure environment within the thorax. The frequency of hiatal hernias increases with age, from 10% in patients younger than 40 years to 70% in patients older than 70 years (Qureshi, 2016). This is because as patients age, the diaphragmatic muscle and surrounding membranes around the hiatus weakens and loses elasticity (Roman & Kahrilas, 2014).

Hiatal hernias can be treated both medically and surgically. Conservative therapy should be initiated at first, particularly lifestyle changes and administration of pharmacologic agents. Surgery is usually reserved for symptomatic hernias that are refractory to pharmacologic therapy, or cases where there is bowel obstruction or ischemia.

Clinical Aspects

ASSESSMENT

Diagnosis is supported by an accurate history and diagnostic tests, whereas physical examination is nonspecific. While taking a patient's history, the registered nurse should assess for symptoms and related aggravating factors that indicate the presence of a hiatal hernia. Patients with sliding hiatal hernias typically endorse gastroesophageal reflux disease (GERD) symptoms like reflux, heartburn, or regurgitation, whereas patients with PEH indicate obstructive symptoms like postprandial fullness, epigastric pain, bloating, nausea, emesis, dysphagia, or retching. Atypical symptoms include cough, dyspnea, laryngitis, vocal hoarseness, dental erosions, or chest discomfort, which may also be related to different health processes. Any sign of acute chest pain and dysphagia in a patient with a known hiatal hernia can suggest incarceration. This is a medical emergency and providers should be notified immediately (Kohn et al., 2013). Auscultating the lungs for rhonchi can imply presence of pulmonary complications. Inquire about recurrent pneumonias, which can be due to silent aspiration. Question the patient regarding any history of anemia, hematochezia, melena, or hematemesis, which can be a result of Cameron's ulcers. A nutritional assessment with attention to unintentional weight loss or signs of dehydration may help identify the need for supplemental nutrition via parenteral nutrition or placement of a temporary feeding tube. In addition, since obesity is a significant risk factor for hiatal hernias, weight should be monitored. Explore the patient's social history, including smoking and alcohol use, as well as any stressors, which can exacerbate GERD symptoms. Medication reconciliation and checking for compliance also helps influence treatment planning.

NURSING INTERVENTIONS, MANAGEMENT, AND IMPLICATIONS

Nursing diagnoses include knowledge deficit about the disorder, diagnostic tests and treatments; acute pain related to dysphagia, reflux, gastric distention, impaired perfusion to herniated stomach; imbalanced nutrition due to inadequate consumption of body requirements related to dysphagia or reflux; and risk for aspiration due to dysphagia or regurgitation.

The most consequential role of a nurse caring for a patient with a hiatal hernia is health teaching. Because obesity is a significant risk factor, weight reduction is paramount. Refraining from wearing constricting clothing around the abdomen also helps decrease intra-abdominal pressure. Encourage patients to chew well, eat slowly, and to eat small amounts to prevent gastric distention. Remaining upright for 1 hour after eating, waiting at least 2 to 3 hours after last meal of the day, and sleeping with head of bed elevated at least 30° helps foster esophageal emptying, prevents aspiration of regurgitated contents, and prevents upward migration of hernia. Advise patients to avoid certain trigger foods (e.g., chocolate, fatty foods, fried foods), which can aggravate symptoms. Because alcohol, nicotine, and caffeine immediately decrease lower esophageal sphincter pressure, encourage patients to stop smoking and eliminate alcohol and caffeine. If psychological stress seems to cause symptoms, discuss coping mechanisms and stress management techniques.

If elective surgery is planned, discuss the benefits of weight loss with the patient before surgery. Obesity is also a risk factor for dehiscence and hernia recurrence postoperatively (Cohn & Soper, 2017). Tobacco abusers should refrain from smoking at least 4 weeks before surgery or as prescribed by the surgeon. Smoking increases the risk of postoperative deep vein thrombosis and, due to the effects of impaired oxygen uptake, cells in the surgical wound receive less oxygen. In turn, this delays wound healing and increases the chance of infection. Reinforce any preoperative instructions and ensure that any blood-thinning agents are documented and held for the appropriate length of time. To ease anxiety, it is helpful to prepare the patient for what to expect after surgery, for example, incisions, presence of tubes, diet, activity, length of stay, and/or postoperative restrictions.

OUTCOMES

As a result of thorough and reinforced health education, patients should increase compliance with therapy and instruction. Execution of nursing interventions postoperatively helps to identify complications early and prevent poor outcomes. Reassessment after nursing interventions are performed is important to determine treatment success or the need for alternative therapy.

Treatment of hiatal hernias is usually indicated for GERD. Proton pump inhibitors (PPIs) are more effective than histamine$_2$ receptor antagonists in healing esophagitis and decreasing the incidence of esophageal strictures, both complications of chronic GERD. Although generally safe, PPIs can cause adverse effects. Long-term PPI use has been associated with decreased bone density. Although the risk for osteoporosis is low, judicious use of PPIs in postmenopausal women who are at risk for hip fractures is recommended. Patients at risk for osteoporosis should have bone mineral density testing; treatment for osteoporosis may be indicated. In addition, PPIs have been linked to decreased intestinal magnesium absorption resulting in low serum magnesium levels. Before treatment with PPIs, patients should have baseline magnesium levels assessed and repeated at intervals. Intermittent studies and meta-analyses have also indicated that PPIs increase likelihood of development and recurrence of *Clostridium difficile* infection (Roman & Kahrilas, 2014). Patients should be instructed to report any persistent diarrhea to the provider. Finally, in 2011, the U.S. Food and Drug Administration (FDA) advised avoiding concurrent use of clopidogrel (Plavix) with omeprazole or esomeprazole because together they significantly reduce the antiplatelet activity of clopidogrel (FDA, 2011).

Summary

Most hiatal hernias are asymptomatic, but in some people hiatal hernia slowly worsen and may eventually require treatment. Rarely, a life-threatening complication may present acutely and require emergent surgery. Modifiable risk factors include maintaining a healthy weight, smoking cessation, and moderate alcohol consumption.

Cohn, T. D., & Soper, N. J. (2017). Paraesophageal hernia repair: Techniques for success. *Journal of Laparoendoscopic and Advanced Surgical Techniques. Part A, 27*(1), 19–23. doi:10.1089/lap.2016.0496

Kohn, G. P., Price, R. R., Demeester, S. R., Zehetner, J., Muensterer, O. J., Awad, Z. T., . . . Fanelli, R. D. (2013). Guidelines for the management of hiatal hernia—A SAGES guideline. Retrieved from https://www.sages.org/publications/guidelines/guidelines-for-the-management-of-hiatal-hernia

Qureshi, W. A. (2016). Hiatal hernia. *Medscape.* Retrieved from http://emedicine.medscape.com/article/178393-overview

Roman, S., & Kahrilas, P. J. (2014). The diagnosis and management of hiatus hernia. *British Journal of Medicine, 349,* g6154. doi:10.1136/bmj.g6154

U.S. Food and Drug Administration. (2011). Safety information—clopidogrel bisulfate tablet. Retrieved from https://www.accessdata.fda.gov/drugsatfda_docs/appletter/2011/020839s055ltr.pdf

■ HUMAN IMMUNODEFICIENCY VIRUS

Scott Emory Moore

Overview

HIV is a retrovirus, most often transmitted through sexual activity or the sharing of needles or syringes, that affects approximately 1.2 million people in the United States (AIDS.gov, 2015; Centers for Disease Control and Prevention [CDC], 2016). The retrovirus attacks its hosts' immune cells (CD4+ T cells among others). There is no known cure for HIV, and, if undiagnosed and untreated, HIV can progress to AIDS. AIDS, the most advanced stage of HIV, results from the suppression of the immune system to the point of failure (Selik et al., 2014). However, with early diagnosis, connection to HIV care, combined antiretroviral therapy (cART), and viral suppression, HIV can be rendered a chronic illness. Nursing care for adults with HIV/AIDS should focus on limiting infections, symptom management, and the psychosocial implications of HIV/AIDS.

Background

In 1981, the illness that would come to be known as AIDS was first discussed as a probable association between a rare *Pneumocystis* pneumonia and homosexual activity among men in Los Angeles, California (CDC, 1981). Since then, AIDS has been shown to develop as a result of HIV infection. HIV is a retrovirus that incorporates its genetic code into the DNA of T-lymphocyte cells. HIV uses its host cell to replicate its genetic code and build new HIV viruses to infect other cells. In some cases, the HIV host cells become dormant making it difficult for the immune system to remove the virus or cART to affect the virus (Gallo & Montagnier, 2003).

There are two types of HIV: HIV-1 and HIV-2. HIV-1 is the most common type of infection in the United States, but there are cases of HIV-2 in the United States, although it is more common in western Africa than the United States. It is also possible to be infected with both HIV-1 and HIV-2. In addition to the two types of HIV, there are multiple groups within each type, and groups can have subtypes. These subtypes each have their own unique nature such as increased resistance to specific drugs, or increased successful transmission rates. In North America, HIV-1, group M, subtype B is the most common virus causing HIV infection (Hemelaar, 2012).

Initial diagnosis of HIV in an adult is usually based on laboratory data using multiple tests. The first type of testing used usually consists of an HIV antibody screening, which if found to be reactive (positive result), leads to confirmatory testing using another type of test that uses a differing mechanism for testing the presence of HIV or HIV antibodies (Selik et al., 2014). HIV-1 viral load testing, for example, would be an acceptable test to confirm a reactive antibody screen. Once diagnosed, staging is the next step of clinical classification of HIV. HIV is classified into one of five possible classifications, 0, 1, 2, 3, or unknown. Stage 0 is the earliest stage of HIV infection, considered to be the first 180 days since the last known negative test until the first positive HIV test. If the time since last negative test is greater than 180 days then HIV staging (stages 1, 2, 3, and unknown) is based on clinical criteria, CD4+ T-lymphocyte count or percentage of total lymphocytes, and/or diagnosis of an opportunistic illness (Selik et al., 2014). When criteria for stage 0 are met, regardless of the presence of clinical criteria for the other stages, the patient is categorized as stage 0. If there is no information for the clinical criteria for staging then the initial stage is unknown, but, as with those with initial staging of 0, the progression of the disease will rely on the CD4+ T-cells and/or the presence of an opportunistic illnesses. Stage 3 is also known as AIDS, and it is defined as having less than 200 CD4+ T-cells, or less than 14% of all lymphocytes are CD4+ and/or an opportunistic illness is present (Selik et al., 2014).

HIV affected approximately 1.2 million people in the United States, and approximately 36.7 million people worldwide at the end of 2015 (CDC, 2016; World Health Organization [WHO], 2016). In the United States in 2015, a total of 39,513 people were diagnosed with HIV and 18,303 people with AIDS (CDC, 2016).

Men who have sex with men continue to make up the majority of new diagnoses, 83% in 2014 (CDC, 2016). HIV disproportionately affects African Americans and Hispanic Americans, accounting for 44% and 24%, respectively of estimated new HIV diagnoses in the United States in 2014 (CDC, 2016). Older adults are a growing group of newly infected individuals, with 17% of new diagnoses in 2014 occurring in people aged 50 years and older. Of those newly diagnosed individuals who are 55 years old and older, 40% are diagnosed with AIDS because of delayed identification of the disease. Other groups at risk for HIV infection include people who are incarcerated, intravenous-drug users, of lower socioeconomic status, and people who trade sex for money or drugs (CDC, 2016).

The age-adjusted death rate for HIV was 2.0 per 100,000 people in 2014, down from 10.2 in 1990. Advanced stage HIV can leave a patient open to opportunistic illnesses ranging from cancers, such as Kaposi sarcoma, lymphoma, and cervical cancer, to microbial infections, including mycobacterium, toxoplasmosis, and candidiasis of the esophagus, bronchi, trachea, or lungs. In addition, the presence of HIV-associated encephalopathy and wasting syndromes can also be hallmarks of AIDS (Selik et al., 2014).

Clinical Aspects

ASSESSMENT

An HIV/AIDS-related assessment should include some disease-specific questions such as length of HIV diagnosis; which providers treat their HIV/AIDS; which cART regimen, if any, the patient is on; what time(s) of day he or she takes the cART; if the patient takes the medication as scheduled; if patient has any history of AIDS-defining illnesses. Other things of note in the assessment of these patients may be related to some of the risk factors for HIV such as substance use/abuse, trading sex for drugs or money, and screening for abuse, depression, malnutrition, and failure to thrive. Although the screening and diagnostic testing for the presence of HIV are important for diagnosis of HIV, CD4+ T-cell count, viral load, hemoglobin, hematocrit, renal function, and white blood cell count results are more useful during the care of HIV+ patients.

NURSING INTERVENTIONS, MANAGEMENT, AND IMPLICATIONS

It is less likely that HIV/AIDS is the principle reason for the patient needing nursing care; however, in addition to monitoring and treatment of the primary condition it is important to be aware of the compounding nature that HIV/AIDS may have on dealing with the presenting illness. The symptoms and features associated with HIV/AIDS can lead to certain complications, including delayed wound healing or inability to fend off infections (local or systemic) related to immune system deficiency, difficulty with participation in physical therapy secondary to fatigue, forgetfulness, and cognitive dysfunction related to the virus. Thus, nurses should be aware of the following: hydration, infection prevention, nutrition, polypharmacy, social support, stigma, and symptom management (e.g., cognitive dysfunction, depression, fatigue, pain, sleep disturbances, wasting). Each of these has specific associations with HIV/AIDS, but for most patients there are not any specific differences for nursing care of HIV/AIDS patients.

Polypharmacy and related complications are concerning for adults living with HIV/AIDS as they may take multiple medications for chronic illnesses or opportunistic infection prophylaxis in addition to their cART. Patients with HIV/AIDS may benefit greatly from a social work consult to ensure that they are aware of the various public services available to them. In addition to need for social support, HIV/AIDS-related stigma must be addressed. Not every HIV+ patient has disclosed his or her status, thus it is imperative for nurses to be informed about which people, if any, know about the patient's HIV status (Relf & Rollins, 2015).

OUTCOMES

The measure of optimal outcomes in patients living with HIV/AIDS are evaluated by whether and how consistently a patient is engaged in HIV care. The HIV care continuum spans levels of engagement ranging from unengaged, undiagnosed HIV through fully engaged, regular HIV-specific care (Gardner, McLees, Steiner, Del Rio, & Burman, 2011). When patients with HIV/AIDS need nursing care, it is important to assess the extent of their engagement in HIV-specific care.

Summary

With cART treatment, people with HIV/AIDS are living longer than they did in the 1980s. Although some patients are being diagnosed at stage 3 (AIDS), the patient's laboratory values may return to stage 1 or 2 levels as a result of treatment of the virus and AIDS-associated illness. Identification and evaluation of HIV/AIDS-related symptoms and patient advocacy are key parts of ensuring the best outcomes.

AIDS.gov. (2015). How do you get HIV or AIDS? Retrieved from http://www.aids.gov/hiv-aids-basics/hiv-aids-101/how-you-get-hiv-aids/index.html

Centers for Disease Control and Prevention. (1981). Pneumocystis pneumonia. *Morbidity and Mortality Weekly Report, 30*(21), 250–252.

Centers for Disease Control and Prevention. (2016). HIV in the United States: At a glance. Retrieved from https://www.cdc.gov/hiv/statistics/overview/ataglance.html

Gallo, R. C., & Montagnier, L. (2003). The discovery of HIV as the cause of AIDS. *New England Journal of Medicine, 349*(24), 2283–2285. doi:10.1056/NEJMp038194

Gardner, E. M., McLees, M. P., Steiner, J. F., Del Rio, C., & Burman, W. J. (2011). The spectrum of engagement in HIV care and its relevance to test-and-treat strategies for prevention of HIV infection. *Clinical Infectious Diseases, 52*(6), 793–800. doi:10.1093/cid/ciq243

Hemelaar, J. (2012). The origin and diversity of the HIV-1 pandemic. *Trends in Molecular Medicine, 18*(3), 182–192. doi:10.1016/j.molmed.2011.12.001

Relf, M. V., & Rollins, K. V. (2015). HIV-related stigma among an urban sample of persons living with HIV at risk for dropping out of HIV-oriented primary medical care. *Journal of the Association of Nurses in AIDS Care, 26*(1), 36–45. doi:10.1016/j.jana.2014.03.003

Selik, R., Mokotoff, E., Branson, B., Owen, S., Whitmore, S., & Hall, H. (2014). Revised surveillance case definition for HIV infection-United States, 2014. *Morbidity and Mortality Weekly Report, 63*(RR03), 1–10.

World Health Organization. (2016). Global summary of the AIDS epidemic 2015. Retrieved from http://www.who.int/hiv/data/epi_core_2016.png?ua=1

■ HYPERTENSION

Marian Soat

Overview

Hypertension (HTN) in adults, if not detected early and treated appropriately, can lead to myocardial infarction (MI), renal failure, stroke, and death (James et al., 2014). According to the Centers for Disease Control and Prevention (Yoon, Fryar, & Carroll, 2015), approximately 77.9 million American adults suffer from HTN, which is defined by the Eighth Joint National Committee (JNC8) as blood pressure (BP) that is equal to or greater than 140/90 mmHg. Because patients with HTN often present with no symptoms, the disease is difficult to diagnose, and controlling HTN is a challenge for health care providers (Wozniak, Khan, Gillespie, & Sifuentes, 2016). Nursing care for adults with HTN is focused on regular monitoring of signs and symptoms, a strict medication regimen, and compliance with lifestyle modifications.

Background

BP is the force exerted by the blood against the walls of the blood vessels. The extent of that force depends on both the cardiac output and the resistance of blood vessels. Optimal BP is generally defined as the level above which minimal vascular damage occurs. High BP is a condition in which the force of the blood against the artery walls is strong enough that, over an extended period of time, it may cause health problems such as heart disease (Hedegaard, Hallis, Rvn-Neilsen, & Kjeldsen, 2016).

Specifically, HTN is equated with BP higher than 140/90 mmHg if the patient is younger than 60 years, and higher than 150/90 mmHg for patients older than 60 years, according to the JNC 8 (2014). The overall occurrence is similar between men and women but differs with age: for those younger than 45 years, HTN is more common in men; for those older than 65 years, it is more common in women.

Worldwide, more than 1 billion adults are afflicted with HTN, causing more than 9 million deaths per year (Ettehad et al., 2016). Many patients are unaware of their elevated BP because they are asymptomatic. Symptoms experienced by patients are in the form of headaches, shortness of breath, or nosebleeds. Unfortunately, these signs and symptoms are not specific to HTN, and often do not occur until HTN has reached a severe or life-threatening stage.

There are two types of HTN. Primary, or essential HTN, tends to develop gradually over many years and for most adults, there is no identifiable cause. Secondary HTN appears suddenly, often caused by an underlying condition, resulting in a higher level BP than that attributed to primary HTN. Various conditions can lead to secondary HTN, including renal disease, obstructive sleep apnea, and thyroid disease. Certain medications, such as birth control pills, cold remedies, decongestants, over-the-counter pain relievers, and some prescription drugs, as well as illegal drugs such as cocaine and amphetamines, may cause an elevation in BP. Alcohol abuse or chronic alcohol use may cause an elevation in BP (Rapsomaniki et al., 2014).

A hypertensive "crisis" is a significant increase in BP that threatens to cause a stroke. Extremely high BP—a systolic pressure of 180 mmHg or higher or a diastolic pressure of 120 mmHg or higher—may damage blood vessels, which become inflamed and may leak fluid or blood and, as a result, the heart may not be able to pump blood effectively. Causes of a hypertensive emergency include noncompliance with antihypertensive medication or interaction between medications. In addition, an adult with HTN may experience a hypertensive crisis while having a stroke, an MI, an aortic rupture, or convulsions.

A hypertensive crisis is divided into two categories: urgent and emergent. In an urgent hypertensive crisis, the BP is extremely high but there is no evidence of end-organ damage. In an emergent hypertensive crisis, the BP is extremely high and resulting organ damage is indicated. An emergent hypertensive crisis can be associated with life-threatening complications. The adult may experience severe chest pain and/or a severe headache, accompanied by confusion and blurred vision, nausea, vomiting, severe anxiety, shortness of breath, seizures, and unresponsiveness. If an adult displays these symptoms along with highly elevated BP, that person will need immediate medical attention, including hospitalization for treatment with oral or intravenous medications (Ettehad et al., 2016).

Clinical Aspects

ASSESSMENT

A crucial component for effective nursing care for the patient with HTN is a comprehensive physical examination and medical history, as well as ongoing assessment, according to NANDA International (formerly the North American Nursing Diagnosis Association) (Herdman & Kamitsuru, 2014). Adults at risk for developing HTN should be noted and reported on regularly. Risk factors for HTN include excess weight, sedentary lifestyle, and noncompliance with medications.

As the patient's history is assessed, the nurse should evaluate reports of extreme fatigue, intolerance for activities, sudden weight gain, swelling of extremities, and progressive shortness of breath. These symptoms may indicate poor ventricular function or impending cardiac failure.

Proper equipment must be used in taking a BP, including a quality stethoscope and BP cuff. The patient should be relaxed, with his or her upper arm at the level of the heart. The nurse should remove any excess clothing that would interfere with the reading and the patient should remain still and quiet during the BP reading.

The nurse should check central and peripheral pulses. Bounding carotid, jugular, radial, or femoral pulses may be a sign of HTN. Pulses in the lower extremities may be diminished, indicating vasoconstriction. When auscultating heart and breath sounds, an S4 sound is common in a patient with HTN due to increased arterial pressure. Presence of crackles and/or wheezing may indicate pulmonary congestion secondary to developing heart failure. The nurse should observe skin color, moisture, temperature, and capillary refill time as pallor may be due to peripheral vasoconstriction. Dependent and general edema may indicate heart failure as well as renal or vascular impairment (Bauer, Briss, Goodman, & Bowman, 2014). The nurse should be sure to check laboratory data, including cardiac markers, complete blood count, electrolytes, arterial blood gases, blood urea nitrogen, and creatinine. Recording and reporting laboratory data can identify contributing factors to HTN, as well as indicate organ damage.

NURSING INTERVENTIONS, MANAGEMENT, AND IMPLICATIONS

Nursing management of the adult with HTN should focus on relieving stress by providing a calm environment while hospitalized. In order to decrease stimulation and promote relaxation, activities should be minimized. If needed, the adult should have scheduled uninterrupted rest times. The adult may need assistance with self-care activities, which will decrease the physical stress that can affect BP (Bauer et al., 2014).

Nursing care for the adult with HTN should emphasize compliance with a therapeutic regimen, lifestyle modifications, and prevention of complications. These restrictions can help manage fluid retention with a hypertensive response, which will decrease cardiac workload. Adults with HTN should be encouraged to quit smoking, reduce sodium intake to a maximum of 2,400 mg/day, and participate in moderate to vigorous activity 3 to 4 days per week, averaging 40 minutes a session per day (James et al., 2014).

Cigarette smoking can significantly increase the risk of cardiovascular disease, including HTN. A full assessment of the adult's smoking activity should be obtained, including identifying and documenting tobacco use. Nursing care involves encouraging the adult to quit smoking with the help of medication as well as a referral to a smoking-cessation counselor. If the adult is not willing to quit smoking immediately, he or she should be provided with smoking-cessation information for future use.

Adults with HTN should be placed on a healthy diet, such as the dietary approaches to stop hypertension (DASH) diet. The DASH diet is plant focused, rich in fruits, nuts, and vegetables. It is low fat, incorporating nonfat dairy, lean meats, fish, and poultry, and including whole grains and heart-healthy fats. The DASH diet emphasizes limiting portion sizes, eating a variety of foods, and ensuring an adequate amount of nutrients. There is also a lower sodium DASH diet, in which the adult can consume up to 1,500 mg of sodium a day. The DASH diet encourages limited alcohol consumption; the Dietary Guidelines for Americans recommend up to two drinks a day for men and one for women.

According to the American Heart Association (Brook et al., 2013), physical activity reduces not only HTN but also the risk of coronary artery disease, stroke, and type 2 diabetes. Adults with HTN should be encouraged to engage in regular physical activity, from moderate to vigorous, which can include brisk walking, swimming, and bicycle riding. Even while hospitalized, adults with HTN should be encouraged to engage in physical activity such as a walking regimen. Long term, the nurse should encourage the adult to maintain this activity, which may be supported by walking with a spouse, a friend, or in a group.

The adult with HTN should be encouraged to participate in activities that help alleviate stress, such as breathing exercises, muscle relaxation, and yoga. Nursing care should encourage long-term stress reduction, such as education in stress management, a plan for balancing work/life activities, and adequate rest (Oza & Garcellano, 2015).

The hypertensive patient may be prescribed one or more of the following initial drugs of choice for HTN, according to the JNC8 guidelines: angiotensin-converting-enzyme (ACE) inhibitor (ACE-I), angiotensin receptor blocker (ARB), calcium channel blocker (CCB), and a thiazide diuretic. Nursing care should emphasize and monitor the adult's strict compliance with his or her medication therapy, which is vital to the success of a program for reducing HTN.

OUTCOMES

Desired outcomes for the adult with HTN include maintaining BP within an individually accepted range as well as a stable cardiac rhythm and rate (James et al., 2014). If goal BP is not reached within a month of treatment, an increase of the dose of the initial drug, or a second drug, may be warranted. Nursing care then involves monitoring BP, ensuring compliance with medication, and noting and reporting any side effects such as increased fatigue or shortness of breath. This care regimen should be maintained until goal BP is reached.

Summary

Adults diagnosed with HTN should be monitored closely, as complications from the disease can escalate. Recommendations for BP control, including treatment levels, goals, and drug therapy, should be based on evidence as well as on considerations specific to the individual. For adults with HTN, the benefits of adopting lifestyle changes, including a healthy diet, weight control, and regular exercise, should be stressed to aid in BP control (James et al., 2014).

Bauer, U. E., Briss, P. A., Goodman, R. A., & Bowman, B. A. (2014). Prevention of chronic disease in the 21st century: Elimination of the leading preventable causes of premature death and disability in the USA. *Lancet, 384*(9937), 45–52.

Brook, R. D., Appel, L. J., Rubenfire, M., Ogedegbe, G., Bisognano, J. D., Elliott, W. J., . . . Rajagopalan, S. (2013). Beyond medications and diet: Alternative approaches to lowering blood pressure: A scientific statement from the American Heart Association. *Hypertension, 61*(6), 1360–1383.

Ettehad, D., Emdin, C. A., Kiran, A., Anderson, S. G., Callender, T., Emberson, J., . . . Rahimi, K. (2016). Blood pressure lowering for prevention of cardiovascular disease and death: A systematic review and meta-analysis. *Lancet, 387*(10022), 957–967. doi:10.1016/S0140-6736(15)01225-8

Hedegaard, U., Hallas, J., Ravn-Nielsen, L. V., & Kjeldsen, L. J. (2016). Process- and patient-reported outcomes of a multifaceted medication adherence intervention for hypertensive patients in secondary care. *Research in Social and Administrative Pharmacy, 12*(2), 302–318. doi:10.1016/J.SAPHARM.2015.05.006

Herdman, T. H., & Kamitsuru, S. (Eds.). (2014). *Nursing diagnoses: Definitions & classification 2015–2017.* Chichester, UK: Wiley Blackwell.

James, P. A., Oparil, S., Carter, B. L., Cushman, W. C., Dennison-Himmelfarb, C., Handler, J., . . . Ortiz, E. (2014). Evidence-based guideline for the management of high blood pressure in adults report from the panel members appointed to the Eighth Joint National Committee (JNC 8). *Journal of the American Medical Association, 311*(5), 507–520. doi:10.1001/jama.2013.284427 Retrieved from http://jamanetwork.com/journals/jama/fullarticle/1791497

Oza, R., & Garcellano, M. (2015). Nonpharmacologic management of hypertension: What works? *American Family Physician, 91*(11), 772–776.

Rapsomaniki, E., Timmis, A., George, J., Pujades-Rodriguez, M., Shah, A. D., Denaxas, S., . . . Hemingway, H. (2014). Blood pressure and incidence of twelve cardiovascular diseases: Lifetime risks, healthy life-years lost, and age-specific associations in 1.25 million people. *Lancet, 383*(9932), 1899–1911.

Wozniak, G., Khan, T., Gillespie, C., & Sifuentes, L. (2016). Hypertension control cascade: A framework to improve hypertension awareness, treatment, and control. *Journal of Clinical Hypertension, 18*(3), 232–239. doi:10.1111/jch.12654. Epub 2015 Sept 4

Yoon, S. S., Fryar, C. D., & Carroll, M. D. (2015). *Hypertension prevalence and control among adults: United States, 2011–2014.* NCHS data brief, no 220. Hyattsville, MD: National Center for Health Statistics.

■ HYPERTHYROIDISM

Colleen Kurzawa

Overview

Hyperthyroidism (HT) occurs as a result of overfunction of the thyroid gland, which leads to an excess of thyroid hormone (TH) in the body (De Leo, Lee, & Braverman, 2016). According to De Leo et al. (2016), 1% to 3% of people in the United States will develop thyroid disease, HT increases with age, and the prevalence of HT is greater in females. TH increases metabolism and protein synthesis, which affects all major organs. Persons with HT may present with mild to severe manifestation depending on the amount and period of time of hypersecretion of TH. Nursing care of persons with HT focuses on prevention and treatment of complications.

Background

HT refers to an excess of TH that is synthesized and secreted by the thyroid gland, and *thyrotoxicosis* refers to excess circulating TH no matter what the source (De Leo et al., 2016). Patients with excessive TH will display an increased basal metabolic rate, increased cardiovascular function, increased gastrointestinal function, and increased neuromuscular function; weight loss; heat intolerance; and problems with fat, protein, and carbohydrate metabolism (Lemone, Burke, Bauldoff, & Gubrud, 2015; Melmed, Polonsk, Larsen, & Kronenberg, 2016). Several factors that cause HT are excessive thyroid-stimulating hormone (TSH) receptor stimulation (Graves' disease), autonomous TH secretion (toxic multinodular goiter), destruction of follicles in the thyroid with release of TH (infection, thyroiditis), and extrathyroidal sources of TH (overmedication; Lemone et al., 2015; Melmed et al., 2016). The most common causes of HT are Graves' disease and toxic multinodular goiter (Ross et al., 2016).

Worldwide, the prevalence of HT varies with the degree of iodine insufficiency in populations; especially at risk are pregnant women, children, and the elderly (De Leo, 2016; Devereaux & Tewelde, 2014). In the United States, the prevalence of HT is 1.2%, with 0.5% overt HT and 0.7% subclinical HT (Devereaux & Tewelde, 2014; Ross et al., 2016). Subclinical HT ranges from 1% to 10% in different populations and increases with age (Mitchell & Pearce, 2016). Grade I subclinical HT results when the TSH is low but detectable, and grade II subclinical HT results when TSH is suppressed (Mitchell & Pearce, 2016). About 76% of grade I subclinical HT goes back to euthyroid state (normal) and only 12.5% of grade II subclinical HT returns to the euthyroid state (Mitchell & Pearce, 2016). Patients with grade II subclinical HT have a 3.1% chance of progressing to a clinical HT in 7 years and patients with grade I subclinical HT have a 0.5% chance of progressing to a clinical HT in 7 years

(Mitchell & Pearce, 2016). According to Ross et al. (2016), subclinical HT populations that are asymptomatic should be treated at 65 years and older when there is cardiac disease and osteoporosis. The percentages of females who develop HT are 1% to 2%, and it is 0.1% to 0.2% for males (Melmed et al., 2016). The prevalence of thyroiditis is 10% to 15% and toxic adenoma is 3% to 5% (Devereaux & Tewelde, 2014).

Graves' disease is caused by thyroid-stimulating autoantibodies (Melmed et al., 2016). Graves' disease typically includes a triad of symptoms: goiter (swelling of the thyroid gland), exophthalmos (protruding eyes), and skin problems. About 80% of all hyperthyroid cases are Graves' disease with an incidence of 1 per 1,000, and it is greater in females 30 to 60 years of age with a family history of thyroid problems (Melmed et al., 2016).

In pregnancy, the most common cause of HT is Graves' disease. The incidence of HT is five to nine per 1,000 pregnant women per year (De Leo et al., 2016). Postpartum thyroiditis in the mother is transient and may develop anywhere from 6 weeks to 6 months after childbirth (Devereaux & Tewelde, 2014). The fetus is also at risk before birth because thyroid antibodies are able to cross the placenta (De Leo et al., 2016).

HT in children is rare but if not treated it may lead to serious complications with growth and development (Srinivasan & Mirsra, 2015). The incidence of HT per 1,000 young children is 0.44 and in adolescents it is 0.26 (Endocrine Society, 2017). Graves' disease accounts for 95% of HT cases (Srinivasan & Mirsra, 2015). Subclinical HT prevalence in children is 0.7% (Endocrine Society, 2017).

Thyroid storm is an uncommon complication of HT but has an extremely high mortality rate (Devereaux & Tewelde, 2014). Thyroid storm is accelerated HT and accounts for 1% to 2% of admissions for HT (Devereaux & Tewelde, 2014; Mohananey et al., 2016). Thyroid storm occurs abruptly in patients being treated incompletely or may be precipitated by infection, trauma, surgical emergency, radiation thyroiditis, diabetic ketoacidosis, and toxemia during pregnancy (Melmed et al., 2016). Manifestations are the result of an extreme metabolic state and include irritability, tachycardia, vomiting, high temperature, profuse sweating, delirium, or psychosis, eventually leading to apathy, stupor, and coma (Lemone et al., 2015; Melmed et al., 2016). According to Mohananey et al. (2016), the mortality rate from thyroid storm has decreased over the past several years (60% in 2003, 21% in 2011).

Clinical Aspects

ASSESSMENT

TH in the body acts to increase metabolism and protein synthesis. Manifestations are similar to problems such as increased sympathetic nervous system stimulation (Lemone et al., 2015; Melmed et al., 2016). Physical manifestations are cardiovascular (hypertension, tachycardia, arrhythmias, and edema); protein, carbohydrate, and lipid metabolism (increased appetite, weight loss, and aggravation of diabetes mellitus); nervous system (nervousness, emotional lia-bility, exaggerated movements, tremors of tongue, hands, eyelids, and fatigue); eyes (blurred vision, photophobia, lacrimation, and exophthalmos); respira-tory (dyspnea); gastrointestinal (diarrhea, hepatomegaly, jaundice, nausea, vomiting); musculoskeletal (muscle weakness, pathologic fractures, increased excretion of calcium and phosphorus, osteoporosis, and osteomalacia); skin (warm and moist, fine hair, soft nails); reproductive (delayed sexual maturity, amenorrhea, reduced fertility, gynecomastia, and erectile dysfunction; Melmed et al., 2016).

Nursing assessments should include a thorough health history and physical examination. The health history should focus on family prevalence of thyroid disease, menstruation history, gastrointestinal problems, weight changes, and medication use (Lemone et al., 2015). Physical assessment should center on vital signs and an examination of skin, eyes, cardiovascular, gastrointestinal, repro-ductive, musculoskeletal system, and other systems (Lemone et al., 2015).

Laboratory results that demonstrate elevated TH, low TSH (elevated pitui-tary tumor), elevated triiodothyronine (T3)/thyroxine (T4), and erythrocyte sed-imentation rate would indicate HT. Other tests may include a protein-binding inhibition assay and bioassay. The radioactive iodine uptake (RAIU) will be elevated. A thyroid ultrasound may indicate the presence of a nodular thyroid gland and a thyroid scan may confirm hyperfunctioning nodules.

Nursing diagnosis for the person with HT should be individualized and take into consideration all possible effects on major organs and metabolism. The most common health problems include cardiovascular, visual, nutrition, and body image (Lemone et al., 2015). Persons may have increased blood pressure, tachycardia, and dyspnea. Vital signs should be monitored, activity and rest need to be balanced, and stress should be decreased with relaxation interventions (Lemone et al., 2015). Disturbed sensory perception due to diplopia, photopho-bia, and eye changes can put the patient at risk for falls. Patients should wear dark glasses, use artificial tears, and elevate the head of bed (Melmed et al., 2016). Imbalanced nutrition (less than body requirements) is due to the hyper-metabolic state induced by HT. The patient should understand the need to check weight daily and keep a record. Collaboration with a dietician is important to help ensure patients consume adequate amounts of carbohydrates and proteins in relation to their metabolic demand (Lemone et al., 2015). Disturbed body image and anxiety are due to changes with eyes, hair loss, perspiration, sexual changes, and mood changes (Lemone et al., 2015). Good communication skills are necessary to build a trusting relationship that allows the person to verbalize her or his feelings and perceptions of the illness. Finally, the nurse needs to clar-ify any misconceptions and provide information.

Summary

There is no cure for HT, and so the primary focus is on maintenance of the disease process and alleviation of related symptoms. Nurses need to assist the patient in the identification of stress-relieving activities and emphasize the need for a trusting relationship with health care professionals. Nursing care is centered on education and health promotion. Patients need to be aware that medication regimens will be lifelong so they will need to be educated on ways to monitor their symptoms and what side effects to report. If radioactive iodine therapy or surgery is required, then postprocedure care is initiated. With treatment for HT, the person must understand signs and symptoms of hypothyroidism and thyroid storm.

De Leo, S., Lee, S. Y., & Braverman, L. E. (2016). Hyperthyroidism. *Lancet, 388*(10047), 906–918.

Devereaux, D., & Tewelde, S. Z. (2014). Hyperthyroidism and thyrotoxicosis. *Emergency Medicine Clinics of North America, 32*(2), 277–292.

Endocrine Society. (2017). Endocrine facts and figures. Retrieved from http://endocrine facts.org/health-conditions/thyroid/4-hyperthyroidism

Lemone, P., Burke, K., Bauldoff, G., & Gubrud, P. (2015). *Medical–surgical nursing: Critical thinking in patient care* (6th ed.). Upper Saddle River, NJ: Pearson.

Melmed, S., Polonsk, K. S., Larsen, P. R., & Kronenberg, H. M. (2016). *Williams textbook of endocrinology* (13th ed.). Philadelphia, PA: Elsevier.

Mitchell, A. L., & Pearce, S. H. (2016). Subclinical hyperthyroidism: First do no harm. *Clinical Endocrinology, 85*(1), 15–16.

Mohananey, D., Villablanca, P., Bhatia, N., Agrawal, S., Murrieta, J. C., Ganesh, M., . . . Ramakrishna, H. (2016). Trends in incidence, management and outcomes of cardiogenic shock complicating thyroid storm in the United States. *Circulation, A18332,* 134. Retrieved from http://circ.ahajournals.org/content/134/Suppl_1/A18332.short

Ross, D. S., Burch, H. B., Cooper, D. S., Greenlee, M. C., Laurberg, P., Maia, A. L., . . . Walter, M. A. (2016). 2016 American Thyroid Association guidelines for diagnosis and management of hyperthyroidism and other causes of thyrotoxicosis. *Thyroid, 26*(10), 1343–1421.

Srinivasan, S., & Misra, M. (2015). Hyperthyroidism in children. *Pediatrics in Review, 36*(6), 239–248.

■ HYPOTHYROIDISM

Karen L. Terry

Overview

Hypothyroidism is an endocrine disorder characterized by insufficient circulating levels of the thyroid hormones thyroxine (T4) and triiodothyronine (T3). Primary hypothyroidism occurs when there is either reduced thyroid hormone or impaired thyroxine synthesis by follicle cells. Central hypothyroidism occurs when the hypothalamic–pituitary axis is damaged. Hypothyroidism consists of two subsets referred to as *secondary* and *tertiary*. Deficient pituitary thyroid-stimulating hormone (TSH) production is considered secondary hypothyroidism. Deficient hypothalamic thyroid-releasing hormone (TRH) production is considered tertiary hypothyroidism (March, 2016).

Hypothyroidism is more prevalent in less developed countries, but has decreased overall due to routine iodine supplementation in salt, flour, and other food staples. Worldwide, insufficient iodine intake is the most common cause of hypothyroidism, whereas autoimmune disease is the most common cause in the Unites States (Orlander et al., 2016). The focus of nursing care for adults with hypothyroidism is on symptom management and the delivery of nursing interventions that prevent or reduce complications during care and recovery as it relates to the severity of the disease at the time of diagnosis.

Background

Hypothyroidism is easily treatable and reversible. If left unchecked, severe hypothyroidism can lead to coma and death. Garber et al. (2012) noted in the American Association of Clinical Endocrinologists (AACE) guidelines that TSH, T3, and T4 levels need to be carefully interpreted to diagnose hypothyroidism. Not all patients with abnormal lab results will be diagnosed with hypothyroidism or be treated with hormones. Most patients need to be symptomatic, have TSH levels greater than 4.5 mIU/L and low levels of thyroid hormone to receive hormone replacements (Garber et al., 2012). In addition, diagnosis of primary or central hypothyroidism will also help determine how medical treatment ensues. Possible causes of primary hypothyroidism could include chronic lymphocytic (autoimmune) thyroiditis, postpartum thyroiditis, subacute (granulomatous) thyroiditis, drug-induced hypothyroidism, and iatrogenic hypothyroidism. Possible causes of central hypothyroidism could include pituitary and hypothalamus tumors, lymphocytic hypophysitis, Sheehan syndrome, history of brain irradiation, medications, congenital nongoiterous hypothyroidism type 4, and thyrotropin-releasing hormone resistance or deficiency (Orlander et al., 2016). Partial or complete surgical removal of the thyroid gland can also result in hypothyroidism.

Hypothyroidism is more prevalent in women with low body mass index during childhood (Orlander et al., 2016). In the landmark National Health and

Nutrition Examination Survey (NHANES) 1999 to 2002, the frequency of hypothyroidism was noted to increase with age and the prevalence was higher in Whites and Mexican Americans than in African Americans, with 3.7% of the U.S. population reporting hypothyroidism or TSH levels exceeding 4.5 mIU/L (Aoki et al., 2007). In the United States, according to the National Institute of Diabetes and Digestive and Kidney Diseases (NIDDKD), 4.6% of the population reported hypothyroidism, and subclinical hypothyroidism affects 1% to 10% of the population (NIDDKD, 2016).

If untreated and allowed to progress, severe hypothyroidism worsens metabolic abnormalities and leads to coma and death in adults. Severe hypothyroidism in infants causes cretinism and irreversible mental retardation. Hypothyroidism and its treatment, if diagnosed before severe advancement and permanent damage, have a good prognosis, and abnormal signs and symptoms reverse fairly well with thyroid hormone replacement. Quality-of-life measures have also been noted to significantly improve in just 6 weeks of treatment (Orlander et al., 2016).

Clinical Aspects

ASSESSMENT

Key to the nursing process in caring for the patient with hypothyroidism is a thorough assessment, including history, physical, laboratory findings, and diagnostic or imaging studies (March, 2016). Early in the disease process, compensatory mechanisms maintain T3 hormone levels, but as time and stressors continue, these mechanisms fail and T3 production or release decreases. Patients present different clinical presentations depending on how long the hypothyroidism has occurred or how severe the suppression of thyroid hormone. Documentation of an accurate timeline is important as well as its onset, duration, and severity of signs and symptoms. Medical, surgical, and family history are obtained, with particular attention to risk factors for hypothyroidism. Common medications that have the potential to cause hypothyroidism include amiodarone, interferon alpha, rifampin, phenytoin, lithium, and carbamazepine (Orlander et al., 2016).

Common symptoms of hypothyroidism include fatigue, weight gain, puffy face, goiter, cold intolerance, joint or muscle pain, constipation, dry skin, dry or thinning hair, heavy or irregular menses, fertility problems, depression, bradycardia, and decreased sweating. Common risk factors for developing hypothyroidism include family history of hypothyroidism, goiter, radiation to neck, past thyroid surgery, Sjögren's syndrome, lupus, rheumatoid arthritis, type 1 diabetes mellitus, 6 months postpartum, and pernicious anemia (NIDDKD, 2016).

During physical examination particular attention to the presence of goiter or delayed relaxation of deep tendon reflexes can be significant indicators of hypothyroidism (March, 2016). Goiter may present as difficulty swallowing or hoarse voice and not necessarily an enlarged neck mass. Common lab abnormalities for hypothyroidism include elevated TSH, with low T3 and/or T4 levels. Imaging studies are used to evaluate lesions/tumors; chest radiography can show enlarged heart/pleural effusions; sinus bradycardia and other electrophysiological changes can be noted with EKG evaluation (March, 2016).

NURSING INTERVENTIONS, MANAGEMENT, AND IMPLICATIONS

Nursing care of the patient is dependent on the severity of hypothyroidism at the time of diagnosis. Patients with long-standing hypothyroidism can present with myxedema, which leads to coma and death. Nursing problems would include mental deterioration, decreased cardiac output, impaired spontaneous ventilation, activity intolerance, and loss of skin integrity (NANDA, n.d.). Assessment of mental and neurological status changes, adequate cardiopulmonary support to maintain tissue perfusion, pressure ulcer prophylaxis, and psychosocial support for the family are priorities. In addition to ventilation and fluid support, nursing would administer proper intravenous dosage of levothyroxine with stress glucocorticoids and perform cardiac assessments. Continued review of laboratory data would determine subsequent levothyroxine dose adjustments.

In less critically ill patients, symptoms are less life threatening and affect quality of life. Nursing-related problems include constipation, disturbed body image, imbalanced body temperature, and knowledge deficits. Focus is on maintaining normal bowel function, addressing altered self-concept due to possible weight gain and hair loss, maintaining temperature control, and addressing knowledge deficit related to lack of information about the disease process and self-care (Belleza, 2016).

Patients need to know to take their thyroid hormone with water 30 minutes prior to any other mediation and food. Levothyroxine drug interactions can occur among many medications, including iron, aluminum, magnesium, calcium carbonate, cimetidine, sucralfate, and caffeine. Teach patients not to stop medication; replacement therapy is usually needed for life. Genetic studies are helping develop combination hormone therapies that promise improved efficacy.

OUTCOMES

Expected outcomes for the proper management of severe hypothyroidism are improved cardiac status and normal breathing patterns, activity participation and return to independence, and intact skin integrity. For patients with less severe hypothyroidism, outcomes would include normal bowel function, improved body image and thought process, maintenance of normal body temperature, and proper administration of medications and self-care (Belleza, 2016). Overall, patients should return to normal metabolic states.

Summary

Hypothyroidism is a common endocrine disorder that is easily treated. Nursing care and interventions are aimed at symptom relief and reduction of complications during recovery. Severity and advancement of the hypothyroidism will affect patient clinical presentation; therefore, nursing interventions and care plans must be individualized to meet the patient's needs at the time of diagnosis. Genetic studies may help in identifying patients who would benefit from pharmacogenomics. Thyroid hormone treatment reverses symptoms, helps return patients to normal metabolic states, and improves quality of life.

Aoki, Y., Belin, R. M., Clickner, R., Jeffries, R., Phillips, L., & Mahaffey, K. R. (2007). Serum TSH and total T4 in the United States population and their association with participant characteristics: National Health and Nutrition Examination Survey (NHANES 1999–2002). *Thyroid, 17*(12), 1211–1223. doi:10.1089thy.2006.0235

Belleza, M. (2016). Hypothyroidism: Nursing care management and study guide. *Nurse Study Guides (medical-surgical nursing)*. Retrieved from http://nurseslabs.com/hypothyroidism

Garber, J. R., Cobin, R. H., Gharib, H., Hennessey, J. V., Klein, I., Mechanick, J. I., . . . Woeber, K. A. (2012). Clinical practice guidelines for hypothyroidism in adults: Cosponsored by the American Association of Clinical Endocrinologists and the American Thyroid Association. *Endocrine Practice, 18*(6), 988–1028.

March, P. (2016). *Quick lesson: Hypothyroidism in adults*. Glendale, CA: CINAHL Information Systems.

NANDA. (n.d.). Nursing diagnosis list for 2015–2017. Retrieved from http://health-conditions.com/nanda-nursing-diagnosis-list-2015-2017

National Institute of Diabetes and Digestive Kidney Diseases. (2016). Hypothyroidism (underactive thyroid). Retrieved from http://www.niddk.nih.gov/health-information/health topics/endocrine/hypothyroidism

Orlander, P. R., Varghese, J. M., Freeman, L. M., Griffing, G. T., Davis, A. B., Bharaktiya, S., . . . Ziel, F. H. (2016). Hypothyroidism. *Medscape*. Retrieved from http://emdecine.medscape.com/article/122393-overview

■ INFLAMMATORY BOWEL DISEASE IN ADULTS

Ronald Rock

Overview

Inflammatory bowel disease (IBD) is a chronic autoimmune disease of unknown etiology characterized by periods of remission and exacerbation. Crohn's disease (CD) and ulcerative colitis (UC), the two chronic conditions of IBD, are characterized by chronic uncontrolled inflammation of the gastro-intestinal (GI) tract causing edema, ulceration, bleeding, and profound fluid and electrolyte losses (Centers for Disease Control and Prevention [CDC], 2016). IBD has been associated with decreased quality of life and extensive morbidity, and often results in complications requiring hospitalization and surgical intervention (CDC, 2016). Overall, an estimated 3.1 million, or 1.3% of U.S. adults are diagnosed with IBD (CDC, 2016). Nursing care of the adult with IBD focuses on management of fluid and electrolyte imbalances, nutritional deficiencies, infections, chronic pain, and body-image disturbances (Burkhalter et al., 2015).

Background

Although the etiology of IBD is unknown, evidence suggests that normal intestinal flora trigger an abnormal immune reaction resulting in an overactive, inappropriate, and sustained inflammatory response. According to the CDC (2016), UC is slightly more common in males, ex-smokers, and nonsmokers, whereas CD is more frequent in women and smokers. Diagnosis of IBD is usually made before age 30 years, with peak incidences from 14 to 24 years and a second smaller peak in the sixth decade. Caucasians, individuals of white-collar occupations, and persons of Ashkenazi Jewish decent are more susceptible to IBD than other racial, occupational, and ethnic subgroups (CDC, 2016). Diet, oral contraceptive use, perinatal and childhood infections, and atypical mycobacterial infections are thought to play a role in developing IBD (CDC, 2016).

CD often presents in adolescence and is more prevalent in women than in men. Although the etiology of CD is unknown, it is associated with a mutation in the NOD2 gene (Wilkins, Jarvis, & Patel, 2011). UC is more common in North America and Europe than in other regions. Risk factors for UC include a history of recent infection with *Salmonella* or *Campylobacter*, and a family history of the disease (Adams & Bornemann, 2013).

Both disorders are characterized by extraintestinal manifestations, most commonly affecting the skin, eyes, mouth, and joints; the hepatobiliary, renal, and pulmonary systems can also be affected. In addition, persons with IBD are at increased risk for developing osteoporosis and colon cancer. CD is characterized by transmural inflammation of the bowel wall and can occur anywhere in the GI tract from the mouth to the anus, but most often involves the terminal ileum and colon. Typically, ulcerations are deep and longitudinal, penetrating between islands of inflamed edematous mucosa, characterized by the classic "skip lesions" and cobblestone appearance. Because the inflammation penetrates the entire bowel wall, microscopic leaks can allow bowel contents to enter the peritoneal cavity, resulting in abscess, fistulae, or peritonitis.

In contrast, UC typically starts in the rectum and moves proximally in a continuous pattern toward the cecum, different than the typical skip lesions of CD. Although there is sometimes mild inflammation in the terminal ileum, UC is primarily a disease of the colon and rectum. In UC, inflammation and ulcerations occur in the mucosal layer of the large intestine, hence fistulae and abscess formation are rare.

IBD is a chronic lifelong condition with significant health and economic costs. Based on data from 2004, IBD accounts for approximately 1,300,000 physician visits and 92,000 hospitalizations in the United States each year (CDC, 2016). In addition, 75% of patients diagnosed with CD and 25% of patients with a diagnosis of UC will require surgery (CDC, 2016). Mortality and morbidity of IBD are more closely linked to acquired coexisting conditions, such as infection, thrombus, or chronic disease, than the disease itself (Kassam et al., 2014). In 2008, direct treatment costs for patients with IBD were greater than $6.3 billion, whereas indirect costs were $5.5 billion, and these are anticipated to rise without a cure (CDC, 2016).

Clinical Aspects

ASSESSMENT

Patients with IBD may present with a variety of unspecific and overlapping features, making the differential diagnosis a challenge compounded by the lack of a single gold standard diagnostic test to distinguish between UC and CD (Tontini, Vecchi, Pastorelli, Neurath, & Neumann, 2015). The first step of diagnosis is a complete patient history addressing the onset, severity, and pattern of symptoms, especially frequency and consistency of bowel movements. The history focused on risk factors and possible alternative diagnoses should include recent travel, exposure to antibiotics, food intolerance, medications, smoking, and family history of IBD. Common symptoms of IBD include abdominal pain, diarrhea, fatigue, fever, GI bleeding, and weight loss. Physical evaluation should include heart rate, blood pressure, temperature, and body weight; abdominal examination may reveal tenderness, distention, or masses. An anorectal examination should be performed as one third of patients have a perirectal abscess, fissure, or fistula at some time during the illness (Wilkins et al., 2011).

Laboratory tests are useful for diagnosing IBD, assessing disease activity, identifying complications, and monitoring response to therapy. Initial testing often includes white blood cell count; platelet count; measurement of hemoglobin, hematocrit, blood urea nitrogen, creatinine, liver enzymes, and C-reactive protein; and erythrocyte sedimentation rate. Stool culture and testing for

Clostridium difficile toxin should also be considered to rule out an infectious cause of diarrhea. Endoscopic or colonoscopic biopsy is valuable in the diagnosis and differentiation of UC from CD.

Treatment goals for patients with IBD are achieving remission and preventing exacerbations and complications. Medical management focuses on relieving symptoms, controlling inflammation, and healing of intestinal mucosa. Pharmacologic treatment is initiated early in the disease and is based on a step-down or step-up approach; medications include biologics (tumor necrosis factor alpha inhibitors), corticosteroids, immunomodulators (azathioprine [AZA] and 6-mercaptopurine [6-MP]), antibiotics, and aminosalicylates. Surgery is indicated to treat complications or when medical management fails to control the disease. Surgical options vary depending on the type and severity of IBD and include drainage of abscesses, fistula repair, strictureplasty, bowel resection (with or without ostomy formation), and colectomy. Patients with CD who undergo multiple resections of the small intestine may develop short bowel syndrome. Short bowel syndrome is associated with several complications, including acid/base and fluid/electrolyte imbalances, malabsorption, vitamin and mineral deficiencies, and renal stones. Persons with CD often experience disease recurrence even with surgical intervention, whereas removal of the diseased colon in UC may be considered curative.

NURSING INTERVENTIONS, MANAGEMENT, AND IMPLICATIONS

An individual with IBD will journey through the health care system at different points, from initial investigation and diagnosis, through emergency care, admission, surgery (planned or emergent), postoperative care and discharge, education regarding management of associated medical conditions, and follow-up care with routine IBD management (Foskett, 2013). Because of systemic involvement, a multidisciplinary team approach is recommended. No single model of care is appropriate for all patients all the time; care may be delivered in hospital, shared between hospital and primary care, or through supported self-managed care (Foskett, 2013). Nursing care of patients with IBD focuses on managing fluid and electrolyte imbalances, malabsorption and nutritional deficiencies, infections, chronic pain, and body-image disturbances specific to the individual needs of patients (Burkhalter et al., 2015).

OUTCOMES

The main goal of treatment of IBD is to improve the patient's condition and health-related quality of life (HRQOL; Peyrin-Biroulet et al., 2016). Unfortunately, the physical well-being of the patient with IBD is not the only nursing concern. The uncertainty and chronicity of the disease and the lack of a definitive cure require nursing to be aware of other HRQOL indictors for this patient population. With the increasing incidence of IBD in the United States, identifying interventions to address the patient's psychosocial and physiologic needs and determining the impact of disease on the individual's activities of daily living (Iglesias-Rey et al., 2014) are essential.

Summary

Adults diagnosed with IBD may experience chronic or acute manifestations of CD or UC. The disease may result in long-term medical management and/or surgery. Evidence-based medical and surgical nursing care is critical in managing this patient population. In combination with physiologic, pharmacologic, and, if needed, psychological therapy, patients suffering with this potentially debilitating disease can be effectively managed.

Adams, S. M., & Bornemann, P. H. (2013). Ulcerative colitis. *American Family Physician, 87*(10), 699–705.

Burkhalter, H., Stucki-Thür, P., David, B., Lorenz, S., Biotti, B., Rogler, G., & Pittet, V. (2015). Assessment of inflammatory bowel disease patient's needs and problems from a nursing perspective. *Digestion, 91*(2), 128–141.

Centers for Disease Control and Prevention. (2016). Prevalence of inflammatory bowel disease among adults aged ≥18 years—United States, 2015. *Morbidity and Mortality Weekly Reports 28;65(42),* 1166–1169. doi:10.15585/mmwr.mm6542a3

Foskett, K. (2013). Inflammatory bowel disease—Patient engagement and experience. *Journal of Community Nursing, 27*(3), 29–32.

Iglesias-Rey, M., Barreiro-de Acosta, M., Caamaño-Isorna, F., Rodríguez, I. V., Ferreiro, R., Lindkvist, B., . . . Dominguez-Munoz, J. E. (2014). Psychological factors are associated with changes in the health-related quality of life in inflammatory bowel disease. *Inflammatory Bowel Diseases, 20*(1), 92–102.

Kassam, Z., Belga, S., Roifman, I., Hirota, S., Jijon, H., Kaplan, G. G., . . . Beck, P. L. (2014). Inflammatory bowel disease cause-specific mortality: A primer for clinicians. *Inflammatory Bowel Diseases, 20*(12), 2483–2492.

Peyrin-Biroulet, L., Panés, J., Sandborn, W. J., Vermeire, S., Danese, S., Feagan, B. G., . . . Rycroft, B. (2016). Defining disease severity in inflammatory bowel diseases: Current and future directions. *Clinical Gastroenterology and Hepatology, 14*(3), 348–354. e17.

Tontini, G. E., Vecchi, M., Pastorelli, L., Neurath, M. F., & Neumann, H. (2015). Differential diagnosis in inflammatory bowel disease colitis: State of the art and future perspectives. *World Journal of Gastroenterology, 21*(1), 21–46.

Wilkins, T., Jarvis, K., & Patel, J. (2011). Diagnosis and management of Crohn's disease. *American Family Physician, 84*(12), 1365–1375.

■ LEUKEMIA

Marisa A. Cortese

Overview

Leukemia is a malignancy of the blood. Cells of the blood develop in the bone marrow. The bone marrow is the site of production for erythrocytes (red blood cells [RBCs]) and leukocytes (white blood cells [WBCs]), as well as thrombocytes (platelets). There were approximately 60,140 new cases of leukemia diagnosed in the United States in 2016 (National Cancer Institute Surveillance, Epidemiology, and End Results Program [NCI SEER], 2017). Leukemia is often treated with chemotherapy, which may cause adverse effects for the patient (National Cancer Institute, 2017).

Background

Leukemia is a malignancy in which immature cells or ineffective WBCs (lymphoblasts) grow rapidly within the bone marrow. These lymphoblasts begin to accumulate in the bone marrow and eventually replace normal cells. This causes anemia, neutropenia, and thrombocytopenia. Leukemia can be classified as either an acute or chronic condition.

There are two types of acute leukemia found in the adult population: acute lymphoblastic leukemia (ALL) and acute myeloid leukemia (AML; National Cancer Institute, 2017). ALL and AML are both aggressive types of leukemia. ALL is caused by the rapid proliferation of lymphoblasts (immature lymphocytes), whereas AML is caused by the rapid growth of myeloblasts (immature myeloid cells; National Cancer Institute, 2017).

Acute leukemia can spread to other parts of the body such as the lymph nodes, spleen, liver, and central nervous system (CNS). Some of the common signs and symptoms found in acute leukemia are fatigue, fever, night sweats, bruising/bleeding easily, unexplained weight loss, swollen lymph nodes, and frequent infections (National Cancer Institute, 2017).

When patients present with symptoms of acute leukemia, a thorough history and physical examination with laboratory tests that include a complete blood count with differential, chemistry panel, and coagulation tests need to be performed. A bone marrow biopsy and aspiration is performed in order to determine the extent of the disease and to test for genetic mutations, which may show prognostic factors (National Cancer Institute, 2017).

A patient's prognosis and treatment plan depends on a number of factors that include age, comorbidities, CNS involvement, and chromosomal abnormalities in the bone marrow (Gaynor et al., 1988; Hoelzer et al., 1988). The standard treatment for patients with acute leukemia is chemotherapy and possible allogeneic hematopoietic stem cell transplantation (HSCT). Allogeneic HSCT is a process in which stem cells are collected from a donor and infused into a patient who has received a combination of chemotherapy and immunosuppressive therapy. This will promote bone marrow recovery (Ezzone, 2013).

There are two types of chronic leukemia found in the adult population: chronic lymphocytic leukemia (CLL) and chronic myelogenous leukemia (CML). CLL and CML are both slow-growing cancers. CLL is caused by bone marrow making too many lymphocytes, whereas CML is caused by a distinct genetic abnormality found on the Philadelphia chromosome (Dighiero & Hamblin, 2008; Goldman & Melo, 2003).

Patients diagnosed with CLL or CML may have symptoms of fatigue, fever, or night sweats. Patients with CLL may develop enlarged lymph nodes (Dighiero & Hamblin, 2008; Goldman & Melo, 2003).

Similar to those patients diagnosed with acute leukemia, a complete medical workup must be performed. The following examinations and testing should be performed: a thorough history and physical examination, laboratory tests, including complete blood count with differential and a chemistry panel. A bone marrow biopsy and aspiration is performed in order to determine the extent of the disease and to test for genetic mutations that may show prognostic factors (National Cancer Institute, 2017).

A patient's prognosis and plan of care are dependent on age, comorbidities, and the presence or absence of specific chromosomal abnormalities found in the blood and/or bone marrow (Dighiero & Hamblin, 2008; Goldman & Melo, 2003). The standard treatment for CLL is chemotherapy. Patients diagnosed with CML are treated with agents called *tyrosine kinase inhibitors*, which stop the enzyme that produces the malignant cells from forming (Dighiero & Hamblin, 2008; Goldman & Melo, 2003).

Clinical Aspects

ASSESSMENT

Patients diagnosed with an acute or chronic leukemia will need to be monitored closely for adverse events during their treatment. It is important to assess patients for potential fever, infection, and other complications that may be found during their initial workup as well as follow-up assessments during active treatment. Patients should be asked during their assessments whether they have had any recent fever, night sweats, chills, bleeding or bruising, abdominal pain, or frequent infections. On physical examination, a patient may appear pale and feverish; have swollen lymph nodes in the neck, armpit, or groin; have swelling of the abdomen; and/or have an enlarged spleen (National Cancer Institute, 2017).

A patient undergoing treatment for leukemia is at risk for infection. The risk factors associated are the lack of mature WBCs, immunosuppression, and bone marrow suppression due to chemotherapy. To prevent infection in patients with leukemia, it is important to educate patients as well as their families on protecting from sources of pathogens or infection. Patients and their families need education on good handwashing techniques to reduce the risk of the patient receiving an infection from others. A neutropenic diet that restricts eating fresh fruits and vegetables should be followed. These foods should be properly washed, peeled, and/or cooked. The patient's temperature should be monitored closely for temperature elevations (Shelton, 2013).

Inability to cope with their diagnosis and treatment can be an issue for many patients diagnosed with leukemia. The patient may express an intense fear or anxiety. Evaluating anxiety and supporting coping mechanisms can help manage a patient's fear and anxiety. Nurses should encourage patients to use stress management techniques such as deep breathing exercises and guided imagery. If needed, a nurse should refer the patient to social work for further assistance (Bush, 2013).

Patients may also develop malnutrition and volume depletion from chemotherapy. This loss may be due to nausea, vomiting, anorexia, and/or fever. Maintaining adequate fluid volume should be managed by monitoring urine input and output. Daily weights should be obtained. Patients should be encouraged to eat and drink to reduce anorexia. Monitor blood pressure (BP) and heart rate (HR) frequently; a change may reflect hypovolemia (Held-Warmkessel, 2013).

OUTCOMES

The expected outcomes for patients undergoing treatment for leukemia are to prevent/reduce the risk of infection and promote a safe environment. Patients need to be educated on preventing dehydration and maintaining adequate fluid volume. Patients should appear relaxed and be able to rest/sleep (Shelton, 2013).

Summary

Leukemia is a blood cancer that is treated by chemotherapy. Whether the leukemia is acute or chronic, nurses need to be aware of the risk factors and potential side effects of chemotherapeutic agents. Identifying infection and deficit volume in a timely manner is important. Proper education regarding treatment, side effects, and potential risks is needed for all patients and their families.

Bush, N. J. (2013). Psychosocial management. In B. H. Gobel, S. Triest-Robertson, & W. H. Vogel (Eds.), *Advanced oncology nursing certification* (pp. 637–631). Pittsburgh, PA: Oncology Nursing Society.

Dighiero, G., & Hamblin, T. J. (2008). Chronic lymphocytic leukaemia. *Lancet, 371*(9617), 1017–1029.

Ezzone, S. A. (2013). Blood and marrow stem cell transplantation. In B. H. Gobel, S. Triest-Robertson, & W. H. Vogel (Eds.), *Advanced oncology nursing certification* (pp. 261–262). Pittsburgh, PA: Oncology Nursing Society.

Gaynor, J., Chapman, D., Little, C., McKenzie, S., Miller, W., Andreeff, M., . . . Gee, T. (1988). A cause-specific hazard rate analysis of prognostic factors among 199 adults with acute lymphoblastic leukemia: The Memorial Hospital experience since 1969. *Journal of Clinical Oncology, 6*(6), 1014–1030.

Goldman, J. M., & Melo, J. V. (2003). Chronic myeloid leukemia—Advances in biology and new approaches to treatment. *New England Journal of Medicine, 349*(15), 1451–1464.

Held-Warmkessel, J. (2013). Cardiac, gastrointestinal, neurologic, and ocular toxicities. In B. H. Gobel, S. Triest-Robertson, & W. H. Vogel (Eds.), *Advanced oncology nursing certification* (pp. 261–262). Pittsburgh, PA: Oncology Nursing Society.

Hoelzer, D., Thiel, E., Löffler, H., Büchner, T., Ganser, A., Heil, G., . . . Rühl, H. (1988). Prognostic factors in a multicenter study for treatment of acute lymphoblastic leukemia in adults. *Blood, 71*(1), 123–131.

National Cancer Institute. (2017). Leukemia. Retrieved from http://www.cancer.gov/types/leukemia

National Cancer Institute Surveillance, Epidemiology, and End Results Program. (2017). Cancer stat facts: Leukemia. Retrieved from http://seer.cancer.gov/statfacts/html/leuks.html

Shelton, B. (2013). Myelosuppression. In B. H. Gobel, S. Triest-Robertson, & W. H. Vogel (Eds.), *Advanced oncology nursing certification* (pp. 261–262). Pittsburgh, PA: Oncology Nursing Society.

■ LIVER CANCER

Shannon A. Rives

Overview

Liver cancer is one of the leading cancers worldwide (Singal & El-Serag, 2015). Liver cancer can be primary or a result of metastasis. A primary tumor originates in the liver. Hepatocellular carcinoma (HCC) is the most common primary tumor and is often the consequence of underlying liver disease (Ryerson et al., 2016). Cholangiocarcinoma is cancer of the bile ducts and may occur in the intrahepatic biliary ducts. A secondary tumor is caused by metastasized tumor cells to the liver from other organs. The liver is a common site for metastases from breast, colon, bladder, kidney, ovarian, pancreatic, and lung cancer. Liver cancer is often found parenthetically because liver-specific symptoms may be absent or overlapping with chronic liver disease. Screening algorithms can be useful for early recognition; treatment options are selected by weighing risks and benefits. Nursing care is influenced by the treatment regimen, but overall education and support for patients and their families is needed throughout the process.

Background

Liver cancer is more common in sub-Saharan Africa and Southeast Asia than in the United States (American Cancer Society [ACS], 2016). Each year, liver cancer affects approximately 31,000 Americans (22,000 men and 9,000 women) and the incidence rate of liver cancer in the United States continues to rise (U.S. Cancer Statistics Working Group, 2017). Worldwide estimates of newly diagnosed events of hepatocellular carcinoma (HCC) exceeded 750,000 cases (Schütte, Balbisi, & Malfertheiner, 2016). Chronic liver disease has affected the incidence rates of HCC in the United States, which have continually increased in recent decades (Singal & El-Serag, 2015; Mittal et al., 2016). Chronic hepatitis B and C (HBV/HCV) infections are prominent risk factors for developing HCC; infection rates in the United States range from 850,000 to 2.2 million and 2.7 million to 3.5 million, respectively (Ryerson et al., 2016). Other risk factors include nonalcoholic steatohepatitis (NASH), type 2 diabetes mellitus, obesity, tobacco use, excessive alcohol use, exposure to aflatoxins (produced by fungi found on crops such as corn and peanuts), male gender, Asian descent, and genetic disorders (hemochromatosis; Ryerson et al., 2016; Schütte, Balbisi, & Malfertheiner, 2016; Schütte, Schulz, & Malfertheiner, 2016).

Five-year survival rates vary based on the stage and type of liver cancer. For persons with localized cancer, the 5-year survival rate is approximately 31%, compared to stage 4 cancer with metastases, for which the 5-year rate is approximately 3% (ACS, 2016). Currently, the average 5-year survival rate is around 15% (Mittal et al., 2016). Early detection is the cornerstone of an optimal treatment plan, but, unfortunately, HCC is not easily detected through objective and subjective data collection. For high-risk patients, screening usually includes an abdominal ultrasound and determination of an alpha-fetoprotein level (AFP; Singal & El-Serag, 2015). A diagnosis can be established based on a combination of factors, including the presence or absence of underlying liver disease, characteristics of the tumor, increased serum markers (AFP greater than 500 ng/mL), CT scan or MRI results, and/or histological findings from biopsy (Pagana & Pagana, 2014; Singal & El-Serag, 2015).

Treatments for liver cancer include surgical intervention (partial hepatectomy or liver transplant), tumor ablation, embolization, targeted therapies, chemotherapy, and radiation. Transarterial chemoembolization (TACE) involves placement of a catheter in the hepatic artery to deliver chemotherapy and embolization agents directly to the tumor. The procedure is performed in interventional radiology and utilizes fluoroscopy and contrast media. Tumor characteristics, such as size, location, grade, and staging and the individual patient condition, are dynamics that impact the course of treatment.

Most cases of HCC are seen in patients with cirrhotic livers (Schütte, Schulz, & Malfertheiner, 2016). In chronic liver disease, the hepatocytes are injured from exposure to harmful agents (excessive fat, alcohol, excessive iron, or viral infection). Hepatocyte destruction activates vitamin A-storing hepatic stellate cells, situated in the space between the capillaries and liver cells, which yield collagen proteins and other elements that assist in creating a fibrin mesh (Benyon & Iredale, 2000). The fibrin mesh is similar to scar tissue that develops in the wound-healing process and lies between the hepatocytes and capillaries that supply oxygenated blood from the hepatic artery and nutrient-rich blood from the portal vein. The liver is a regenerative organ and will attempt to repair itself; if the offending agent is removed, there is potential for the scar tissue to be broken down and the fibrosis may resolve to some degree.

In patients with cirrhosis, continuous injury and inflammation lead to the development of a thick and tough fibrin mesh. Over time, the fibrin mesh will disrupt the normal architecture of the liver, producing nodular structures (this gives the liver a bumpy surface). Even in this altered state, the liver will still attempt to repair itself by producing more hepatocytes, but these new cells may have mutations.

Clinical Aspects

ASSESSMENT

Although signs and symptoms of liver cancer may be ambiguous or absent, accurate collection of objective and subjective data is still an essential part of patient care. As the tumor increases in size, the patient may report a feeling of fullness after eating or pain in the right side of the abdomen. An increase in the symptoms associated with the patient's underlying liver disease may be the first sign of liver cancer. A thorough patient history is important to identify potential risk factors for liver disease such as exposure to viruses, alcohol consumption, intravenous drug use, components of the metabolic syndrome, and genetic disorders. If the patient has an established diagnosis of cirrhosis, it is important to determine the cause and stage, as well as the presence of symptoms. Transition from compensated cirrhosis to decompensated cirrhosis can be hastened by the presence of a tumor. The patient should be assessed for any personal or family history of cancer, nutritional status, changes in appetite, unintentional weight loss, presence of abdominal pain, changes in bowel activity, and any respiratory symptoms. Objectively, a focused physical assessment should include inspecting for signs of liver disease, abdominal distention and other physical abnormalities of the abdomen, auscultating bowel sounds, and palpating and percussing for hepatomegaly and masses.

In the tertiary setting, the patient's treatment regimen will impact the nurse's daily focus. For example, postprocedural assessment of lower extremity pulses is relevant for a patient following chemoembolization. Following surgical resection, patients should have pain levels and respiratory status monitored, while evaluating for organ rejection is pertinent for transplant recipients. In general, monitoring for signs and symptoms of respiratory problems, infection, hypoglycemia, bleeding, weight gain, fluid and electrolyte imbalances, and cognitive changes is ongoing. Laboratory results can also offer some clues into the patient's condition. Trending liver enzymes, bilirubin, prothrombin time, and albumin levels all assess liver function. A compromised liver can cause a decrease in renal function so blood urea nitrogen (BUN) and creatinine levels are followed.

NURSING INTERVENTIONS, MANAGEMENT, AND IMPLICATIONS

Nursing has the opportunity to utilize primary and secondary prevention strategies to decrease the risk of liver disease and liver cancer whether in the community, ambulatory office, or acute care setting. Health-promotion strategies should include teaching the patient how to avoid HBV, including sex safe practices, stressing the avoidance of needle sharing, promoting HBV vaccination for at-risk populations, and adhering to safety measures that prevent transmission in the hospital. Current recommendations suggest persons born between 1945 and 1965 should be tested for HCV (Ryerson et al., 2016). For the patient who tests positive, treatment with antivirals should be discussed. High-risk patients should also be encouraged to keep any follow-up appointments with the medical team.

OUTCOMES

Decreasing a patient's risk factors for developing HCC should be an expected outcome. The HBV vaccine can offer a defense from the virus and can reduce the rate of HCC cases (Schütte, Balbisi, & Malfertheiner, 2016). Currently, there is no vaccine for HCV; however, achieving sustained virological response using HCV antiviral medication therapy lessens the risk of HCC (Schütte, Balbisi, & Malfertheiner, 2016). An increase in testing for HCV will identify infected people and treatment can be offered.

Summary

Liver cancer is a cause of cancer deaths worldwide. A diagnosis of liver cancer drastically decreases life expectancy and can be devastating to a patient and the family. Nursing plays a vital role in caring for patients with liver cancer by providing education and psychosocial support. Identifying patients at risk, particularly persons with a history of chronic liver disease, is the first step in early recognition and treatment of liver cancer. Prevention and surveillance through education and testing are interventions that can be integrated across the continuum of care.

American Cancer Society. (2016). Liver cancer survival rates. Retrieved from https://www.cancer.org/cancer/liver-cancer/detection-diagnosis-staging/survival-rates.html

Benyon, R. C., & Iredale, J. P. (2000). Is liver fibrosis reversible? *Gut, 46*(4), 443–446.

Mittal, S., Kanwal, F., Ying, J., Chung, R., Sada, Y. H., Temple, S., . . . El-Serag, H. B. (2016). Effectiveness of surveillance for hepatocellular carcinoma in clinical practice: A United States cohort. *Journal of Hepatology, 65*(6), 1148–1154.

Pagana, K. D., & Pagana, T. J. (2014). *Mosby's manual of diagnostics and laboratory tests* (5th ed.). St. Louis, MO: Elsevier Mosby.

Ryerson, A. B., Eheman, C. R., Altekruse, S. F., Ward, J. W., Jemal, A., Sherman, R. L., . . . Kohler, B. A. (2016). Annual report to the nation on the status of cancer, 1975–2012, featuring the increasing incidence of liver cancer. *Cancer, 122*(9), 1312–1337.

Schütte, K., Balbisi, F., & Malfertheiner, P. (2016). Prevention of hepatocellular carcinoma. *Gastrointestinal Tumors, 3*(1), 37–43.

Schütte, K., Schulz, C., & Malfertheiner, P. (2016). Nutrition and hepatocellular cancer. *Gastrointestinal Tumors, 4*(2), 188–194. doi:10.1159/000441822

Singal, A. G., & El-Serag, H. B. (2015). Hepatocellular carcinoma from epidemiology to prevention: Translating knowledge into practice. *Clinical Gastroenterology and Hepatology, 13*(12), 2140–2151.

U.S. Cancer Statistics Working Group. (2017). *United States cancer statistics: 1999–2014 incidence and mortality web-based report*. Atlanta, GA: Department of Health and Human Services, Centers for Disease Control and Prevention, and National Cancer Institute. Retrieved from http://www.cdc.gov/uscs

■ LUNG CANCER

Helen Foley

Overview

Lung cancer is the leading cause of cancer death in the United States for both men and women (Seigel, Miller, & Jemal, 2016). If detected in its early stages, lung cancer can be cured surgically. Yet, lung cancer is commonly diagnosed only after it has spread to other sites within the lung or body. Lung cancer has been widely associated with cigarette smoking, although other risk factors, such as exposure to radon, various occupational chemical exposures, and secondhand smoke, play a role, which has resulted in stigma and the misconception that all lung cancer patients have a history of smoking. In fact, lung cancer is a disease of advanced age. The median age of a lung cancer patient at diagnosis has been estimated at 71 years, and two thirds of all patients diagnosed are between the ages of 65 and 84 years (National Cancer Institute Surveillance, Epidemiology, and End Result Program [NCI SEER], 2016).

Nursing care of the patient with lung cancer focuses on support of the patient through diagnosis and treatment. This includes symptom management for symptoms arising from the disease itself or the treatment. Nurses play important roles in primary and secondary prevention, treatment, and symptom management. Nurses are also instrumental in addressing quality-of-life issues, coordinating the care delivery team, and preparing patients and families for end of life. Nurses are the primary caregivers at end of life and are an important part of every hospice care team.

Background

According to the American Cancer Society, lung cancer is the most prevalent cancer in men, after prostate cancer, and the second most prevalent cancer in women (ACS, 2016a). Histology or cell type is important for both prognosis and treatment. Lung cancers are divided into two main groups, non-small cell lung cancer (NSCLC) and small cell lung cancer (SCLC). Mesothelioma is often grouped with lung cancer, but it is actually a malignancy of the pleura, or lining of the lungs, associated with asbestos exposure, and will not be discussed here.

NSCLC, primarily adenocarcinoma cell type, accounts for more than 80% of all lung cancers, and almost 100% of lung cancer found in nonsmokers (Sherry, 2017). Staging matters for both survival and treatment. Early-stage lung cancers are amenable to surgery or surgery and radiation (stages 1 and 2) and carry a 5-year survival rate of 49% for stage 1 and 30% for stage 2. Stage 3 cancers may be treated with a combination of chemotherapy and radiation and have a 5-year survival rate of 14% or less. Stage 4 lung cancer, which has spread to other organs or the opposite lung at the time of diagnosis, also treated with chemotherapy and radiation, has a 5-year survival rate of 1% (ACS, 2016b).

New treatments, such as immune therapy and targeted therapies for NSCLC, are offering increasing survival for some patients. Immune therapies utilize immune checkpoint inhibitor antibodies to help harness the body's own immune system to fight the cancer (Knoop, 2016). Although less toxic overall, they have their own set of side effects resulting from the activation of the body's immune system, and currently are very expensive. Scientists are still determining which patients are most likely to benefit from these treatments. Like chemotherapy, they require intravenous infusion in a specialized treatment center. Targeted therapies are directed at particular biomarkers in the cancer and include agents such as epidermal growth factor receptor (EGFR) mutations and anaplastic lymphoma kinase (ALK) gene fusions. Targeted therapies are generally oral agents reserved for the small percentage of patients who have a particular mutation in their cancer (Knoop, 2016) and require genetic testing of the tumor. These mutations are more often found in female nonsmokers (Sherry, 2017).

SCLC makes up less than 20% of all lung cancers, but is considered a rapidly growing cancer, and is almost always associated with a smoking history. Seventy-five percent of patients with SCLC are diagnosed with extensive, late-stage disease (Knoop, 2016). Treatment of limited-stage and extensive-stage SCLC is generally chemotherapy with and without radiation therapy. Prophylactic cranial radiation is almost always recommended due to the high frequency of metastasis to the brain. Median survival for limited-stage SCLC is 14 to 20 months; median survival for extensive-stage SCLC is 9 to 11 months, but can be as short as a few weeks (Knoop, 2016).

Clinical Aspects

ASSESSMENT

Nurses in every setting have a role in secondary prevention by identifying patients who are current smokers. Nurses should assess the patient's readiness to quit, provide motivation, and help the patient find appropriate resources for smoking-cessation strategies. The American Lung Association and National Comprehensive Cancer Network (NCCN) have excellent resources and guidelines to help patients stop smoking (American Lung Association, 2016; NCCN, 2017). Nurses also have a role in identifying patients who meet the current lung cancer screening criteria established by the U.S. Preventive Services Task Force and supported by the American Cancer Society and the NCCN network. Screening criteria are adults aged 55 to 80 years with a 30-pack-year smoking history, current smokers, or those who have quit in the last 15 years. The current recommendation is annual screening using low-dose CT scan of the chest (U.S. Preventive Services Task Force, 2016).

Nurses play a key role in educating patients about various aspects of treatment and assessing their tolerance of the treatment. Early identification and treatment of side effects will contribute to increased quality of life. Neutropenia, esophagitis, swallowing issues, taste alterations, hair loss, and skin erythema and breakdown are especially common in patients receiving concurrent chemotherapy and radiation.

OUTCOMES

Nurses also provide symptomatic treatment and palliative care for patients with lung cancer. These symptoms, including pain, cough, dyspnea, fatigue, and poor appetite, affect quality of life for the patient and cause distress for family members. Accurate assessment, appropriate referrals, and supportive counseling by the nurse can improve the quality of life for the patient and family. A lung cancer diagnosis is a crisis for both the patient and family members. Lung cancer patients are likely to experience physical, spiritual, psychological, and social distress. Appropriate identification of disturbance in one or more of these quality-of-life domains and timely intervention or referral by the nurse can lead to improved patient outcomes. The importance of palliative care in lung cancer patients should not be underestimated. A study of lung cancer patients showed that when lung cancer patients had palliative care service provided in conjunction with standard cancer care, they had higher satisfaction with their care and lived an average of almost 3 months longer than those who received standard care alone (Temel et al., 2010).

Nurses play a vital role in helping patients with advanced care planning and identifying their goals for care and end-of-life preferences. Nurses are often relied on to communicate these issues to the health care team, and serve as advocates for patients and families. This requires the nurse to have good communication skills and comfort in addressing sensitive issues. Oncology nurses benefit from end-of-life training through such programs as those offered by the American Association of Colleges of Nursing's End-of-Life Nursing Education Consortium (ELNEC).

Summary

Lung cancer is a devastating diagnosis for patients and their families. Eighty percent of patients diagnosed with lung cancer will die from their disease (NCI SEER, 2016). Lung cancer is associated with significant symptom and treatment burdens that have long-standing impact on the patient's quality of life. The development of new treatments in the last few years offers hope for patients for prolonged survival and some even have a better side-effect profile than chemotherapy and radiation.

Patients benefit from good nursing care along the disease continuum, from diagnosis to death. Nurses play a vital role in assessing and managing bothersome side effects, educating patients, monitoring treatment and treatment-related problems, and coordinating the care team. Lung cancer patients benefit when nurses are able to comfortably and openly discuss goals of care and end-of-life issues with patients and their families.

American Cancer Society. (2016a). Facts and figures. Retrieved from https://www .cancer.org/cancer/non-small-cell-lung-cancer/detection-diagnosis-staging/survival -rates.html

American Cancer Society. (2016b). Non-small cell lung cancer survival rates by stage. Retrieved from http://www.cancer.org/cancer/non-smallcelllungcancer/detection diagnosis-staging/survival-rates.html

American Lung Association. (2016). Stop smoking. Retrieved from http://www.lung.org/stop-smoking

Knoop, T. (2016). Lung cancer. In C. H. Yarbro, D. Wujcik, & B. H. Holmes (Eds.), *Cancer nursing: Principles and practice* (8th ed., pp. 1679–1720). Burlington, MA: Jones & Bartlett.

National Cancer Institute Surveillance, Epidemiology, and End Result Program. (2016). Cancer of the lung and bronchus cancer stat facts. Retrieved from http://seer.cancer.gov/statfacts/html/lungb.html

National Comprehensive Cancer Network. (2017). Clinical practice guidelines in oncology. Smoking cessation. Version 1.2017. Retrieved from http://www.nccn.org/professionals/physician_gls/pdf/smoking.pdf

Sherry, V. (2017). Lung cancer: Not just a smoker's disease. *American Nurse Today, 12*(2), 16–21.

Siegel, R. L., Miller, K. D., & Jemal, A. (2016). Cancer statistics, 2016. *CA: A Cancer Journal for Clinicians, 66*(1), 7–30.

Temel, J. S., Grier, J. A., Muzicansky, A., Gallagher, E. R., Admane, S., Jackson, V. A., . . . Lynch, T. J. (2010). Early palliative care for patients with metastatic non-small cell lung cancer. *New England Journal of Medicine, 363*(8), 733–742.

U.S. Preventive Services Task Force. (2016). Final update summary: Lung cancer screening. Retrieved from http://www/uspreventativeservicestaskforce.org/Page/Document/Update Summary Final/Lung-cancer-screening

■ LYMPHOMA

Marisa A. Cortese
Jane F. Marek

Overview

Lymphoma is a cancer of the lymphatic system and can appear anywhere in the body. The primary purpose of the lymphatic system is to fight infection. Both B- and T-lymphocytes play a key role in fighting infection by regulation of the immune system and production of cytokines and antibodies. B-lymphocytes are produced in the bone marrow and T-lymphocytes are produced by the thymus gland. Lymphomas are divided into two types: Hodgkin's lymphoma (HL) and non-Hodgkin's lymphoma (NHL), named after the British pathologist Thomas Hodgkin who described the disease in 1832. Both of these lymphomas can occur in children and adults.

There were approximately 81,080 new cases of lymphoma diagnosed in the United States in 2016 (National Cancer Institute [NCI], 2017a). The 5-year survivor rate for HL is approximately 85%, for NHL 69%; the 10-year survival rate decreases for both lymphomas (80% and 58%, respectively; Rummel, 2015). HL is generally considered a curable disease, but treatments may cause profound adverse effects for the patient.

Background

Genetic and environmental factors contribute to the development of lymphomas. Environmental influences include exposure to pesticides, benzenes, or radiation; occupations at increased risk include farmers, chemists, and persons employed in the rubber, petroleum, plastics, and synthetic industries (Rummel, 2015). Both lymphomas are more common in Caucasians than in any other racial group. Persons who have received an organ transplant or are being treated with immunosuppressive drugs are at increased risk for developing the disease.

HLs are caused by alterations in lymphocytes resulting in large, abnormal lymphocytes in the lymph nodes called *Reed–Sternberg cells*; most HLs are derived from B-lymphocytes. Most persons with HL are diagnosed between the ages of 15 and 35 years or over 65 years. Risk factors for developing HL include male gender, history of infection with Epstein–Barr or HIV, or having a first-degree relative with HL. The common signs and symptoms of HL are lymphadenopathy, hepatomegaly or splenomegaly, unexplained fever, night sweats, unintentional weight loss, pruritus, and fatigue (Rummel, 2015). Patients often experience pain in the enlarged lymph nodes after alcohol intake.

NHL refers to a group of lymphatic cancers derived from B-lymphocytes, T-lymphocytes, or natural killer cells; the majority of NHL originates from B-cells.

NHL can be indolent or aggressive. Indolent lymphoma tends to spread slowly and has few signs and symptoms. Aggressive lymphoma spreads quickly, and the patient may have many signs and symptoms, some of which can be severe. Most lymphomas are diagnosed in persons aged 65 to 74 years. Additional risk factors include a history of any of the following: organ transplant; previous cancer treatment; inherited immune disorder; autoimmune disease; or infection with HIV/AIDS, human T-lymphotropic virus type I, Epstein–Barr virus, or *Helicobacter pylori*.

The most common sign of NHL is lymphadenopathy anywhere in the body. Other clinical manifestations include hepatomegaly or splenomegaly, unexplained fever, fatigue, unintentional weight loss, decreased appetite, and skin rash or pruritus (Shankland, Armitage, & Hancock, 2012). Patients with lymphomas may also present with symptoms specific to the tumor location, for example, a chest lesion may cause respiratory problems or chest pain.

Patients diagnosed with lymphoma require a complete medical workup. A thorough history and physical examination and laboratory tests, including complete blood count with differential and chemistry panel, should be performed. Other causes of lymphadenopathy and symptoms of lymphoma must be ruled out. A lymph node biopsy is necessary for diagnosis; bone marrow aspiration and biopsy may be performed to check for metastasis. Following biopsy, staging is done to determine the extent of the disease and to guide treatment. A PET or CT scan can be useful in determining the extent of disease.

A patient's prognosis is dependent on age, comorbidities, staging, and the presence or absence of specific chromosomal abnormalities found in the blood and/or bone marrow (Rummel, 2015). The prognosis is also dependent upon the presence of systemic symptoms, or B-symptoms. B-symptoms include fever more than 38°C for 3 consecutive days, unintentional weight loss of more than 10% body weight in 6 months, and drenching night sweats (Carbone, Kaplan, Musshoff, Smithers, & Tubiana, 1971).

The standard treatment is chemotherapy, immunotherapy, or radiation therapy, alone or in combination. Patients with indolent NHL may be followed and monitored closely, rather than undergo treatment. Patients with relapsed/refractory disease may undergo a hematopoietic stem cell transplant (NCI, 2017b).

Clinical Aspects

ASSESSMENT

The nurse should assess the patient for risk factors and specific symptoms associated with lymphoma, including a history of viral illness or cancer treatments; fever; night sweats; chills; bleeding or bruising; and abdominal pain or frequent infections. A thorough medication history should be elicited, paying particular attention to immunosuppressant use, which may increase the risk of lymphoma. On physical examination, a patient may appear pale and feverish, and have enlarged lymph nodes in the neck, armpit, or groin or present with a rash (Rummel, 2015).

Patients with a large tumor burden and certain types of high-grade NHL are at increased risk for tumor lysis syndrome (TLS). TLS occurs as a result of cancer treatments, which cause rapid destruction of neoplastic cells resulting in hyperkalemia, hypocalcemia, hyperphosphatemia, and hyperuricemia. TLS can occur with the administration of chemotherapy, radiation therapy, biotherapy, glucocorticoids, or general anesthesia. This is a potentially life-threatening condition that can cause metabolic disturbances such as acute kidney injury, seizures, cardiac arrhythmias, metabolic acidosis, or death (Cope, 2013). An elevated lactate dehydrogenase, renal insufficiency, or dehydration before therapy can indicate an increased risk for developing TLS (Ikeda, Jaishankar, & Krishnan, 2016).

Prevention of infection is a nursing priority; patients with lymphoma are at increased risk for infection due to the disease process and also as an adverse effect of treatment. Interventions should focus on preventing infection, preventing injury, decreasing fatigue, and promoting optimal nutrition. The patient and family should be included in the teaching, so they can continue preventive strategies at home.

The nurse/patient navigator is an important resource to support and guide patients and their families across the cancer continuum (Rummel, 2015). The nurse navigator functions as part of a multidisciplinary team to assist patients in dealing with the financial, communication, treatment, psychosocial, and logistical barriers faced when dealing with cancer. They play a key role in patient education and support patients after treatment as they transition to survivorship (Rummel, 2015). The role of the nurse navigator is supported by the Academy of Oncology Nurse & Patient Navigators and the American College of Surgeons Commission on Cancer (Rummel, 2015).

The goal of treatment is to achieve a cure and maintain the patient's quality of life. The desired outcomes for patients undergoing treatment for lymphoma are to prevent/reduce the risk of infection and complications. Patients must be carefully monitored during and after care treatment for adverse effects and realize the importance of follow-up care.

Summary

The prognosis for patients with lymphoma varies depending on the individual patient, type of lymphoma, and stage of disease. Advances in treatment have led to increased survivorship for patients with both NHL and HL. Nurses working in any setting may encounter patients with lymphoma along any stage of the cancer continuum. Knowledge of the risk factors, disease process, and treatment modalities can enable nurses to provide quality and evidence-based care to these patients.

Carbone, P. P., Kaplan, H. S., Musshoff, K., Smithers, D. W., & Tubiana, M. (1971). Report of the Committee on Hodgkin's Disease Staging Classification. *Cancer Research, 31*(11), 1860–1861.

Cope, D. G. (2013). Metabolic emergencies. In B. H. Gobel, S. Triest-Robertson, & W. H. Vogel (Eds.), *Advanced oncology nursing certification* (pp. 568–574). Pittsburgh, PA: Oncology Nursing Society.

Ikeda, A. K., Jaishankar, D., & Krishnan, K. (2016). Tumor lysis syndrome. *Medscape.* Retrieved from http://emedicine.medscape.com/article/282171-overview#a5

National Cancer Institute. (2017a). Cancer stat facts: Lymphoma. Retrieved from http:// seer.cancer.gov/statfacts/html/nhl.html

National Cancer Institute. (2017b). Lymphoma. Retrieved from http://www.cancer.gov/ types/lymphoma

Rummel, M. (2015). Non-Hodgkin lymphoma and Hodgkin lymphoma: The role of the nurse navigator in improving patient outcomes. *Journal of Oncology Navigation & Survivorship, 6*(3), 3–10.

Shankland, K. R., Armitage, J. O., & Hancock, B. W. (2012). Non-Hodgkin lymphoma. *Lancet, 380*(9844), 848–857.

■ MULTIPLE SCLEROSIS

Alaa Mahsoon

Overview

According to the National Multiple Sclerosis Society (2016), multiple sclerosis (MS) is a chronic condition that damages the myelin sheath (demyelination) that surrounds nerve fibers in the brain, spinal cord, and optic nerves. Demyelination causes impaired nerve conduction that creates neurological problems. According to Alroughani, Akhtar, Ahmed, Behbehani, and Al-Hashel (2016), MS is an immune-mediated disease because the immune cells in the central nerves system (CNS) are attacked by an unknown antigen. Clinical pictures of patients with MS differ from person to person. However, early symptoms might involve numbness, tingling, or weakness in the extremities; visual changes; impaired balance; and urinary frequency and urgency. Besides physical deterioration of the disease, MS can be psychologically destructive for patients and their families. Therefore, nursing care is crucial for patients' physical and psychological stability and well-being.

Background

According to the National Multiple Sclerosis Society (2016), MS prevalence among the U.S. population is not well studied because health care providers are not required to report cases of MS; because of its invisible symptoms individuals have MS and do not know it. However, there are 2.3 million reported cases worldwide. MS is more prevalent in women and Whites. The rate of MS is also high among individuals between the ages of 40 and 59 years as well as non-Hispanics in the United States. The Centers for Disease Control and Prevention indicate that in the United States the rate varies from 58 to 95 cases per 100,000 population (Dobson et al., 2016). However, the prevalence rate varies among regions and ages worldwide. Variation in ultraviolet (UV) radiation exposure among regions accounts for the geographic difference between MS prevalence estimates. Disparately, adults between the ages of 40 and 59 years have higher chances of contracting the disease compared to children.

Social, environmental, and biological factors contribute to the development of MS. MS is regarded as a significant cause of disability in young people. The etiology of the disease is unknown. Genetic factors increase an individual's risk by 2% to 4% and are present in 30% of individuals without MS. Thus, relatives of patients with MS have an increased chance of getting the disease due to their genetic predisposition (Moccia et al., 2016). Environmental factors, such as radiation exposure, are also likely to influence disease susceptibility. Despite the lack of data demonstrating a link between exposure to bacteria and development of MS, an association is known to exist (Moccia et al., 2016).

Social determinants are also linked with race; MS is more prevalent in Whites with higher socioeconomic status than in Hispanics and other ethnic groups. Research further indicates that the prevalence and incidence of MS increases with age (Jelinek et al., 2016). The rise in the prevalence rate is influenced by prolonged survival of patients with MS, whereas the incidence rate is affected by the risk factors identified. MS is often regarded as a highly variable illness and poses a fundamental challenge to health care providers. More than 50% of people who have MS experience clinical symptoms such as brain lesions.

Clinical Aspects

The etiology of MS is not clear; however, clinical manifestations often link complex interactions between the immune system and environmental and genetic factors. The associated negative impact affects patients' disability over time, primarily when the onset of treatment is late or when clinicians are not familiar with the immunopathogenesis, natural course, and symptoms of the disease. MS also reduces the quality of life, causing premature disability and an increased mortality rate (Dilokthornsakul et al., 2016).

Nursing process or care, as well as quality-improvement processes, has a significant role in reducing the adverse effects of the clinical condition in context. MS creates the need for increased efficacy and safety of the treatment methods provided. Nurses have a critical role in facilitating the start and management of the treatment options in MS. However, the nurse's role has evolved over the years as they are now required to establish collaborative partnerships with patients and other health care providers. Nurses also have a vital role in helping the patients understand the available treatment options as well as understanding their diseases. They also help encourage the patient's adherence and management of treatment to promote positive outcomes (Riemann-Lorenz et al., 2016).

MS nurses have also expanded their role and training or set of skills due to increased changes in the treatment paradigm. MS also requires a broad range of clinical options, dosing schedules, and addressing the risk factors, which has created the need for nurses and other health care providers to enhance their professional training and development. Nursing care and process improvement should be based on a patient-centered approach that addresses the patient needs to improve positive outcomes. The process of care provided can include different steps such as assessment stage, problem identification, nursing intervention, and outcomes evaluation.

ASSESSMENT

The assessment phase includes a stage during which nurses will be involved in identifying the relevant history of the patients because genetic factors are key risk factors in MS. Patient history presents a chance to understand the association between risk of MS and genetics. This information helps to shape the intervention methods adopted. The patient's physical condition is evaluated so as to provide diagnostic data to the nursing care and process improvement teams to promote positive outcomes (Jelinek et al., 2016).

NURSING INTERVENTIONS, MANAGEMENT, AND IMPLICATIONS

The nursing-related problems that are responsive to nursing interventions or process change may include communication problems and teamwork issues. As such, the care model that should be adopted for MS patients includes a collaborative approach to care that involves both the patients and other care providers to promote positive outcomes. The approaches are also responsive to process change because they are influenced by patient needs and available interventions.

MS has no cure; however, care providers can use their positions to reduce the adverse effects or patient suffering by providing nursing interventions that address identified needs. The most appropriate nursing interventions and management options necessary to address MS include the provision of patient-centered care and a collaborative approach to care. The methods offer a chance to include both the care providers and the patients in their care. The methods serve as evidence-based interventions that promote the likelihood of shaping patient outcomes. Nurses can also support the implementation of early treatment of the disease. The evidence-based approaches used provide an opportunity to reduce the associated adverse effects and provide the health care institutions an opportunity to shape patient care (Jelinek et al., 2016).

OUTCOMES

In most cases, the use of a collaborative approach to patient-centered care among other evidence-based practices promotes positive outcomes. However, given the fact that MS is not curable, the available interventions provide a chance to manage the condition, especially when early intervention is provided. Hence, the expected outcomes of the proposed interventions for MS include a reduction in the overall mortality rate, improved quality and safety of care provided, and positive results for patients.

Summary

MS is a critical health condition that often leads to negative outcomes such as patient disability. Research has identified key risk factors of genetic and environmental issues. Although MS does not have a cure, care providers can utilize different interventions to manage the condition based on the disease pathogenesis. The evolution of treatment options has created the need to have an active collaboration between care providers and the patients. Nurses have a fundamental role in helping patients understand the available treatment options as well as their medical condition. They are expected to improve their professional skills to ensure expertise in the ever-changing therapies for MS. Future trends may influence the delivery of nursing care and improve patient outcomes and treatment options or therapies. Therefore, the role of MS nurses will continue to evolve over time; better management can be shaped by involving patients in their care and establishing a collaborative approach among care providers.

Alroughani, R., Akhtar, S., Ahmed, S., Behbehani, R., & Al-Hashel, J. (2016). Is time to reach EDSS 6.0 faster in patients with late-onset versus young-onset multiple sclerosis? *PLOS ONE, 11*(11), e0165846.

Dilokthornsakul, P., Valuck, R. J., Nair, K. V., Corboy, J. R., Allen, R. R., & Campbell, J. D. (2016). Multiple sclerosis prevalence in the United States commercially insured population. *Neurology, 86*(11), 1014–1021.

Dobson, R., Ramagopalan, S., Topping, J., Smith, P., Solanky, B., Schmierer, K., . . . Giovannoni, G. (2016). A risk score for predicting multiple sclerosis. *PLOS ONE, 11*(11), e0164992.

Jelinek, G. A., De Livera, A. M., Marck, C. H., Brown, C. R., Neate, S. L., Taylor, K. L., & Weiland, T. J. (2016). Lifestyle, medication and socio-demographic determinants of mental and physical health-related quality of life in people with multiple sclerosis. *BMC Neurology, 16*(1), 235.

Moccia, M., Palladino, R., Lanzillo, R., Carotenuto, A., Russo, C. V., Triassi, M., & Brescia Morra, V. (2017). Healthcare costs for treating relapsing multiple sclerosis and the risk of progression: A retrospective Italian cohort study from 2001 to 2015. *PloS One, 12*(1), e0169489.

The National Multiple Sclerosis Society. (2016). Multiple sclerosis. Retrieved from http://www.nationalmssociety.org/What-is-MS

Riemann-Lorenz, K., Eilers, M., von Geldern, G., Schulz, K.-H., Köpke, S., & Heesen, C. (2016). Dietary interventions in multiple sclerosis: Development and pilot-testing of an evidence based patient education program. *PLOS ONE, 11*(10), e0165246. doi:10.1371/journal.pone.0165246

■ MYASTHENIA GRAVIS

Jennifer Gonzalez

Overview

Myasthenia gravis (MG) is an acquired autoimmune disease characterized by fluctuating skeletal muscle weakness and fatigability that increases with exercise and improves with rest (Drachman & Amato, 2014). MG can develop into a lifelong chronic neuromuscular disease resulting in periods of exacerbation, remission, and sometimes crises of bulbar, ocular, facial, and respiratory muscles requiring medication adjustment and immunotherapy treatments (Drachman & Amato, 2014). MG occurs in both genders and all ethnic groups, although it is more common in women under the age of 40 years and men older than 60 years (National Institute of Neurological Disorders and Stroke [NINDS], 2010). Nursing care of adults with MG should focus on symptom identification, psychosocial assessment, patient education on medication regimens, and airway management during MG crises.

Background

MG is the most common disorder involving the neuromuscular junction (NMJ). There are approximately 36,000 to 60,000 cases of MG in the United States with a prevalence of 14 to 20 cases per 100,000 people (Howard, 2015); MG affects more than 700,000 people worldwide (Sanders et al., 2016). Over time, the ability to understand functions of the NMJ, autoimmunity, and role of the thymus gland has been attributed to an increase in survival rates and overall life span of patients with MG (NINDS, 2010). An international task force convened by the Myasthenia Gravis Foundation of America created a consensus guide for treatment goals, minimal manifestations, remission, crises, and additional statements to guide clinicians in the management of MG (Sanders et al., 2016).

In many cases of MG, muscle weakness and fatigability occur from a decrease or lack of acetylcholine receptors (ACh-Rs) available at the NMJ during normal muscle contraction (Drachman & Amato, 2014). ACh, released by neurons at the NMJs, produces action potentials that stimulate contraction of skeletal muscles by depolarizing the muscle membrane (Drachman & Amato, 2014). In some forms of MG, ACh-R antibodies are released as an immune response causing rapid turnover of ACh-Rs, blockage of ACh-R sites, and impairment to the post-synaptic muscle membrane where depolarization occurs (Drachman & Amato, 2014). Symptoms generally become apparent when the number of ACh-Rs is approximately 30% of normal.

The thymus gland is responsible for immune development in childhood and is believed to play a role in the immune response in certain subtypes of MG (NINDS, 2010). Conditions of the thymus, such as hyperplasia or thymomas, may be an indication for thymectomy, resulting in realignment of the immune system and the potential for symptom reduction or cure (NINDS, 2010). Early-onset MG is characterized by positive ACh-R antibodies, thymic hyperplasia, and onset of symptoms younger than 40 years (Livesay, 2012). Persons with late-onset MG are typically diagnosed after age 40 years; have a normal thymus gland; and have positive antibodies for ACh, titin, and ryanodine receptors (Livesay, 2012). Most persons with MG have anti-ACh-R antibodies. Patients without anti-ACh-R antibodies are classified as having seronegative myasthenia gravis (SNMG). Many patients with SNMG have antibodies against muscle-specific tyrosine kinase (MUSK). The MUSK receptors are another component in the NMJ needed for successful neurotransmission for muscle contraction. Patients with this subtype of MG are usually female, diagnosed before age 40, and have normal thymus glands (Livesay, 2012).

Clinical Aspects

ASSESSMENT

The Myasthenia Gravis Foundation classified MG into five main types and several subtypes based on severity of symptoms, ranging from Class I with ocular muscle weakness to Class V with respiratory muscle weakness requiring intubation. Clinical manifestations of MG include muscle weakness that fatigues with repetitive movement and improves with rest. Muscle weakness is usually symmetrical with normal sensory function and deep tendon reflexes. As previously discussed, there are different subtypes of MG with varying clinical presentation. There are two clinical forms, referred to as ocular myasthenia gravis (OMG) and generalized myasthenia gravis (GMG). Approximately 85% of patients have OMG and present with fluctuating ocular involvement that does not progress to other muscles (Drachman & Amato, 2014). Other ocular symptoms include ptosis, diplopia, ocular palsy, and nystagmus (Smith, 2016). Within 2 years of OMG diagnosis, 50% of patients will progress to the GMG form with involvement of bulbar, facial, and limb muscles (American Association of Neuroscience Nursing [AANN], 2013). An adult with bulbar dysfunction will have symptoms such as dysphagia, dysphonia, and dysarthria (Smith, 2016). Snarling or expressionless face and flattening of the nasolabial fold are characteristic of facial muscle involvement (AANN, 2013). Persons with extremity involvement display weakness in the neck and upper extremities (AANN, 2013). Respiratory muscle involvement can cause dyspnea, hypoventilation, and respiratory failure requiring intubation and mechanical ventilation.

Diagnosis of MG is based on the patient's history and physical examination and bedside and serologic testing. Bedside testing includes the ice test and edrophonium test, but these tests should not be used as the sole means of diagnosis. The ice test can be useful for patients with ptosis in differentiating MG from other disorders. In the ice test, an ice pack is placed over the patient's eyes for 2 to 5 minutes; the cold should limit anticholinesterase activity, allowing for more availability of ACh. The test is considered positive if the eyelid elevates 2 mm following application of ice (Nair, Patil-Chhablani, Vankatramani, & Gandhi, 2014). The administration of intravenous edrophonium will show a rapid relief of symptoms if the MG type is responsive to acetylcholinesterase (ACh-E; AANN, 2013).

Serum laboratory tests include anti-ACh-R antibodies; 80% of patients with GMG will test positive (Nair et al., 2014). Adults with OMG may have negative anti-ACh-R antibody results but it is thought to be related to low detectable levels and should not be used to confirm the diagnosis (Drachman & Amato, 2014). Other laboratory testing includes antistriated muscle antibody testing, present in the majority of patients younger than 40 years of age with thymoma, and anti-MUSK antibody testing.

Other diagnostics may be indicated based on the patient's symptoms. A new onset of ocular symptoms may require a head CT scan or MRI to rule out brain lesions (Drachman & Amato, 2014). CT and MRI may also be performed to evaluate the thymus gland. Vital capacity is used to measure lung function when respiratory muscles are involved. Muscle strength and EMG (electromyography) should be included in the clinical workup.

NURSING INTERVENTIONS, MANAGEMENT, AND IMPLICATIONS

Nursing care of the adult with MG should focus on symptom management, psychosocial support, and medication compliance and administration. ACh-E inhibitors, such as pyridostigmine (Mestinon), can slow the degradation of ACh, allowing more availability of the neurotransmitter at the NMJ, thereby improving muscle activity (AANN, 2013). Excess ACh can result in cholinergic crisis, so it is important for nurses to teach patients the importance of taking their medications as prescribed, and also the side effects and signs and symptoms of overdose. Immunosuppression through administration of azathioprine (Imuran) or cyclosporine can also be used for immune-mediated MG. Patient education regarding immunosuppressives is required to ensure safety. The side effects associated with immunosuppressive therapy, including infection, nephrotoxicity, hepatotoxicity, and bone marrow suppression, warrant the need for close physician monitoring when initiating these medications (AANN, 2013).

Priority nursing problems related to the care of patients with MG include the management and identification of myasthenia crisis. Myasthenia crisis is a life-threatening complication characterized by severe respiratory muscle weakness and frequent bulbar weakness that may necessitate intubation and mechanical ventilation. Patients are at increased risk for aspiration due to excessive drooling and muscle weakness. Symptoms of MG may be potentiated by stress, surgery, or medications such as certain antibiotics, beta blockers, and muscle relaxers (Drachman & Amato, 2014). During MG crisis, immune-modulating therapy and plasmapheresis to remove circulating antibodies can aid in symptom management. Administration of intravenous immunoglobulin G (IVIG) is used to bind antibodies, permitting an increased availability of ACh during crisis (AANN, 2013). In addition to understanding the therapies used during crises, nurses should also consider the psychosocial aspects of the patient experiencing the crisis and during other uncertain periods of the disease such as exacerbations. Education points should include energy conservation, identification of triggers, when to seek medical attention, and information about professional organizations that may provide additional support.

OUTCOMES

Patients in remission with minimal ocular symptoms, such as eyelid weakness, may have their medication dose decreased or discontinued (Sanders et al., 2016). Mortality rates in adults with MG are between 4% and 8% and have continued to improve; the highest mortality rates occur within the first 2 years of diagnosis (AANN, 2013; Livesay, 2012). Prognosis is better in those whose disease remains restricted to ocular involvement; less favorable prognoses are associated in persons with thymomas (AANN, 2013).

Summary

MG can be accurately identified by clinical assessment, serological testing, and clinical diagnostic testing, although adults with mild weakness may require an extensive workup due to the need for differential diagnosis to rule out other causes of muscle weakness (NINDS, 2010). Medications that increase availability of ACh are a key component of symptom management in persons with MG. Many adults with MG can have a normal life. Immune-modulating therapies have allowed for treatment of MG crisis and have been attributed to improved prognosis (Sanders et al., 2016). Nurses should provide holistic care that involves chronic disease management such as medication coaching, symptom relief and prevention, community support, and patient and family education.

American Association of Neuroscience Nursing. (2013). Care of the patient with myasthenia gravis. AANN Clinical Practice Guidelines Series. Retrieved from http://www .myasthenia.org/LinkClick.aspx?fileticket=I2Imja5gU4s%3D&tabid=101

Drachman, D. B., & Amato, A. A. (2014). Myasthenia gravis and other diseases of the neuromuscular junction. In D. Kasper, A. Fauci, & S. Hauser (Eds.), *Harrison's principles of internal medicine*. Retrieved from http://access medicine.mhmedical.com/content.aspx?bookid=1130&sectionid=79756727

Howard, J. F. (2015). Clinical overview of myasthenia gravis. Retrieved from http:// www.myasthenia.org/HealthProfessionals/ClinicalOverviewofMG.aspx

Livesay, S. (2012). Neurologic problems. In J. G. W. Foster & S. S. Prevost (Eds.), *Advanced practice nursing of adults in acute care* (pp. 223–227). Philadelphia, PA: F. A. Davis.

Nair, A. G., Patil-Chhablani, P., Vankatramani, D. V., & Gandhi, R. A. (2014). Ocular myasthenia gravis: A review. *Indian Journal of Ophthalmology, 62*(10), 985–991. doi:10.4103/0301-4738.144987

National Institute of Neurological Disorders and Stroke. (2010). Myasthenia gravis fact sheet (Publication No. 10-768). Washington, DC: DHHS. Retrieved from https://www.ninds.nih.gov/Disorders/Patient-Caregiver-Education/Fact-Sheets/ Myasthenia-Gravis-Fact-Sheet

Sanders, D. B., Wolfe, G. I., Benatar, M., Evoli, A., Gihus, N. E., Illa, I., . . . Narayanaswami, P. (2016). International consensus guidance for management of myasthenia gravis. *Neurology, 87*(4), 419–425. doi:10.1212/WNL.0000000000002790

Smith, D. (2016). The neurologic system. In H. Craven (Ed.), *Core curriculum for medical–surgical nursing* (5th ed., pp. 407–460). Pitman, NJ: Academy of Medical–Surgical Nurses.

■ OBESITY

Kelly Ann Lynn

Overview

Obesity is a chronic metabolic disease that is associated with considerable morbidity and mortality. Obesity has been identified as a contributing factor for the development of several significant diseases, including type 2 diabetes mellitus (DM), hypertension (HTN), coronary artery disease (CAD), peripheral vascular disease, nonalcoholic fatty liver disease (NAFLD), osteoarthritis (OA), obstructive sleep apnea (OSA), and many cancers (colon, breast, ovarian; Hahler, 2002; Lobstein et al., 2015; Ng et al., 2014). Obesity also contributes to fertility and reproductive issues, depression, and dementia. Rates of obesity are rising in virtually all populations: in adults and children, and in developed and developing countries. Underscoring the significant impact of obesity on population health, the incidence of obesity is rising and has been described as a *global pandemic* (Ng et al., 2014). Nursing care of patients with obesity must focus on prevention, early intervention, and effective interventions that reduce morbidity and mortality associated with obesity and resultant disease.

Background

Obesity is defined as having a body mass index (BMI) greater than 30; a BMI between 25 and 29.9 is considered overweight. According to the Centers for Disease Control and Prevention (CDC), approximately 69% of adults in the United States are overweight, with more than one third (78.6 million) of these considered obese (CDC, 2015). Worldwide, obesity has more than doubled since 1980. The World Health Organization (WHO) statistics for 2014 are shocking: nearly 39% of adults or 1.9 billion people were overweight or obese; 41 million children younger than the age of 5 were overweight or obese (WHO, 2016). These statistics are very alarming, particularly when considering the propensity for illnesses and morbidity, disability, and mortality attributed to obesity and high BMI.

BMI is a universally accepted scale for assessing healthy weight and it refers to weight in kilograms divided by height in meters squared (BMI = kg/m^2). It is important to note that BMI is not an exact measurement. Muscle weighs more than fat and thus someone with a high muscle mass may have a deceptively high BMI. Likewise, someone with low muscle mass may have a misleading BMI. Waist circumference is another metric that is essential to assessing for obesity. Men should have a waist circumference less than or equal to 40 inches and women should have a waist circumference less than or equal to 35 inches.

Obesity is a complex disease and often has several contributing factors; obesity may be the result of genetic, metabolic, hormonal, and/or emotional issues. Emerging research suggests obesity may result from sleep deprivation, infection, exposure to endocrine-disrupting chemicals (EDCs), certain medications, and changes to the gut microbiome, among others (McAllister et al., 2009). Obesity is a major health concern because it is a precursor to other serious health conditions. The burden of disease-related obesity is massive. Nurses must address BMI, diet, and lifestyle with patients to prevent the devastating sequelae related to obesity.

Clinical Aspects

ASSESSMENT

A thorough nursing assessment is essential for all patients with obesity. This includes a comprehensive patient history with targeted questions related to eating habits, activity level, and reproductive/menstrual history. Physical assessment should be thorough and address vital signs, particularly height, weight, waist circumference, heart rate, and blood pressure. To evaluate circulation and identify areas of skin breakdown or infection, a thorough skin assessment is essential. It is imperative that nurses perform a comprehensive psychosocial assessment to identify underlying or associated mental health conditions, specifically depression. Moreover, a review of essential laboratory values is of utmost importance. The urinalysis will help detect for the presence of glucose in the urine; serum chemistry will assess for electrolyte imbalances, cholesterol and lipid panel, fasting blood sugar, hemoglobin A1c for blood sugar control, serum albumin and vitamin B_{12} levels for malnutrition, blood urea nitrogen (BUN) and creatinine levels to evaluate renal function, thyroid function tests, liver enzymes and liver panel, and erythrocyte sedimentation rate (ESR or sed rate) to detect inflammation.

The review of medications is an essential part of the nursing assessment as some medications can contribute to obesity. These include psychotropic medications, antidiabetic drugs, antihypertensives, steroid hormones and contraceptives, antihistamines, and protease inhibitors (McAllister et al., 2009).

Nursing assessment of obesity must include all three components: comprehensive, in-depth history; a physical examination with evaluation and interpretation of laboratory and diagnostic tests; and medication review. Any encounter with patients with an elevated BMI (greater than or equal to 25) should address all of these issues.

NURSING INTERVENTIONS, MANAGEMENT, AND IMPLICATIONS

Nursing care of obese and overweight patients should focus on lifestyle and weight management. Prevention of the serious consequences related to obesity, specifically diabetes, cancer, and cardiovascular events, is the goal of care. Partnering with patients and championing their efforts will contribute to their success. Patients should be counseled on all available treatment options, including medical management, bariatric surgery, and endoscopic procedures that will help them be successful in reversing obesity. Patients must be encouraged to approach their care as a series of lifestyle changes rather than a diet, exercise, and medication program. Lowering BMI will reduce the incidence of diabetes, cardiovascular disease, urinary retention, and urinary sepsis. Nursing care must include comprehensive education and emotional support for patients and their families.

Nursing interventions will vary based on the clinical presentation, the treatment course, and the long-term objectives for a given patient. All patients will need considerable education about healthy lifestyle, their disease process, treatment options, and the side effects of medications that may be offered.

Some patients will be offered medical management to facilitate weight loss. These patients will require in-depth education about the medications, side effects, and potential interactions with other medications taken. Patients who choose bariatric surgery will need to be educated about the planned surgery and specific issues related to the various surgical options (gastric bypass, sleeve gastrectomy, laparoscopic adjustable band, duodenal switch). The details of the postoperative diet, management of nausea, and the signs and symptoms of infection need to be reviewed in detail. Similarly, patients opting for endoscopic intervention (endoscopic gastroplasty, endoscopic balloon) will need to be educated specific to these procedures.

Obese patients need guidance to adopt healthier lifestyle behaviors. They need to make healthier food choices by reducing sugar and simple carbohydrates in favor of nonstarchy vegetables and high-quality lean protein. Nurses should help patients develop a healthy relationship with food by discouraging emotional eating and disordered eating patterns (i.e., binging and craving). Food should be seen as a source of life. It must be emphasized to obese patients that every meal offers an opportunity to nourish their physical being.

Patients are encouraged to increase their activity level, starting off slowly and gradually increasing in intensity. Also, patients should be encouraged to adopt effective stress management techniques to reduce emotional eating and promote wellness. Walking, yoga, and meditation are all excellent stress reducers.

In addition, patients must be encouraged to improve their sleep habits. Adults should get 7 hours of sleep per night; children and adolescents need more. Sleep is essential to weight loss and overall health. This may be particularly difficult for obese people because they often suffer from OSA as a comorbidity of their obesity. Patients with OSA will need more intervention to ensure that they get the recommended amount of sleep.

Obese patients are often marginalized. Nurses must advocate for this vulnerable patient group to ensure that they get the appropriate care needed. All treatment areas must have appropriate seating and equipment (blood pressure cuffs, gowns) to ensure the safety and dignity of these patients.

Obesity is a multifaceted disease that affects not only patients, but also their partners and families. Nurses must offer patients and families an opportunity to process the complex emotions surrounding this disease.

OUTCOMES

The expected outcomes of evidence-based nursing care for patients with obesity are the prevention of serious consequences associated with the progression of this disease (diabetes, cancer, cardiovascular disease) so as to increase the patient's quality of life, and decrease the incidence of developing comorbid conditions.

Summary

Obesity medicine is a new specialty that recognizes that the condition is a disease, and that treating obesity is the best way to prevent diabetes. Early intervention and initiation of appropriate nursing care can prevent significant morbidity and result in better quality of life. Nurses must partner with their patients to develop customized care plans to reduce weight, improve health, and prevent progression of disease. Nursing support and education can help patients to choose healthier lifestyle behaviors and ease their distress and to promote compliance with their care plans.

Centers for Disease Control and Prevention. (2015). Adult obesity facts. Retrieved from http://www.cdc.gov/obesity/data/adult.html

Hahler, B. (2002). Morbid obesity: A nursing care challenge. *Medsurg Nursing, 11*(2), 85–90.

Lobstein, T., Jackson-Leach, R., Moodie, M. L., Hall, K. D., Gortmaker, S. L., Swinburn, B. A., . . . McPherson, K. (2015). Child and adolescent obesity: Part of a bigger picture. *Lancet, 385*(9986), 2510–2520. doi:10.1016/S0140-6736(14)61746-3

McAllister, E. J., Dhurandhar, N. V., Keith, S. W., Aronne, L. J., Barger, J., Baskin, M., . . . Allison, D. B. (2009). Ten putative contributors to the obesity epidemic. *Critical Reviews in Food Science and Nutrition, 49*(10), 868–913.

Ng, M., Fleming, T., Robinson, M., Thomson, B., Graetz, N., Margono, C., . . . Abraham, J. P. (2014). Global, regional, and national prevalence of overweight and obesity in children and adults during 1980–2013: A systematic analysis for the Global Burden of Disease Study 2013. *Lancet, 384*(9945), 766–781. doi:10.1016/S0140-6736(14)60460-8

World Health Organization. (2016). Obesity and overweight fact sheet. Retrieved from http://www.who.int/mediacentre/factsheets/fs311/en

■ OSTEOARTHRITIS

Mary Variath

Overview

Osteoarthritis (OA) is characterized as a chronic, degenerative, inflammatory disease that can affect any joint or structural component of a joint (Gomes et al., 2016; Kang et al., 2016). OA is the most common form of arthritis, and a leading cause of pain and disability globally. Middle-aged adults and the elderly are likely to experience symptoms of OA, which is consistent with the increased prevalence of OA among persons aged 45 years and older (Kapoor, 2015). Although OA can affect any joint, the hip and knee joints are commonly affected and can contribute to significant reductions in quality of life among those affected by OA. Nursing care for persons living with OA should consider nonpharmacological therapies in combination with pharamaceuticals to minimize pain and maintain the physical functioning of the affected joint (Uthman et al., 2014).

Background

In the United States, OA is a prevalent and disabling chronic condition. According to the Organization for Economic Cooperation and Development, about 28.5% men and 27.9% women in the United States are affected with OA (Kang et al., 2016). Advanced age is a factor associated with OA. In fact, it is estimated that individuals who are aged 70 years and older have a higher likelihood of having OA than persons aged 50 to 60 years (Kang et al., 2016). The incidence of OA has also been linked to obesity. Obesity has shown to drastically increase the incidence of OA of the knee in men and women (Kapoor, 2015). Thus, advanced age and obesity have been established as major risk factors for the development and progression of OA. Other risk factors include gender, race and ethnicity, genetics, nutrition, smoking, traumatic injury, and type 2 diabetes mellitus (Frey, Hügle, Jick, Meier, & Spoendlin, 2016; Huebner et al., 2016; Kang et al., 2016; Kapoor, 2015).

The relative significance of certain risk factors may differ from joint to joint, for early versus end-stage OA, for development as opposed to progression of disease, and for radiographic versus symptomatic disease. Although it is well established that the risk of developing OA increases dramatically with age; age is not the sole determinant of developing the disease.

Genetic, environmental, metabolic, and biochemical factors or a combination of these may result in more severe outcomes. Furthermore, inactivity of the joint may result in accelerated cartilage degradation. Sometimes the progressive loss of articular cartilage can be accompanied by alterations of the underlying structures, such as subchondral bone alteration. Besides, synovial tissue inflammation may be observed leading to synovitis, resulting in the initiation and/or progression of OA. Together, these structural changes produce the symptoms of joint pain, restriction of motion, crepitus with motion, joint effusions, and deformity.

Clinical Aspects

ASSESSMENT

Symptoms of OA are localized and not systemic, and include pain, bony enlargement, crepitation, tenderness to palpation, reduced range of movement, deformities, and overall functional limitation. Distal interphalangeal nodes called *Heberden's nodes* are a bony enlargement that are classic signs of hand OA; Bouchard's nodes in proximal interphalangeal joints are common in women. In advanced hip OA, leg length discrepancy and muscular atrophy, secondary to joint splinting for pain relief, may be noticed.

With spine OA, weakness and/or numbness in the arms and legs may result from nerve root impingement due to osteophytes. Localized warmth, an indication of inflammation, such as synovitis, may be noted in knee or hand OA. Individuals may experience one or more of these symptoms leading to pain and disability.

Joint pain and joint disability are the dominant symptoms of OA and the primary reason individuals seek medical help. The pain generally is described as mechanical in nature with a gradual onset, that increases with increased joint use but is relieved by rest in early stages. Pain, even at rest, especially at night, indicates severity of the condition. Joint stiffness, especially early-morning stiffness due to prolonged periods of inactivity, is another typical sign of OA. However, stiffness associated with OA is relieved with increased activity unlike persistent stiffness in rheumatoid arthritis. Together, pain and stiffness result in functional impairment of the joint.

In addition to assessing for local symptoms, diagnostic investigations such as diagnostic imaging, including radiographic assessment and MRI, which play a pivotal role in ruling out OA, also help. These tests assist in early diagnosis, grading, and monitoring of OA. CT, ultrasound, and nuclear medicine are also used to assess OA, although the role these play is very limited (Salat, Salonen, & Veljkovic, 2015).

These methods are generally used to stage the severity of the disease condition. Although there are no specific blood tests to rule out OA, an elevated erythrocyte sedimentation rate (ESR) indicates synovitis. Synovial fluid assessment can be performed to differentiate between OA and other forms of arthritis.

NURSING INTERVENTIONS, MANAGEMENT, AND IMPLICATIONS

Because OA is a chronic progressive disease with localized symptoms, primary nursing care should focus on assessing for the severity of pain, extent of deformity, functional disability, and examination of diagnostic imaging and laboratory data to confirm OA. The next step is to choose the appropriate steps to help slow the disease progression, damage, and disability, while managing the symptoms at the same time. Although there is no cure for OA, there are myriad treatment options to manage the symptoms, which include pharmacological and nonpharmacological options (Sepriano et al., 2015).

The pharmacological management of OA is currently based on a wide spectrum of therapeutic options to relieve pain, improving the physical function and quality of life. The American College of Rheumatology guidelines recommend topical capsaicin; topical nonsteroidal anti-inflammatory drugs (NSAIDs); oral NSAIDs, including cyclooxygenase inhibitors; and tramadol (Roubille, Pelletier, & Pelletier, 2015). However, the rapid-acting symptomatic treatments for OA consist mainly of analgesics and NSAIDs. Among them, acetaminophen remains the first-line therapeutic agent because of its cost-effectiveness, efficacy, and safety. Opioids and duloxetine are two other often-used agents. If the symptoms are not severe, topical NSAIDs, such as capsaicin and lidocaine patches, are reported to be effective (Roubille et al., 2015). The non-NSAIDs, such as corticosteroids that are anti-inflammatory drugs, and hyaluronic acid, which is a glycosaminoglycan component for the maintenance of joint homeostasis, are administered as intra-articular treatments in severe conditions (Roubille et al., 2015).

Other OA drugs with disease-modifying properties are being developed, such as slow-acting drugs for OA that are believed to reduce joint pain and slow structural disease progression in the joint. In addition, cartilage changes, bone remodeling, and synovial inflammation control are the types of studies in progress. Furthermore, a few promising therapies might emerge, such as platelet-rich plasma, bone remodeling modulators, and inflammatory inhibitors (Roubille et al., 2015).

Nonpharmacological intervention is directed toward self-management programs. Examples include muscle strengthening, low-impact aerobic exercises on land and in water; weight loss; physical therapy; and neuromuscular education (Schachar & Ogilvie-Harris, 2015). Surgery may be considered for individuals whose function and mobility remain compromised and are refractory to pharmacological and nonpharmacological interventions. Surgical interventions for OA include arthroscopy, osteotomy, arthrodesis, and total joint arthroplasty.

OUTCOMES

The intended outcomes of any type of intervention include pain management, providing comfort, minimizing activity intolerance, and ineffective functional and role performance.

Affected individuals learn self-management therapies, including land and/or water aerobic exercises, to improve activities of daily living and provide coping mechanisms.

Summary

OA is a chronic degenerative disorder, causing pain and limitation of movements due to gradual deterioration and inflammation of articular cartilage and joints, resulting in major physical and functional limitations. OA can affect any joint; however, hip and knee joints have a higher prevalence, with higher incidence of OA of the knee due to its weight-bearing function, resulting in a declining quality of life of the individual. Individuals older than 45 years are most often affected. The incidence of OA has risen with the escalation of obesity in the population. Because there is no cure for OA, the primary focus is symptomatic management using pharmacological or nonpharmacological therapies. Pain management, disease-progression control, and deformity prevention are the expected outcomes.

Frey, N., Hügle, T., Jick, S. S., Meier, C. R., & Spoendlin, J. (2016). Type II diabetes mellitus and incident osteoarthritis of the hand: A population-based case-control analysis. *Osteoarthritis and Cartilage, 24*(9), 1535–1540.

Gomes, W. F., Lacerda, A. C., Brito-Melo, G. E., Fonseca, S. F., Rocha-Vieira, E., Leopoldino, A. A., . . . Mendonça, V. A. (2016). Aerobic training modulates T cell activation in elderly women with knee osteoarthritis. *Brazilian Journal of Medical and Biological Research, 49*(11), e5181.

Huebner, J. L., Landerman, L. R., Somers, T. J., Keefe, F. J., Guilak, F., Blumenthal, J. A., . . . Kraus, V. B. (2016). Exploratory secondary analyses of a cognitive-behavioral intervention for knee osteoarthritis demonstrate reduction in biomarkers of adipocyte inflammation. *Osteoarthritis and Cartilage, 24*(9), 1528–1534.

Kang, K., Shin, J. S., Lee, J., Lee, Y. J., Kim, M. R., Park, K. B., & Ha, I. H. (2016). Association between direct and indirect smoking and osteoarthritis prevalence in Koreans: A cross-sectional study. *BMJ Open, 6*(2), e010062.

Schachar, R., & Ogilvie-Harris, D. (2015). Osteoarthritis: Joint conservation strategies. In M. Kapoor & N. N. Mohammad (Eds.), *Osteoarthritis* (pp. 155–169). Cham, Switzerland: Springer International.

Sepriano, A., Roman-Blas, J. A., Little, R. D., Pimentel-Santos, F., Arribas, J. M., Largo, R., . . . Herrero-Beaumont, G. (2015). DXA in the assessment of subchondral bone mineral density in knee osteoarthritis—A semi-standardized protocol after systematic review. *Seminars in Arthritis and Rheumatism, 45*(3), 275–283.

Toupin April, K., Rader, T., Hawker, G. A., Stacey, D., O'Connor, A. M., Welch, V., . . . Tugwell, P. (2016). Development and alpha-testing of a stepped decision aid for patients considering nonsurgical options for knee and hip osteoarthritis management. *Journal of Rheumatology, 43*(10), 1891–1896.

■ OSTEOMYELITIS

Mary Variath
Jane F. Marek

Overview

Osteomyelitis (OM) is inflammation of the bone caused by a variety of infectious organisms (i.e., bacteria, fungi, or viruses) that results in tissue destruction of the affected bone. OM is a complex disease in its pathophysiology, clinical presentation, and management, making accurate diagnosis and treatment a challenging process. The symptoms of OM include history of local inflammation, erythema, and/or swelling. In addition, patients with OM may present with low-grade fever, malaise, and fatigue, along with nonspecific chronic pain at the site of infection (Malhotra, Schulz, & Kallail, 2015). OM may affect any bone, resulting in progressive bone destruction and the formation of sequestra. OM can be acquired through contiguous spread from adjacent soft tissue, joint, and blood infections or direct inoculation of microorganisms into the bone as a result of trauma or surgery (Malhotra et al., 2015). Other risk factors include diabetes, vascular insufficiency, dialysis treatment, intravenous drug use, and immunosuppression. If untreated, OM can become a life-threatening illness due to bacteremia and sepsis. Therefore, early diagnosis, identification of the causative organism, and prompt treatment can prevent recurrent infection, chronic disease, and complications.

Background

OM is an ancient disease and is one of the most difficult infectious diseases to diagnose and treat (Malhotra et al., 2015). OM can affect people of all ages. Major causative bacterial organisms include *Pseudomonas aeruginosa*, *Staphylococcus aureus*, *Streptococcus pyogenes*, and *Streptococcus pneumoniae*. Infection with drug-resistant organisms is of particular concern. For unknown reasons, *Haemophilus influenzae* type B is shown to affect joints rather than bones alone. In addition, fungal or mixed bacteria are associated with skull, vertebral, and/or long bone OM. In fact, about 75% to 95% of skull OM is reported to be of fungal origin (Johnson & Batra, 2014; Peltola & Pääkkönen, 2014).

Bacteria can reach the bone through direct inoculation from traumatic wounds, open fractures, or implanted hardware; by spreading from adjacent tissue affected by various infections, such as cellulitis and septic arthritis; or by hematogenous spread following bacteremia. OM resulting from hematogenous spread is more common in children; boys are more commonly affected than girls. In developed countries, approximately eight in 100,000 children are affected with OM annually; in developing countries, the incidence is higher, especially in resource-poor places where patients present with advanced disease and survivors experience serious and long-lasting complications (Peltola & Pääkkönen, 2014).

Salmonella species are reported to be a common cause of OM in developing countries as well as in patients with sickle cell disease. OM usually results from adjacent tissue inflammation and infection, as in the case of OM of the skull as a result of contiguous spread from an infected sinus or penetrating trauma (Malhotra et al., 2015). Skull base OM, although rare, is associated with a 10% to 20% mortality rate and primarily affects patients with diabetes and/or immunocompromised men in their 60s (Conde-Diaz et al., 2017).

Pyogenic vertebral OM generally occurs as an acute OM infection in patients older than 55 years. The estimated incidence of vertebral OM has increased in recent years to four to 10 per 100,000 persons annually in high-income countries, increasing the economic burden of the disease (Bernard et al., 2015).

Treatment depends on the etiology of the infection. Debridement of the affected bone was once considered the primary method of treatment; however, long-term systemic antimicrobial therapy has since replaced debridement as the first-line therapy (Conde-Diaz et al., 2017; Johnson & Batra, 2014). In severe cases, antimicrobial therapy needs to be continued for several weeks to avoid recurrent or chronic infection.

Surgical intervention is indicated if the patient does not respond to antimicrobial treatment or has persistent soft tissue infection, joint infection, or bony abscess. Goals of surgical management are debridement of necrotic bone and tissue, management of dead space, restoration of vascular supply, and adequate wound closure. Surgical techniques include bone debridement and resection, stabilization using an external fixator (including the Ilizarov technique), revascularization procedures, and, as a last resort, amputation. Infection following fracture fixation and prosthetic joint infection may result in removal of the hardware, systemic antibiotic therapy, and fracture fixation or joint revision after resolution of infection. Local antibiotic therapy with antibiotic-impregnated beads (antibiotic bead pouch) and spacers may be considered with joint infections and open fractures complicated with OM. In persons with extensive soft tissue involvement, hyperbaric oxygen treatment, vacuum-assisted wound closure (VAC), and skin grafting may be indicated.

Clinical Aspects

ASSESSMENT

Long-bone OM is classified by the Cierny–Mader system that is used to guide treatment. Symptoms of OM may include pain, persistent sinus tract or wound drainage, poor wound healing, and presence of fever. Bony necrosis may not occur for 6 weeks after the onset of infection (Spencer, 2015). Further, if signs and symptoms are less severe, the individual may be slow to seek medical care, in which case bone deterioration may continue without treatment. Therefore, a thorough history and physical assessment are critical to determine the initial injury, infection, or precipitating event.

OM can be classified as acute if the duration of the illness has been less than 2 weeks, subacute for a duration of 2 weeks to 3 months, and chronic for duration longer than 3 months. Classic clinical manifestations in children include inability to walk, fever and focal tenderness, visible redness and swelling around the affected bone. Symptoms are dependent on the affected bone. For example, spinal OM in adults is characteristically manifested as back pain, whereas pain on a digital rectal examination suggests sacral OM.

Diagnosis is determined by the patient's history and clinical presentation and diagnostic testing. Laboratory testing is nonspecific to OM and includes complete blood count and differential, C-reactive protein, and erythrocyte sedimentation rate. Bone biopsy and wound and blood cultures are performed to identify the causative organism and to develop the antibiogram (Peltola & Pääkkönen, 2014). Selection of imaging techniques is based on clinical findings. In some cases, plain radiographs may be sufficient for diagnosis. If plain films are normal or inconclusive, MRI is most sensitive for OM; CT or scintigraphy can also be used, especially if a long bone is affected or if symptoms are not localized.

OUTCOMES

Nursing interventions include managing pain, monitoring neurovascular status of the affected extremity, administering antibiotic therapy, preventing further infection, supporting and immobilizing the affected area, preventing further injury, teaching the patient and family about medications, antibiotic therapy, treatments, prognosis, and rehabilitation therapy. Nurses can take an active role in infection-control education, which will help to control OM development and prevent complications (Spencer, 2015).

Summary

OM usually involves long-term treatment, and recurrence rates are high. Prompt identification of the offending organism and appropriate antibiotic therapy are key in optimizing patient outcomes. Because of the complexity of the illness, a multidisciplinary team approach is necessary. Physical and occupational therapy referrals are often indicated and the patient may require help with activities of daily living and the use of assistive devices until weight-bearing is permitted. Due to the length of treatment, psychosocial support of the patient and family is an important intervention. Treatment goals include limb preservation and prevention of complications, including pathologic fracture and further injury, flexion contractures and muscle atrophy, and systemic complications. Identification of persons at risk and prevention of infection are important nursing considerations.

Bernard, L., Dinh, A., Ghout, I., Simo, D., Zeller, V., Issartel, B., . . . Therby, A. (2015). Antibiotic treatment for 6 weeks versus 12 weeks in patients with pyogenic vertebral osteomyelitis: An open-label, non-inferiority, randomised, controlled trial. *Lancet, 385*(9971), 875–882.

Conde-Díaz, C., Llenas-García, J., Grande, M. P., Esclapez, G. T., Masiá, M., & Gutiérrez, F. (2017). Severe skull base osteomyelitis caused by *Pseudomonas aeruginosa* with successful outcome after prolonged outpatient therapy with continuous infusion of ceftazidime and oral ciprofloxacin: A case report. *Journal of Medical Case Reports, 11*(1), 48.

Johnson, A. K., & Batra, P. S. (2014). Central skull base osteomyelitis. *Laryngoscope, 124*(5), 1083–1087.

Malhotra, B., Schulz, T., & Kallail, K. J. (2015). When anemia, atypical plasma cells, and a lytic bone lesion are not myeloma: An unusual presentation of osteomyelitis. *Kansas Journal of Medicine*, 151–152.

Peltola, H., & Pääkkönen, M. (2014). Acute osteomyelitis in children. *New England Journal of Medicine, 370*(4), 352–360.

Spencer, D. (2015). Implications of underlying pathophysiology of osteomyelitis in diabetics for nursing care. MSN StudentScholarship. Paper 68. Retrieved from http:// digitalcommons.otterbein.edu/stu_msn/68

■ OSTEOPOROSIS

Maria A. Mendoza

Overview

Osteoporosis is a chronic, progressive disease characterized by low bone mass density resulting in bone fragility and predisposition to fracture. Approximately 12 million people have osteoporosis in the United States, a number that is expected to rise to 14 million in 2020, of whom 80% are women (Cosman et al., 2015). One and a half million Americans have osteoporotic fractures (Jeremiah, Unwin, Greenawald, & Casiano, 2015), resulting in disability and decreased quality of life and the need for long-term nursing home care (Jeremiah et al., 2015).

Osteoporosis is considered a "silent" disease because it is asymptomatic, with many patients going undiagnosed and untreated until a fracture occurs (Cosman et al., 2015; Lorentzon & Cummings, 2015). The major role of nursing in caring for patients with osteoporosis is in fracture prevention (Smeltzer & Qi, 2014). The impact of osteoporosis is significant, both in the effects on the patient and the economic burden. Assessing risk, assisting the patient to identify modifiable factors, and collaborating on a plan for lifestyle modification to help maintain bone health are important nursing interventions.

Background

Bone health is maintained by a dynamic process of formation and resorption. In osteoporosis there is imbalance in these processes caused by decreased bone formation, increased resorption, or both. Bone loss may be localized or generalized due to disuse or immobilization. Osteoporosis is divided into three types. Type I is related to aging and has two forms: postmenopausal (occurring in women after menopause) and senile (occurring in both genders age 65 and older). Type II usually occurs in younger individuals secondary to an underlying disease such as hyperthyroidism or multiple myeloma. Type III is found in women with amenorrhea associated with eating disorders. This section only discusses type I osteoporosis.

The most common sites for osteoporotic-related fractures (fragility fractures) are the hip, spine, and distal radius (Colles' fracture). Fractures are treated with surgical intervention, open reduction and internal fixation, or total or hemiarthroplasty for hip fractures; kyphoplasty or vertebroplasty for vertebral compression fractures; and closed or open reduction for Colles' fractures. Patients are at increased risk for another fracture following an osteoporotic fracture.

The nonmodifiable risk factors of osteoporosis include age (50 years and older), female gender, family history of osteoporosis, previous fracture (increase in risk by 86%), ethnicity (Caucasian and Asian), menopause/hysterectomy (due to decreased estrogen), inflammatory bowel disease, rheumatoid arthritis, systemic lupus erythematosus, hyperparathyroidism, hyperthyroidism, thin body frame, and primary/secondary hypogonadism (androgen deficiency) in men. Modifiable risk factors include long-term glucocorticoid therapy, excessive alcohol consumption, smoking, poor nutrition, vitamin D deficiency, gastric bypass surgery, eating disorders, insufficient weight-bearing exercise, low dietary calcium intake, certain medications (e.g., antiseizure, thyroid replacement, and selective serotonin reuptake inhibitors), and frequent falls (Cosman et al., 2015; Jeremiah et al., 2015).

Fracture risk assessment can be accomplished in a variety of ways. The fracture risk assessment tool (FRAX) is a valid online assessment tool that assesses the 10-year risk of osteoporotic fracture based on the individual's risk factors. There are limitations to this tool and it should be used in conjunction with clinical judgment. Other methods include bone mineral density (BMD) by dual-energy x-ray absorptiometry (DXA), quantitative computerized tomography (QCT), and hip structure analysis (HSA; Imai, 2014). BMD testing is the most common method used to identify fracture risk and evaluate the patient's response to treatment. The bone density in the hip and spine is measured and compared against established norms (peak BMD of a healthy 30-year-old adult) to give a T-score. The World Health Organization has established criteria for T-scores. A normal T-score is within +1 to −1 standard deviation (SD). Low bone density is between 1 and 2.5 (−1 to 12.5 SD). A level of 2.5 SD or lower is diagnostic of osteoporosis and more than 2.5 SD plus one or more osteoporotic fractures is considered severe osteoporosis (Cosman et al., 2015). BMD is recommended for women at age 65 years or may be done before 65 years on those who are at an increased risk for fractures (Cosman et al., 2015). There is no strong evidence to recommend biennial frequency of testing and no evidence to recommend DXA testing in men (Cosman et al., 2015).

The process of bone remodeling produces biochemical markers such as serum C-telopeptide, urinary telopeptide, serum bone-specific alkaline phosphatase, and aminoterminal propeptide (Jeremiah et al., 2015). These biochemical markers can predict fracture risk and rapidity of bone loss. They can also predict the magnitude of BMD and patient adherence to osteoporosis therapy.

Clinical Aspects

ASSESSMENT

In addition to assessing for the risk factors listed earlier, the nurse should also include an evaluation of the patient's nutritional status, dietary intake of calcium and vitamin D, alcohol consumption, smoking, and exercise habits (weight-bearing and resistive-type exercise and walking). Physical assessment includes height/weight; body mass index (BMI); vital signs, including orthostatic blood pressure and pulse; posture and balance; functional status (mobility, activities of daily living [ADL] abilities); and neurological and cardiovascular status. Physical findings include increased thoracic kyphosis; loss of height over time generally due to fractures of the vertebrae; and fractures in the wrist, hips, and other sites that may occur as disease progresses. Pain from a hip fracture is usually manifested by a report of groin pain, whereas vertebral compression fracture is characterized by acute localized pain after a fall/lifting episode. The area of the spine palpated will be tender to touch.

Diagnostic laboratory tests, such as alkaline phosphatase, calcium, liver and kidney function tests, complete blood count, thyroid-stimulating hormones, parathyroid hormone, total testosterone (men), estradiol (women), 25-hydroxyvitamin D, and urinary calcium, are usually done to diagnose primary and secondary causes of osteoporosis (Jeremiah et al., 2015).

NURSING INTERVENTIONS, MANAGEMENT, AND IMPLICATIONS

Applicable nursing diagnoses for the patient with osteoporosis include risk for injury/falls, acute pain, impaired mobility, and deficient knowledge.

The following interventions are based on the recommendations by the National Osteoporosis Foundation (Cosman et al., 2015) developed by an expert committee regarding prevention, risk assessment, diagnosis, and treatment of osteoporosis.

Risk assessment and counseling on risk of osteoporosis and fractures. The nurse should obtain a history of risk factors listed earlier. Patient engagement to understand the implications of the risk factors and to plan a lifestyle modification regimen to decrease risk is imperative for success. The nurse can play a major role in multidisciplinary teams or programs that increase awareness of osteoporosis screening and treatment in the community and long-term care facilities (Smeltzer & Qi, 2014).

Nutritional and lifestyle counseling to maintain healthy bone. The recommended calcium intake from food and supplements is 1,200 mg daily for women 51 years and older and 1,000 mg daily for all adults aged 19 to 50 and men 51 years and older. The best source for calcium is from food; calcium supplements may cause constipation and increase the risk for kidney stones. The data regarding the association between cardiovascular disease and calcium supplementation are controversial. There does not appear to be an association between calcium supplementation (up to 2,000–2,500 mg/day) and cardiovascular disease risk in healthy adults (Chung, Tang, Fu, Wang, & Newberry, 2016). Patients should be advised not to take calcium supplements in doses over 500 mg at one time to maximize absorption. Vitamin D recommendation is 800 to 1,000 IU per day for adults aged 50 years and older. The major dietary source of vitamin D is vitamin D-fortified milk (400 IU/quart). Fortification with vitamin D may also be found in other foods such as soy milk, juices, and cereals. The nurse should recommend reading food labels for nutritional information. The nurse should also provide information about the effects of smoking and alcohol on bone health and counsel the patient regarding smoking cessation and moderate alcohol intake.

OUTCOMES

The nurse should encourage patients to engage in a lifelong, regular, weight-bearing and muscle-strengthening exercise regimen to increase bone density and improve balance, posture, strength, and agility. Examples of beneficial exercises include walking, jogging, Tai Chi, stair climbing, dancing, and yoga. Patients should be cautioned not to begin a vigorous exercise program before being evaluated by their provider.

The goal of patient education is behavior change. To increase the effectiveness of education, the nurse can personalize the information to make it more relevant and to motivate the patient toward behavior change. For example, using the significance of the patient's BMD score in tailoring lifestyle changes or monitoring the progress of bone health would be more effective than merely providing information (Smeltzer & Qi, 2014).

Fall prevention. There are numerous risk factors for falls. They can be categorized into environmental (e.g., loose rugs, poor lighting, and lack of assistive devices), medical (e.g., age, anxiety, agitation, sensory impairment, cardiac dysfunction, medications, and malnutrition), and neurological/musculoskeletal (e.g., kyphosis and impaired balance, transfer, and mobility). The nurse should identify patients who are at risk for falls and implement safety measures for fall prevention.

Pharmacologic therapy. The role of the nurse in pharmacologic therapy is primarily providing medication education, monitoring for adverse effects and the effectiveness of treatment, and patient adherence. Bisphosphonates are the first-line therapy for postmenopausal women to reduce the risk for hip and vertebral fractures. There are many other medications to treat osteoporosis, including calcitonin, estrogens, selective estrogen receptor modifiers (SERM), tissue-selective estrogen complex, and parathyroid hormone. The nurse is responsible for becoming familiar with the patient's medications, her or his pharmacokinetics, administration, adverse effects, and nursing implications.

Summary

Osteoporosis is the most common metabolic bone disease and is caused by low bone mass density, progressive deterioration of bone tissue, and microarchitecture resulting in bone fragility and predisposition to fracture. Osteoporosis is a common problem worldwide and its prevalence is increasing. There are an estimated 200 million women in the world with osteoporosis and a fragility fracture occurs every 3 seconds (Tabatabaei-Malazy, Salari, Khashayar, & Larijani, 2017). It is a silent disease that generally affects older women with increased incidence after menopause. The nurse plays a major role as a member of the interdisciplinary team who focuses on prevention, detection, and treatment of osteoporosis. Education regarding bone health is an important health-promotion topic for at-risk adults, as well as for younger individuals to develop healthy bones and prevent osteoporosis.

Chung, M., Tang, A. M., Fu, Z., Wang, D. D., & Newberry, S. J. (2016). Calcium intake and cardiovascular disease risk: An updated systematic review and meta-analysis. *Annals of Internal Medicine, 165*, 856–866. doi:10.7326/M16-1165

Cosman, F., de Beur, S. J., LeBoff, M. S., Lewiecki, E. M., Tanner, B., Randall, S., & Lindsay, R. (2015). Erratum to: Clinician's guide to prevention and treatment of osteoporosis. *Osteoporosis International, 26*(7), 2045–2047.

Imai, K. (2014). Recent methods for assessing osteoporosis and fracture risk. *Recent Patents on Endocrine, Metabolic, & Immune Drug Discovery, 10*(2), 48–59. doi:10.2174/1872214808666140118223801

Jeremiah, M. P., Unwin, B. K., Greenawald, M. H., & Casiano, V. E. (2015). Diagnosis and management of osteoporosis. *American Family Physician, 92*(4), 261–268.

Lorentzon, M., & Cummings, S. R. (2015). Osteoporosis: The evolution of a diagnosis. *Journal of Internal Medicine, 277*(6), 650–661.

Smeltzer, S. C., & Qi, B. B. (2014). Practical implications for nurses caring for patients being treated for osteoporosis. *Nursing: Research and Reviews, 4*, 19–33. doi: 10.2147/NRR.S36648

Tabatabaei-Malazy, O., Salari, P., Khashayar, P., & Larijani, B. (2017). New horizons in treatment of osteoporosis. *Daru, 25*(1), 2.

■ PAGET'S DISEASE

Jacqueline Robinson

Overview

Paget's disease of the bone, or osteitis deformans, is a metabolic bone disease that is characterized by both excessive bone resorption and subsequent compensatory bone formation. However, because both processes occur at such an accelerated rate, the bone that forms is exaggerated, more vascular, and fragile. This bone growth leads to deformities and complications if left untreated and these complications are often the presenting symptoms that lead to the diagnosis of the disease itself. The risk for Paget's disease increases with age; in fact, the disease is very uncommon in patients younger than 40 years (National Institutes of Health [NIH], 2011). Nursing care of the patient with Paget's disease is focused on the prevention of complications, the importance of follow-up care once a diagnosis is made, and ongoing education of the patient and family members.

Background

The exact prevalence of Paget's disease is unknown due to the fact that it is often not diagnosed until complications occur or until visible signs manifest. Of those cases that are diagnosed, the disease is more common in men and individuals with increasing age (Nebot Valenzuela & Pietschmann, 2017). However, there are cases when patients who are in their teens and 20s have Paget's disease with a familial inheritance, which affects the bones of the skull, face, and hands, as well as increasing the person's risk for hearing loss (NIH, 2011). The disease is most common in those of Northwest European decent, particularly those from Britain (NIH, 2011).

Unlike other metabolic, noninflammatory diseases of the bone, Paget's disease does not affect the entire skeleton; rather, it affects one or several bones in an area. If a single bone is affected, it is monostotic; if multiple bones are affected, it is polystotic. The most common sites include the skull, femur, tibia, spine, and thorax. There is an increase in both osteoclast and osteoblast activity in the affected area. First, the osteoclasts cause accelerated bone resorption; to compensate for this loss, osteoblasts then accelerate formation. However, this rate is grossly accelerated and leads to highly vascular, disorganized, fibrotic bone that results in overgrowth and deformity (Nebot Valenzuela & Pietschmann, 2017).

Although the exact cause of Paget's disease is unknown, there are studies that suggest both a genetic and environmental component. The familial form of Paget's disease that accounts for one third of cases is linked to a gene mutation of sequestosome-1 (SOSTM-1) in 46% of patients with the disease within the same family (Audet et al., 2016). Other studies suggest a link to a virus, some even suggest the measles virus. Due to a decline in the virus in certain areas, environmental influences have also been suggested as an influence on development (Audet et al., 2016). Viral components have been obtained from the nuclei of osteoclasts from patients positively diagnosed with Paget's disease (Nebot Valenzuela & Pietschmann, 2017).

Although many patients with Paget's disease of the bone are asymptomatic, many suffer from complications that lead them to seek treatment and subsequent diagnosis. In addition, the potential deformity to the affected area(s) not only affects quality of life from an aesthetic point of view but also from a functional standpoint.

Clinical Aspects

ASSESSMENT

The signs and symptoms of Paget's disease of the bone range from a complete absence of symptoms to symptoms specific to a particular affected body area, all the way to systemic manifestations. The patient may simply complain of bone pain in the affected area or surrounding joint space. The systemic manifestations include the potential for high cardiac output heart failure. Due to the fact that the lesions that develop are highly vascular and that this constant cycle of osteoclast and osteoblast activity leads to an increase in metabolic demand, there is an increase in the workload of the heart (Nebot Valenzuela & Pietschmann, 2017).

If the skull is involved, the entire cranium will increase in size; therefore, the face will look smaller. Due to the potential for increased pressure on the cranial nerves, the patient may suffer from hearing loss. The patient may have other neurologic complications, including headaches, tinnitus, and, in rare cases, a buildup of cerebrospinal fluid (Muschitz, Feichtinger, Haschka, & Kocijan, 2016). The patient with lower extremity involvement will have an altered gait with a waddling appearance. The long bones may bow and the patient will appear bowlegged even at rest. If the area is extensive, the surrounding joints can be affected, causing stress on the cartilage leading to osteoarthritis (Muschitz et al., 2016). Rigidity of the thorax and spine is also possible if they are involved in the pathology. Paralysis has been reported as well as pinched spinal nerves (NIH, 2011). Osteosarcoma is a rare complication that can be diagnosed via bone biopsy (NIH, 2011). Fractures are the most common presenting symptom and complication of Paget's disease.

Diagnosis of Paget's disease is made by simple radiograph of the area. Early lesions are osteolytic, whereas older lesions that are more progressed are sclerotic and bone growth is as much as 8 mm/year (Muschitz et al., 2016). A bone scan may be ordered to determine the extent of the disorder and the activity of the cells. Finally, a bone biopsy will be done to confirm osteosarcoma.

The gold standard in terms of diagnosis as well as follow-up on the progression of the disease and treatment outcomes is serum levels of alkaline phosphatase (ALP). This enzyme is produced by bone cells and thus is in excess in patients with Paget's disease as osteoblasts continue to produce incompetent bone. A level twice the normal serum level is considered positive for Paget's disease (NIH, 2011). The serum ALP is sent after treatment is implemented and family members of persons with Paget's disease should also have serum ALP levels sent every 2 to 3 years after the age of 40 (NIH, 2011). The frequency of serum ALP levels after initiation of treatment is based upon the regimen chosen for the patient, with the most potent therapy requiring less frequent follow-up.

Bisphosphonates are the treatment of choice for Paget's disease. These medications prevent fractures and halt disease progression but do not reverse the damage that has already occurred (Kumar, Selviambigapathy, Kamalanathan, & Sahoo, 2016). They work by inhibiting osteoclasts and promoting apoptosis (Muschitz et al., 2016). The ideal bisphosphonate is intravenous zoledronate (Muschitz et al., 2016). This medication is highly nephrotoxic and has also been known to cause flu-like side effects. However, it holds the highest efficacy and therefore requires the least follow-up care. Other bisphosphonates are not as potent and will continue to need more frequent ALP levels.

NURSING INTERVENTIONS, MANAGEMENT, AND IMPLICATIONS

Pain management is a focus of nursing care for some patients, not only with the diagnosis of Paget's disease but also with the complication of osteoarthritis and the pinched nerves that are possible. Nursing must encourage weight-bearing activity to prevent disuse and promote full range of motion. Weight-bearing activity also inhibits bone resorption. Pain may also be relieved by altering hot and cold soaks and emersion therapy. Finally, administration of ordered non-steroidal antiinflammatory medications and acetaminophen may be necessary. Nurses must also encourage their patients to maintain a healthy weight to reduce the burden on the joints and bones.

Safety is another top priority for nursing care of the patient with Paget's disease. The goal is to avoid fractures. A key is to prevent falls. Encourage the use of assistive devices when warranted such as walkers and canes, focusing education on their proper use. Grab bars, hand rails, nonskid mats, and proper lighting must be installed in the home for safety. A thorough evaluation of the home environment for anything that could place a patient at risk for tripping or loss of balance, such as throw rugs, power cords, and clutter, must be done with the patient, also including the patient's family and/or significant others.

Communication is a focus for the patient with hearing impairment. Although bisphosphonates have shown to halt disease progression and prevent fractures, not all hearing issues have reversed. Thus, nursing interventions aimed at improving communication is key for day-to-day functioning of the hearing-impaired patient with Paget's disease.

Finally, the nurse must stress the importance of follow-up care. Testing serum ALP levels for patients diagnosed with the disease is necessary to determine the progression of the disease as well as the efficacy of treatment efforts. It is also crucial that family members of the patient also be tested due to the clear familial link that has been identified.

OUTCOMES

The expected outcomes of nursing care focus on the prevention of complications and pain management. The need for follow-up care as well as an evaluation of the patient's home environment for safety and health promotion is also paramount. Maintaining safety and self-esteem in the home environment is the goal. If a patient does suffer a complication, the nursing care will be reprioritized based on the specific problem.

Summary

The diagnosis of Paget's disease of the bone is often made after a complication has occurred or a radiograph of an adjacent area has revealed the characteristic findings of the disease. It is confirmed with serum ALP levels being twice the normal range. Although there is no specific cause known and there is no cure, there are therapies aimed at halting progression and preventing complications, with bisphosphonates being the primary pharmacologic choice. Nurses play a key role in the prevention of complication and the maintenance of safety as well as encouraging patients to remain compliant with follow-up care.

Audet, M. C., Jean, S., Beaudoin, C., Guay-Bélanger, S., Dumont, J., Brown, J. P., & Michou, L. (2016). Environmental factors associated with familial or non-familial forms of Paget's disease of bone. *Joint Bone Spine, 84*(6), 719–723. doi:10.1016/j.jbspin.2016.11.010

Kumar, R., Sevianbigapathy, J., Kamalanathan, S., & Sahoo, J. (2016). Stress fractures healing with bisphosphonates in Paget's disease. *Joint Bone Spine, 84*, 91. doi: 10.1016./j/jbspin.2016.01.010

Muschitz, C., Feichtinger, X., Haschka, J., & Kocijan, R. (2017). Diagnosis and treatment of Paget's disease of bone: A clinical practice guideline. *Wiener medizinische Wochenschrift, 167*(1–2), 18–24.

National Institute of Health. (2011). Questions and answers about Paget's disease of bone. Retrieved from http://www.bones.nih.gov

Nebot Valenzuela, E., & Pietschmann, P. (2017). Epidemiology and pathology of Paget's disease of bone—A review. *Wiener medizinische Wochenschrift, 167*(1–2), 2–8.

■ PANCREATIC CANCER

Jennifer E. Millman

Overview

Pancreatic cancer is one of the most aggressive malignancies. Although it accounts for just 3% of all cancers in the United States and 7% of all cancer-related deaths (American Cancer Society [ACS], 2016), it is particularly problematic because patients are usually diagnosed with advanced stage cancer that is refractory to aggressive medical care. The only curative treatment for pancreatic cancer is surgical resection. However, more than 80% of patients have nonresectable lesions at the time of diagnosis (De La Cruz, Young, & Mack, 2014). Nursing care of patients with pancreatic cancer should focus on the delivery of holistic care for the patients and their family system.

Background

The incidence of pancreatic cancer ranges between one and 10 cases per 100,000 people worldwide and is more common in men and in developed countries (Ryan, Hong, & Bardeesy, 2014). In the United States, it is the eighth leading cause of cancer death among men and ninth among women (Ryan et al., 2014). The risk of developing pancreatic cancer increases with age; the median age at diagnosis is 71 years (Ryan et al., 2014). Almost all patients are diagnosed after age 45 years, and two thirds of cases are diagnosed after age 65 years (ACS, 2016). The ACS (2016) estimates there were 53,070 new cases of pancreatic cancer and approximately 41,780 deaths due to the disease, annually (ACS, 2016). The lifetime risk of developing pancreatic cancer is about 1.49% or one in 67 persons (Becker, Hernandez, Frucht, & Lucas, 2014).

Pancreatic cancer is notable for its unique biological features. Characteristics include the presence of KRAS (Ki-ras2 Kirsten rat sarcoma viral oncogene homolog) oncogene mutation (greater than 90%), progression from a precursor lesion, and an affinity for local invasion and distant metastasis (Ryan et al., 2014). Most pancreatic cancers arise from microscopic precursor lesions called *pancreatic intraepithelial neoplasia* (PanIN), which is a noninvasive epithelial lesion arising in the pancreatic ducts (Jaloudi & Kluger, 2017). Many pancreatic cancers begin as precancerous growths in the pancreas. With more advanced imaging techniques, it is possible to identify more pancreatic cysts before they develop into cancer. Precancerous growths, such as mucinous neoplasms (MCNs) and intraductal papillary mucinous neoplasms (IMPN), warrant monitoring as they may progress to cancer over time (ACS, 2016). Rapidly growing lesions or lesions connecting to the main pancreatic duct are suggestive of malignancy and may lead to surgical resection.

The pancreas is made up of exocrine and endocrine cells. The islets of Langerhans are endocrine cells that produce insulin and glucagon and regulate blood glucose levels. Most of the pancreas consists of acinar cells that secrete the digestive enzymes lipase, amylase, and protease. The majority of pancreatic tumors are exocrine in origin; 95% of exocrine pancreatic cancers are pancreatic adenocarcinoma (ACS, 2016). Pancreatic endocrine tumors account for less than 5% of pancreatic cancers (ACS, 2016).

Smoking is strongly associated with pancreatic cancer; 20% to 30% of pancreatic cancers may be caused by smoking (ACS, 2016). Other modifiable risk factors include overweight or obesity and workplace exposure to chemicals used in dry cleaning and metal-working. Unmodifiable risk factors include increased age, male gender, African American race, family history of pancreatic cancer, and inherited genetic disorders (ACS, 2016). Up to 10% of pancreatic cancers have a hereditary component and 20% of those have a genetic mutation (Becker et al., 2014). Genetic risk factors include hereditary breast and ovarian cancer syndrome (BRCA1), Lynch syndrome, familial adenomatous polyposis, hereditary pancreatitis, cystic fibrosis, and familial atypical multiple mole melanoma syndrome (Becker et al., 2014).

Diabetes, chronic pancreatitis, cirrhosis of the liver, and *Helicobacter pylori* infection may increase the risk of pancreatic cancer (ACS, 2016). More research is needed regarding the role of alcohol, diet, and physical inactivity in the development of pancreatic cancer. Health-promotion teaching should focus on smoking cessation, maintaining a healthy weight, limiting alcohol intake, and limiting exposure to toxic chemicals (ACS, 2016).

Clinical Aspects

ASSESSMENT

More than two thirds of pancreatic cancer tumors originate in the head of the pancreas, resulting in biliary obstruction (De La Cruz et al., 2014). Presenting symptoms caused by biliary obstruction include abdominal pain, jaundice, pruritus, dark urine, and pale stools. Other more nonspecific symptoms caused by tumors of the tail or body include anorexia, weight loss, early satiety, nausea, and dyspepsia (De La Cruz et al., 2014).

Practitioners should keep in mind that physical findings of pancreatic cancer can vary based on the stage of cancer at diagnosis. Patients who present in the early stages of pancreatic cancer may have no abnormal physical findings on examination. In contrast, patients with advanced pancreatic cancer with liver involvement may present with a palpable gallbladder with mild, painless jaundice (Courvoisier's sign); migratory thrombophlebitis (Trousseau's sign of malignancy), or supraclavicular lymphadenopathy (Virchow node), which is indicative of metastatic abdominal malignancy (De La Cruz et al., 2014).

The pancreas CT protocol, a triphasic cross-sectional imaging, is the standard for diagnosis and staging when patients present with a high suspicion of pancreatic cancer. In cases for which a CT scan is contraindicated, MRI or magnetic resonance cholangiopancreatography (MRCP) can be useful. If a pancreatic mass is seen on imaging, an endoscopic ultrasound with fine-needle aspiration or biopsy is indicated for tissue diagnosis (National Comprehensive Cancer Network [NCCN], 2017). If no obvious mass is seen on cross-sectional imaging and there is no evidence of metastatic disease, then further workup should include endoscopic ultrasound, endoscopic retrograde cholangiopancreatography (ERCP), MRI, and MRCP (NCCN, 2017). Cancer antigen 19-9 (Ca 19-9), a tumor marker clinically significant in pancreatic ductal adenocarcinoma, can be used for diagnosis and prognosis and to monitor the patient's response to treatment. Ca 19-9 is not tumor specific and is not a sufficient screening tool (De La Cruz et al., 2014); it is elevated with several other conditions, including pancreatitis, cirrhosis, biliary tract disease, and other malignancies (De La Cruz et al., 2014).

Surgical resection is the primary treatment method for pancreatic adenocarcinoma. However, only 15% to 20% of patients are candidates for surgical resection when diagnosed (NCCN, 2017). Even with surgery, the prognosis is poor; the 5-year survival rate of patients who undergo surgical resection is only 20% (NCCN, 2017). The decision of whether or not a patient is a candidate for surgical resection should be determined by a multidisciplinary board at a large volume center (NCCN, 2017). Prognosis depends on the tumor grade and staging at the time of diagnosis. Contraindications to surgical resection include the presence of metastatic liver disease or direct involvement of the superior mesenteric artery, inferior vena cava, aorta, celiac axis, or hepatic artery (Jaloudi & Kluger, 2017).

The choice of surgical procedure depends on the location of the tumor. Surgical options include pancreaticoduodenectomy (with or without pylorus sparing), total pancreatectomy, and distal pancreatectomy. Pancreaticoduodenectomy, or Whipple procedure, is indicated for tumors of the head of the pancreas. Tumors of the body and tail are rarely resectable as they cause fewer presenting symptoms and at diagnosis are typically discovered at a more advanced stage. These types of tumors are better treated by distal pancreatectomy. Endoscopic procedures for nonresectable pancreatic cancer include radiofrequency ablation of the bile duct and celiac plexus neurolysis for pain management. Endoscopic retrograde pancreaticoduodenectomy for stent placement and biliary decompression may be indicated for patients with jaundice or cholangitis due to biliary tract obstruction.

Chemotherapy and radiation can be used as adjuvant or neoadjuvant therapy and to treat patients with nonresectable disease. The key chemotherapeutic agents used for patients with advanced pancreatic cancer are gemcitabine (Gemzar), FOLFIRINOX regimen (5-fluorouracil, leucovorin, irinotecan, and oxaliplatin), and nab-paclitaxel (Abraxane). In 2011, treatment with the FOLFIRINOX regimen was shown to prolong overall survival by more than 4 months than treatment with gemcitabine alone (Hronek & Reed, 2015).

Nurses are present during administration of chemotherapy and typically provide care and support when patients experience adverse events (Hronek & Reed, 2015). Thus, it is imperative that nurses know how to manage toxicities from chemotherapy. Toxicities include pancytopenia, peripheral neuropathy, fatigue, anorexia, stomatitis, nausea, and vomiting. Nurses should also monitor patients for depression.

OUTCOMES

Nurses must have a comprehensive understanding of surgical complications and adverse events from chemotherapy as well as an understanding of the psychosocial implications of the diagnosis of pancreatic cancer.

Perioperative nursing considerations for the patient undergoing Whipple procedure include interventions to prevent respiratory complications, hemorrhage, venous thromboembolic events, infection, hepatorenal failure, fluid volume deficit, and nutritional deficits (Jaloudi & Kluger, 2017). Patients who present with jaundice are at risk for coagulopathies, malabsorption, malnutrition, and pruritus (Jaloudi & Kluger, 2017). Pruritus will improve with biliary decompression and symptoms may be managed with an antihistamine. Blood glucose levels should be monitored and some patients may require insulin supplementation. Patients with pancreatic cancer may be at risk for developing pancreatic exocrine insufficiency, which can be managed with pancreatic enzyme supplements.

Summary

Treatment of pancreatic cancer remains challenging. Nurses play a crucial role in educating patients about the disease and supporting patients and families as they cope with the diagnosis of pancreatic cancer. It is essential that nurses are knowledgeable regarding presenting symptoms of pancreatic cancer, treatment modalities, supportive care, and symptom management. Health-promotion teaching should be geared toward risk reduction strategies, especially smoking cessation. Goals for future research include improving screening methods and early detection of pancreatic cancer, especially for high-risk populations.

American Cancer Society. (2016). Pancreatic cancer. Retrieved from https://old.cancer .org/acs/groups/cid/documents/webcontent/003131-pdf.pdf

Becker, A. E., Hernandez, Y. G., Frucht, H., & Lucas, A. L. (2014). Pancreatic ductal adenocarcinoma: Risk factors, screening, and early detection. *World Journal of Gastroenterology, 20*(32), 11182–11198.

De La Cruz, M. S., Young, A. P., & Ruffin, M. T. (2014). Diagnosis and management of pancreatic cancer. *American Family Physician, 89*(8), 626–632.

Hronek, J. W., & Reed, M. (2015). Nursing implications of chemotherapy agents and their associated side effects in patients with pancreatic cancer. *Clinical Journal of Oncology Nursing, 19*(6), 751–757.

Jaloudi, J., & Kluger, M. D. (2017). Pancreatic cancer. In G. Nandakumar (Ed.), *Evidence based practices in gastrointestinal & hepatobiliary surgery* (pp. 566–588). New Delhi, India: JP Medical.

National Comprehensive Cancer Network. (2017). NCCN clinical practice guidelines in oncology: Pancreatic adenocarcinoma. Retrieved from https://www.nccn.org/ professionals/physician_gls/pdf/pancreatic.pdf

Ryan, D. P., Hong, T. S., & Bardeesy, N. (2014). Pancreatic adenocarcinoma. *New England Journal of Medicine, 371*(11), 1039–1049.

■ PARKINSON'S DISEASE

Peter J. Cebull

Overview

Parkinson's disease (PD) is a progressive neurodegenerative condition character-ized by a lack of the neurotransmitter dopamine, which regulates movements and emotions. According to the Michael J. Fox Foundation for Parkinson's Research, more than 60,000 new cases are diagnosed each year with no definitive cure available. Though the exact cause of this disease remains unknown, genetics and environmental factors play a role in the development and progression of PD.

The definitive characteristic of PD is the progressive death of dopaminer-gic neurons in the brain. The resulting lack of sufficient dopamine in the basal ganglia leads to the classic Parkinsonian movements most commonly associated with the disease, although numerous nonmotor symptoms can manifest earlier in the disease course. Research indicates that other neurotransmitters outside the basal ganglia are also affected during disease progression (Kalia & Lang, 2015).

PD results from both a genetic predisposition and environmental influences on susceptible genes. The only definitive diagnostic tool used to confirm PD is postmortem histological analysis to identify the degraded dopaminergic neurons or the presence of abnormal groupings of proteins called *Lewy bodies*. The exact role Lewy bodies play in PD and some forms of dementia is being investigated. Because the treatments for PD are largely symptomatic rather than curative, symptoms are treated after onset and modified as they progress. A diagnosis of exclusion is usually made based on various criteria that contribute to an overall compelling clinical picture (Kalia & Lang, 2015).

Globally, PD is the most prevalent neurodegenerative disease following Alzheimer's disease. Gender is regarded as a major risk factor; three males are affected by the disease for every two females. The most significant factor in PD risk is age; there is an exponential increase of prevalence and incidence in persons younger than 80 years, with the peak age at onset occurring in a per-son's 70s. As the U.S. population ages, the number of Americans affected by this disease is projected to increase by as much as 50% by 2030. For this reason, a working understanding of this disease is of considerable importance to nurses who will be caring for older Americans.

Clinical Aspects

ASSESSMENT

When assessing a person with PD, it is important to understand the key signs asso-ciated with the disease: bradykinesia, rigidity, and resting tremor. Bradykinesia, or slow movements, characterize this disease. Often, the first motion in an action is the most challenging, such as taking the first step when walking or swallowing food later in the disease course. Speech can also be affected for the same reason, causing decreased volume of voice and dysarthria. Other manifestations of this sign occur when walking: a person's arms will often stop swinging as they normally would and facial muscles do not move as easily as they once did, creating a baseline mask-like expression.

Muscle rigidity occurs with decreased use; muscles stiffen, resulting in resistance to both passive and active range of motion throughout the body, especially in the knee and elbow joints. The classic tremor associated with PD is a resting tremor, which occurs while the person is not using a particular muscle group for a specific task. For example, asking a person with a Parkinsonian tremor to write his or her name will reduce the hand tremor once the person is holding the pen; however, the tremor will still interfere with the ability to conduct the smooth fine-motor movements needed for handwriting. In addition to assess for the motor symptoms of PD, it is important to also screen for depression, cognitive difficulties, and issues with the bladder, digestion, and circulation as these also manifest at various stages throughout the disease course (U.S. National Library of Medicine [NLM], 2015).

NURSING INTERVENTIONS, MANAGEMENT, AND IMPLICATIONS

Providing nursing care for a person with PD requires anticipating and understanding the various problems the disease can present. Because of the impaired, disordered movements, there is an increased risk for falling. The lack of control over fine motor and possible cognitive dysfunctions later in the disease course can impair a person's ability to complete activities of daily living (ADL). The treatments of the disease can be both surgical (deep-brain stimulation) and nonsurgical. Medications used to treat the motor symptoms of PD include levodopa (precursor to dopamine), dopamine agonists, catechol-O-methyltransferase (COMT) inhibitors, monoamine oxidase (MAO) B inhibitors, and anticholinergics. Other medications may be prescribed for sleep disorders, dementia, and depression, which are common in persons with PD. Hallucinations and psychosis may be treated by reducing or stopping the dose of one of the medications used to treat the motor symptoms of PD. Levodopa is the most effective medication used to treat bradykinesia, tremor, and rigidity. To improve efficacy of the levodopa, it is combined with carbidopa (Sinemet). The patient must be carefully monitored for the adverse effects associated with long-term therapy with levodopa–carbidopa and dopamine agonists.

The person with PD is at increased risk for falling and injury due to slowing of movements and even "freezing" of movement altogether. A common gait associated with PD is a propulsive, shuffling, small-stepped gait that makes tripping over small objects, such as rugs, or climbing stairs a major hazard and risk for serious injury related to falls. A nurse can conduct a thorough environmental review and work with a patient and his or her caregivers to reduce these hazards.

Lack of fine-motor control is characteristic of this disease because of bradykinesia, tremor, and stiffness. A person who experiences these symptoms, which are typically worse in the mornings and just before the next dose of medications, can have significant difficulty with ADL. Planning ADL and arranging for assistance as needed can be a key nursing intervention to improve the quality of life for a person with PD.

Speech and swallowing can be affected, creating a potential communication barrier and risk for aspiration. The nurse can offer more time and alternative methods of communication when necessary. Dysphagia can be identified by a simple swallowing test. If swallowing difficulty is detected, the nurse can refer the patient for more advanced testing and consult with a nutritionist to recommend dietary modifications to reduce the risk of aspiration. This is a simple but potentially life-saving intervention as one choking incident can result in serious lifelong deficits and even death.

Adverse effects of dopamine agonist therapy are a problem commonly experienced by almost all patients with this disease who take any one of a number of dopamine agonist medications. The most widely used medication to treat PD is levodopa–carbidopa (Sinemet). As therapy continues and the disease progresses, higher doses of the medication are necessary. The nurse needs to monitor the patient for adverse effects such as orthostatic hypotension, hallucinations, excessive daytime sleepiness, dyskinesia, and increased impulsivity or atypical behavior (NLM, 2015). These effects of dopamine-agonist treatment can significantly affect the life of the patient and his or her family. A nurse can intervene by recognizing and educating the patient and caregivers about adverse effects and to notify the prescribing health care provider if they occur.

Summary

PD is a progressive neurodegenerative disorder characterized by a lack of the neurotransmitter dopamine. PD primarily affects older adults, a rapidly increasing population in the United States. Nurses are in a unique position to assess, identify problems, and intervene to improve the quality of life for patients with PD. Although deaths from the disease itself are rare, the common causes of PD-related death are complications related to symptoms such as impaired gait and dysphagia (NLM, 2015).

OUTCOMES

It is important for nurses to understand the stages of disease progression and that patients may go undiagnosed for a significant period of time before the classic motor signs of PD appear. In addition to neuromuscular symptoms, including tremors, bradykinesia/akinesia, and rigidity, the patient's mood and cognition may be affected. The pathophysiology of this disease has also been related to dementia (Lewy body), and depression is an even more common manifestation of patients who are faced with this progressive, life-altering diagnosis (NLM, 2015). All patients with PD should be screened for depression. Although the motor symptoms are often the first and most emphasized feature, these other problems can prove just as debilitating and dangerous, warranting an equal emphasis from health care providers. Through informed, evidence-based nursing care of persons with PD, patient outcomes and morbidity and mortality can be positively influenced.

Kalia, L. V., & Lang, A. E. (2015). Parkinson's disease. *Lancet, 386*(9996), 386, 896–912. doi:10.1016/S0140-6736(14)61393

The Michael J. Fox Foundation Parkinson's Disease. (n.d.). Understanding Parkinson's disease. Retrieved from https://www.michaeljfox.org/understanding-parkinsons/index.html?navid=understanding-pd

U.S. National Library of Medicine. (Ed.). (2015). Parkinson's: Overview. Retrieved from https://www.ncbi.nlm.nih.gov/pubmedhealth/PMH0076679

■ PEPTIC ULCER DISEASE

Lisa D. Ericson
Deborah R. Gillum

Overview

Peptic ulcer disease (PUD) is inflammation of the gastrointestinal mucosa of the stomach and/or duodenum, which can lead to gastric or duodenal ulcers. The major causes of PUD are *Helicobacter pylori* infections and the chronic use of nonsteroidal anti-inflammatory drugs (NSAIDs). Although the prevalence of PUD has declined significantly since 1992, it still affects 4.5 million people in the United States, with an additional half a million newly diagnosed cases each year (Anand, 2017; Lee, 2014). Treatment goals include eradication of *H. pylori*, discontinuation of NSAID use, promotion of ulcer healing, and control of other precipitating risk factors.

Background

PUD is a disruption of the mucosal and submucosal layers of the stomach and/ or duodenum, which results in the body's inability to adequately protect the epithelium from the effects of gastric acid and pepsin. Under normal conditions, a physiologic balance exists between gastric acid secretion and mucosal defense, but PUD develops when there is an imbalance between the body's protective factors and aggressive factors that can damage the gastric mucosa (Anand, 2017; Ignatavicius & Workman, 2016; Konturek & Konturek, 2014). PUD includes three types of ulcers: (a) gastric ulcers that develop in the antrum of the stomach near the acid-secreting mucosa and which usually are the result of *H. pylori* infection, (b) duodenal ulcers that occur within 2 cm of the pylorus and are related to high gastric acid secretion, and (c) stress ulcers that typically occur secondarily to an acute medical crisis or trauma (Ignatavicius & Workman, 2016; Lee, 2014).

Contributing PUD risk factors can be endogenous, such as gastric acid and pepsin, or exogenous, such as *H. pylori* infection, NSAIDs, alcohol consumption, smoking, obesity, or stress (Anand, 2017; Chuah et al., 2014; Konturek & Konturek, 2014). *H. pylori* and NSAID use are the most common causes of PUD. *H. pylori* colonizes in the gastric mucosa and is typically transmitted via the fecal–oral route during early childhood. This bacterium can remain dormant for decades, and although it does not cause illness in most people, it can lead to mucosal inflammation and epithelial cell necrosis, resulting in PUD (Anand, 2017; Ignatavicius & Workman, 2016). Ulcers with an indeterminate cause are termed *idiopathic* and tend to occur with older age, multimorbidity, recent surgery, sepsis, and medications other than NSAIDs (Konturek & Konturek, 2014).

Approximately 4.5 million people in the United States are affected annually by PUD, accounting for more than 507,000 hospitalizations and costing $4.85 billion yearly (Anand, 2017; Laine, 2016). In the United States, the prevalence of *H. pylori* among patients older than 60 years ranges between 40% and 60%, whereas 20-year-olds have a prevalence of 20%. It is rarely diagnosed in children (Anand, 2017; Fashner & Gitu, 2015; Lee, 2014). An additional contributing factor that increases the risk of PUD in older adults includes the number of high-risk medications they are prescribed (e.g., antiplatelet drugs, warfarin, and selective serotonin reuptake inhibitors; Fashner & Gitu, 2015). Although in the past PUD occurred more frequently in males, recent trends show that the gap is narrowing; males have an 11% to 14% lifetime occurrence rate, whereas females have an 8% to 11% lifetime occurrence rate (Anand, 2017; Lee, 2014). People of lower socioeconomic status also have higher rates of PUD, possibly related to higher rates of *H. pylori* infection (Lee, 2014).

PUD prognosis is excellent once the cause of the ulcer is identified. With eradication of *H. pylori* infection, avoidance of NSAIDs, and the appropriate use of antisecretory therapy, most patients are successfully treated (Anand, 2017). First-line therapy of *H. pylori* eradicates more than 80% of infections (Fashner & Gitu, 2015). The mortality rate has decreased modestly in the past 20 years and is approximately 1 death per 100,000 cases. Including all patients with duodenal ulcers, the mortality rate due to ulcer hemorrhage is 5%. If the ulcer should perforate and surgery is required, the mortality risk is 6% to 30%. Several factors are associated with higher mortality rates, including location of the ulcer (perforated gastric ulcers have twice the mortality than perforated duodenal ulcers), shock at the time of admission, immunocompromised state, cirrhosis, renal insufficiency, age older than 70 years, delay of initiation of surgery for more than 12 hours after presentation, and comorbidities (e.g., cardiovascular disease or diabetes mellitus; Anand, 2017).

Clinical Aspects

ASSESSMENT

On history and physical examination, the most common symptoms include nausea and vomiting; hematemesis (vomiting of blood); melena (passage of dark, "tarry" stools that contain blood); pyrosis (heartburn); dyspepsia (indigestion) described as sharp, burning, or gnawing; pain or tenderness in the mid- or upper-epigastric region; pain in the epigastric region after eating; and hyperactive bowel sounds initially that become hypoactive as the disease progresses (Anand, 2017; Ignatavicius & Workman, 2016; Konturek & Konturek, 2014).

Common complications of PUD are perforation, hemorrhage, and pyloric obstruction. Perforation is a medical emergency and clinical manifestations may include sudden, sharp pain; tender, rigid, board-like abdomen (associated with peritonitis); fetal positioning; and absent bowel sounds (Ignatavicius & Workman, 2016).

The current standard for diagnosing PUD is an esophagogastroduodenoscopy (EGD). Endoscopy provides an opportunity to view the ulcer to determine active bleeding and to attempt hemostasis, if necessary. EGD also allows for biopsy of the gastric mucosa to detect the presence of *H. pylori* (using a rapid urease test) and cytologic studies to rule out cancerous cells (Anand, 2017; Ignatavicius & Workman, 2016; Konturek & Konturek, 2014). A nuclear medicine scan may be ordered if perforation or hemorrhage is suspected (Ignatavicius & Workman, 2016).

NURSING INTERVENTIONS, MANAGEMENT, AND IMPLICATIONS

Interventions for nursing include four goals: (a) eliminate *H. pylori* infections, (b) reduce pain, (c) heal ulcers, and (d) prevent reoccurrence. No single medication has been successful in treating *H. pylori*, thus a combination of agents is used. This combination, referred to as *PPI-triple therapy*, includes a proton pump inhibitor (PPI), such as pantoprazole, and two antibiotics (clarithromycin and tetracycline or metronidazole; Fashner & Gitu, 2015). These medications are prescribed for 10 to 14 days. Some providers add bismuth (Pepto-Bismol) to the PPI-triple therapy, which prevents *H. pylori* from binding to the mucosal lining to stimulate mucosal protection. Hyposecretory medications are used to reduce pain by reducing gastric acid secretions. These medications include PPIs (pantoprazole, omeprazole) and histamine blocking agents (H2 receptor antagonist), such as ranitidine and famotidine. Antacids, such as aluminum hydroxide and magnesium hydroxide, can also be used to buffer gastric acid and prevent the formation of pepsin. Mucosal barrier protectors, such as sucralfate, can be used to reduce pain, heal ulcers, and prevent reoccurrence (Ignatavicius & Workman, 2016).

Patient teaching should address peptic ulcer reoccurrence. Patients should avoid alcohol and tobacco as they stimulate gastric acid secretion. During the acute phase of the illness, patients ought to adhere to a bland diet and avoid foods that cause an increase in symptoms. The role of nutrition therapy in PUD management is controversial and no evidence exists to support dietary restrictions. Treatment other than medications is focused on stress reduction, which can be promoted through yoga, guided imagery, and hypnosis (Ignatavicius & Workman, 2016). Other nursing care will include measures to reduce anxiety, maintain nutritional requirements, and help the patient become knowledgeable about the management and prevention of ulcer recurrence (Belleza, 2016).

OUTCOMES

The prognosis for patients with PUD is excellent. Patients are treated successfully with *H. pylori* eradication, avoidance of NSAIDs (lifestyle triggers), and antisecretory therapy. Safety issues are addressed with patient education regarding medication adherence and lifestyle modifications (Ignatavicius & Workman, 2016).

Summary

H. pylori and chronic NSAID use remain the most common contributing factors associated with PUD (Lee, 2014). Quality of life and expected outcomes are excellent for those diagnosed with PUD with appropriate teaching regarding risk factors to prevent reoccurrence (Ignatavicius & Workman, 2016). Successful patient outcomes are promoted through thorough patient education, including the role of *H. pylori* and NSAIDs in PUD development, the importance of adhering to the medical treatment, and avoidance of lifestyle triggers (Lee, 2014).

Anand, B. S. (2017). Peptic ulcer disease. *Medscape.* Retrieved from http://emedicine .medscape.com/article/181753-overview#a5

Belleza, M. (2016). Peptic ulcer disease. Retrieved from https://nurseslabs.com/ peptic-ulcer-disease

Chuah, S. K., Wu, D. C., Suzuki, H., Goh, K. L., Kao, J., & Ren, J. L. (2014). Peptic ulcer disease: Genetics, mechanism and therapies. *BioMed Research International, 2014,* 898349. doi:10.1155/2014/898349

Fashner, J., & Gitu, A. C. (2015). Diagnosis and treatment of peptic ulcer disease and *H. pylori* infection. *American Academy of Family Physicians, 91*(4), 236–242.

Ignatavicius, D. D., & Workman, M. L. (2016). *Medical-surgical nursing: Patient-centered collaborative care.* St. Louis, MO: Elsevier.

Konturek, P. C., & Konturek, S. J. (2014). Peptic ulcer disease. In E. Lammert & M. Zeeb (Eds.), *Metabolism of human diseases* (pp. 129–135). Vienna: Springer Publishing. doi:10.1007/978-3-7091-0715-7_21

Laine, L. (2016). Upper gastrointestinal bleeding due to a peptic ulcer. *New England Journal of Medicine, 374*(24), 2367–2376. doi:10.1056/NEJMcp1514257

Lee, L. (2014). First consult: Peptic ulcer disease. *ClinicalKey.* Retrieved from https:// www.clinicalkey.com/#!/content/medical_topic/21-s2.0-1014794

■ PERICARDITIS

Heidi Youngbauer

Overview

Acute pericarditis is an inflammation of the pericardium with or without pericardial effusion (Adler & Charron, 2015), and is diagnosed in approximately 5% of patients with nonischemic chest pain in North America and Western Europe (Imazio, Gaita, & LeWinter, 2015). The true incidence and prevalence of acute pericarditis are difficult to measure, as low-risk patients are rarely admitted to hospitals (Doctor, Shah, Coplan, & Kronzon, 2016), and many cases may resolve without a diagnosis (Imazio et al., 2015). Acute pericarditis most commonly affects middle-aged individuals (Doctor et al., 2016; Imazio et al., 2015), with the mean age of patients ranging from 41 to 60 years, and is responsible for 0.1% (Adler & Charron, 2015) to 0.2% (Imazio et al., 2015) of hospital admissions.

Patients with acute pericarditis typically present with clinical symptoms of precordial chest pain, worse on inspiration and when the patient is placed supine. A physical assessment may reveal a pericardial friction rub and diffuse ST segment elevation on electrocardiogram (Cremer et al., 2016; Doctor et al., 2016). Depending on the underlying etiology of the disease process, orthopnea, palpitations, mild fever, weakness, and cough may also be reported by patients with acute pericarditis (Adler & Charron, 2015). Therefore, this entry provides information on evidence-based nursing care to optimize the outcomes of patients presenting with pericarditis.

Background

Pericarditis is an inflammation and irritation of the membrane surrounding the heart and may be defined as acute, incessant, recurrent, or chronic depending on recurrence and duration of symptoms (Adler & Charron, 2015; Cremer et al., 2016). According to Cremer et al. (2016), acute pericarditis is common and responsive to appropriate treatment; however, up to 30% of patients will develop complications or recurrent attacks.

The pericardium is a double-walled avascular sac that functions to protect the heart against infection and spread of malignancy (Doctor et al., 2016), provides lubrication, and secures the heart to the mediastinum (Adler & Charron, 2015). The pericardium is composed of a fibrous outer layer called the *parietal pericardium* and a mesothelial inner layer called the *visceral pericardium*, which adheres to the epicardium (Hoit, 2016). The pericardial space between the two layers normally contains 25 mL to 50 mL of fluid, which serves as a lubricant to reduce friction on the epicardium as the heart pumps (Doctor et al., 2016), as well as to equalize forces over the surface of the heart (Hoit, 2016).

The pericardium has a relatively simple structure, with the response to injury limited to the exudation of fluid, fibrin, and inflammatory cells (Hoit, 2016). This inflammatory response leads to the classic symptoms of sharp, pleuritic chest pain relieved with a forward-leaning position (Doctor et al., 2016). Complications of acute pericarditis result when fluid continues to accumulate, leading to a pericardial effusion or a life-threatening condition called *cardiac tamponade*, which compresses the heart, preventing it from normal function (Adler & Charron, 2015). Chronic recurrences and long-term inflammation can result in another complication called *constrictive pericarditis* in which the pericardium loses elasticity and constricts the heart, causing a form of heart failure secondary to a noncompliant pericardium (Miranda & Oh, 2016).

The typical classification of pericardial disease is according to etiology, which may be infectious or noninfectious (Cremer et al., 2016; Doctor et al., 2016), as the pericardium may be affected by infectious, autoimmune, neoplastic, iatrogenic, traumatic, and metabolic disease (Adler & Charron, 2015). Patients should be screened and considered for specific etiology according to their epidemiological background, as the etiology of pericarditis varies depending on geographic location (Doctor et al., 2016). The majority of pericarditis cases in developing countries have an infectious cause, whereas the majority of cases in Western Europe and North America are categorized as idiopathic and are presumed to be viral after unremarkable diagnostic workup (Imazio et al., 2015). Tuberculosis accounts for about 70% of pericarditis diagnoses in developing countries, with a 25% to 40% mortality rate at 6 months postdiagnosis, as many have a concomitant diagnosis of HIV (Imazio et al., 2015). In developed countries, when the specific etiology of pericarditis is identified, the underlying causes include neoplastic disease (5%–10%), systemic inflammatory diseases and pericardial injury syndromes (2%–7%), tuberculous pericarditis (4%), and purulent pericarditis (less than 1%; Imazio et al., 2015, p. 1499). The increasing use of cardiovascular interventions in developed countries, combined with the aging population, also increases the possible risk of pericardial complications, as even minor intracardial bleeding can lead to pericarditis (Imazio et al., 2015).

Clinical Aspects

ASSESSMENT

Meticulous history and physical examination are necessary to differentiate pericarditis in the patient with acute chest pain (Doctor et al., 2016). The most common presentation of pericarditis is chest pain (Adler & Charron, 2015; Doctor et al., 2016; Imazio et al., 2015), typically sudden in onset and sharp in nature (Doctor et al., 2016). The clinical diagnosis of acute pericarditis may be made with two of the following criteria: precordial chest pain that is worse with inspiration and improved with upright position, pericardial friction rub, electrocardiogram changes that include widespread ST elevation, and pericardial effusion (Adler & Charron, 2015; Cremer et al., 2016). Additional supportive findings include elevated inflammatory markers, including C-reactive protein (CRP), erythrocyte sedimentation rate (ESR), and white blood cell (WBC) count, and evidence of inflammation by imaging (Adler & Charron, 2015; Cremer et al., 2016).

Echocardiography is an important imaging technique to detect pericardial fluid as well as the effects on the heart (Doctor et al., 2016), and is recommended in all patients with acute pericarditis (Adler & Charron, 2015). Patients with acute pericarditis and no additional signs and symptoms that predict higher risk of complications are often successfully treated as outpatients (Cremer et al., 2016). However, those patients with high-risk features, including fever, history of immunosuppression, history of trauma, or evidence of severe pericardial effusion, should be hospitalized for more intensive monitoring of possible complications (Doctor et al., 2016).

Pericarditis is categorized according to the duration of symptoms, with the first attack of pericardial inflammation considered acute pericarditis (Cremer et al., 2016; Doctor et al., 2016). Acute pericarditis has a good long-term prognosis, with risks of adverse events or the development of complicated pericarditis relatively rare (Adler & Charron, 2015). Hemodynamic compromise, such as cardiac tamponade, develops rarely and more often in patients with underlying etiology of malignancy or tuberculosis (Adler & Charron, 2015). Myocardial involvement occurs in about 15% of patients with acute pericarditis, although usually it has a benign course (Cremer et al., 2016). The risk of developing constrictive pericarditis is low (less than 1%) for idiopathic and viral pericarditis, intermediate (2%–5%) for autoimmune and malignant etiologies, and high for bacterial (20%–30%) etiologies (Adler & Charron, 2015; Hoit, 2016).

Recurrence of pericarditis, or pericarditis lasting longer than 4 to 6 weeks, is considered a complicated form of the disease (Cremer et al., 2016). Risk for developing complicated pericarditis is associated with early use of corticosteroids, a lack of response to nonsteroidal anti-inflammatory drugs (NSAIDs), and elevated CRP levels (Cremer et al., 2016). The absence of colchicine as treatment is also associated with an increased risk of developing a complicated or recurrent form of pericarditis (Cremer et al., 2016).

OUTCOMES

Patients diagnosed with acute pericarditis have acute pain, anxiety related to the diagnosis, and a risk for activity intolerance due to the disease process of pericarditis. Recommended treatment includes aspirin or NSAIDs, along with gastric protection with colchicine recommended as adjunct therapy to reduce recurrence rates (Adler & Charron, 2015; Imazio et al., 2015). In the presence of acute pain, patients should be assisted to a position of comfort. Education should include information regarding medications and side effects as well as instruction to avoid strenuous exercise until resolution of symptoms and normalization of CRP, electrocardiogram changes, and echocardiogram findings (Adler & Charron, 2015). Steroids are infrequently prescribed and not recommended as first-line therapy for acute pericarditis, although they may be used in cases of pericarditis refractory to NSAIDs or contraindications to the use of aspirin,

NSAIDs, or colchicine (Adler & Charron, 2015). Patients should be assured that outcomes are generally positive when pericarditis is diagnosed promptly and the treatment regimen and recommendations are followed.

Summary

The most recent guidelines regarding diagnosis and treatment of pericarditis emphasize the importance of a thorough physical examination and history in diagnosing acute pericarditis, as the criteria for diagnosis may be obtained with an initial physical examination and electrocardiogram (Adler & Charron, 2015). Although the etiology of pericarditis is varied, the majority of cases in Western Europe and North America are presumed viral, with an unremarkable diagnostic workup (Imazio et al., 2015). The recommended treatment of acute pericarditis can typically be outpatient based and includes aspirin or NSAIDs with adjunct colchicine and exercise restriction (Adler & Charron, 2015). Nursing interventions include nonpharmacologic approaches to relieve pain, education, and support. Overall, the long-term prognosis for patients with acute pericarditis is good with rare complications when the recommended treatment regimen is followed (Doctor et al., 2016).

Adler, Y., & Charron, P. (2015). The 2015 ESC guidelines on the diagnosis and management of pericardial diseases. *European Heart Journal, 36*(42), 2873–2874.

Cremer, P. C., Kumar, A., Kontzias, A., Tan, C. D., Rodriguez, E. R., Imazio, M., & Klein, A. L. (2016). Complicated pericarditis: Understanding risk factors and pathophysiology to inform imaging and treatment. *Journal of the American College of Cardiology, 68*(21), 2311–2328.

Doctor, N. S., Shah, A. B., Coplan, N., & Kronzon, I. (2016). Acute pericarditis: Review. *Progress in Cardiovascular Diseases, 59(2017)*, 349–359. doi:10.1016/j.pcad.2016 .12.001

Hoit, B. D. (2016). Pathophysiology of the pericardium. *Progress in Cardiovascular Diseases, 59(2017)*, 341–348. doi:10.1016/j.pdad.2016.11.001

Imazio, M., Gaita, F., & LeWinter, M. (2015). Evaluation and treatment of pericarditis: A systematic review. *Journal of the American Medical Association, 314*(14), 1498–1506.

Miranda, W. R., & Oh, J. K. (2016). Constrictive pericarditis: A practical clinical approach. *Progress in Cardiovascular Diseases, 59(4)*, 369–379. doi:10.1016/ j.pcad.2016.12.008

■ PERIPHERAL ARTERY DISEASE

Gayle M. Petty

Overview

Peripheral artery disease (PAD), previously referred to as *peripheral vascular disease, peripheral arterial occlusive disease*, or *arteriosclerosis obliterans*, is a varying vascular disease primarily caused by aneurysmal, atherosclerotic, and thromboembolic pathophysiologic processes. These pathophysiologic processes alter the normal structure and function of the arteries. PAD is a common, acute, and chronic condition that affects a large proportion of the adult population worldwide (Hirsch et al., 2006). Patients present with a range of signs and symptoms, and often require emergent revascularization, surgical interventions, or amputation.

Background

Commissioned by the American Heart Association in 2008, the Atherosclerotic Peripheral Vascular Disease Interdisciplinary Working Group came together with the goal to develop programs that will facilitate prevention and treatment of peripheral atherosclerotic diseases (Creager et al., 2008). As a result, definitions for vascular disease nomenclature were recommended. The term *vascular diseases* should refer to all diseases of arteries, veins, and lymphatic vessels. *Atherosclerotic vascular disease* refers to diseases of arteries caused by atherosclerosis (Creager et al., 2008). The 2011 American College of Cardiology (ACC)/American Heart Association (AHA) focused update of the guideline for the management of patients with PAD (updating the 2005 guideline) refers to PAD as peripheral "artery" disease and anatomically identifies lower extremity, renal and mesenteric arteries, and abdominal aortic as the arteries referenced when discussing PAD (Rooke et al., 2011).

The major cause of PAD is atherosclerosis (Hirsch et al., 2006). Risk factors are age related and include a history of cigarette smoking, diabetes, dyslipidemia, hypertension, and hyperlipidemia (Gerhard-Herman et al., 2016). The prognosis of patients with PAD is characterized by an increased risk for cardiovascular ischemic events, such as myocardial infarction or stroke, due to concomitant coronary artery disease and cerebrovascular disease (Gerhard-Herman et al., 2016). Etiologies for PAD beyond atherosclerosis and thromboembolic processes include familial, acquired, inflammatory, or aneurysmal. Establishment of an accurate etiology is necessary if individual patients are to receive ideal treatment (Hirsch et al., 2006).

Clinical Aspects

PAD can involve the aorta, renal and mesenteric arteries, and arteries of the lower extremities. Patients with PAD should receive a comprehensive program of guideline-directed medical therapy (GDMT), including structured exercise and lifestyle modification, to reduce cardiovascular ischemic events and improve functional status (Gerhard-Herman et al., 2016). Smoking cessation is a vital component of care for patients with PAD who continue to smoke (Gerhard-Herman et al., 2016). Patients with PAD should be prescribed a guideline-based program customized to each patient's risk profile that includes pharmacotherapy to reduce cardiovascular ischemic events and limb-related events (Gerhard-Herman et al., 2016). Prescribed pharmacotherapy classifications may include antiplatelets, statins, antihypertensives, oral anticoagulants, and cilostazol (Gerhard-Herman et al., 2016).

ASSESSMENT

Identification and prevention of disease progression before ischemic symptoms become severe are the health care goals for patients with PAD. Patient assessment should focus on any reports of ischemic rest pain, exertional limitation, or a history of walking impairment (Gerhard-Herman et al., 2016). Patients may describe walking limitation characteristics such as fatigue, aching, numbness, or pain in the buttock, thigh, calf, or foot (Hirsch et al., 2006).

Several key physical examination assessment components for PAD include the following: auscultation of both femoral arteries for the presence of bruits; palpation of the femoral, popliteal, dorsalis pedis, and posterior tibial pulse sites; and evaluation of lower extremity pulse intensity. The pulse intensity should be recoded numerically as follows: 0, when the pulse is absent; 1, when the pulse is diminished; 2, when the pulse is normal; and 3, when the pulse is bounding (Gerhard-Herman et al., 2016). As part of the physical examination, patients' shoes and socks should be removed and the feet should be inspected, noting the color, temperature, and integrity of the skin. An abnormal lower extremity pulse examination, a vascular bruit, a nonhealing lower extremity wound, and lower extremity gangrene are all suggestive of PAD (Gerhard-Herman et al., 2016). Additional findings may include lower extremity color changes, including pallor, when elevated and dependent rubor (Gerhard-Herman et al., 2016).

The most cost-effective, low-risk tool for detecting PAD is the resting ankle–brachial index (ABI; Aboyans et al., 2012). The resting ABI is obtained by measuring systolic blood pressure (SBP) at the arms (brachial arteries) and ankles (dorsalis pedis and posterior tibial arteries) in the supine position using a Doppler device (Gerhard-Herman et al., 2016). The ABI is the ratio of the ankle SBP—the numerator of the ratio—to either arm's highest brachial artery SBP—the denominator for the ratio. The numerator for the calculation of the ABI incorporates the SBP of the posterior tibial or the dorsalis pedis artery separately or is the average of both. It can be performed quickly for each lower extremity and has high validity and good reproducibility (Diehm et al., 2012; Gerhard-Herman et al., 2016). An ABI can be an indicator of atherosclerosis at other vascular sites and can serve as a prognostic marker for cardiovascular events and functional impairment, even in the absence of PAD symptoms.

Individuals performing the ABI should have basic knowledge of vascular anatomy, physiology, and the clinical presentation of PAD, as well as a basic understanding of how a Doppler device functions. The normal ABI ranges from 1.00 to 1.40; findings less than or equal to 0.90 are abnormal and values of 0.91 to 0.99 are considered borderline. Values greater than 1.40 indicate noncompressible arteries (Diehm et al., 2012; Gerhard-Herman et al., 2016).

NURSING INTERVENTIONS, MANAGEMENT, AND IMPLICATIONS

Patients with asymptomatic PAD can acutely progress to a situation requiring emergent interventions. Acute limb ischemia arises when a rapid or sudden decrease in limb perfusion threatens tissue viability (Gerhard-Herman et al., 2016). This may be the first manifestation of artery disease in a previously asymptomatic patient.

The hallmark clinical symptom and physical examination signs of acute limb ischemia include the six "Ps": pain, pallor, pulselessness, poikilothermia, paresthesias, and paralysis (Gerhard-Herman et al., 2016; Hirsch et al., 2006). Determining whether a patient with acute limb ischemia has a salvageable or nonviable extremity is crucial. An urgent evaluation is necessary to preserve the limb and prevent systemic illness or death as a result of the metabolic abnormalities associated with tissue necrosis. The ACC/AHA acute limb ischemia guidelines should be followed when performing the evaluation (Gerhard-Herman et al., 2016).

OUTCOMES

Patients with acute limb ischemia and a salvageable extremity should undergo an emergent evaluation leading to prompt endovascular or surgical revascularization. Patients with acute limb ischemia and a nonviable extremity will most likely require an amputation of the diseased limb (Gerhard-Herman et al., 2016).

Summary

Peripheral arterial diseases encompass diseases of the aorta, renal and mesenteric, and the lower extremity arteries. Etiologies may vary, but the majority of PAD is caused by atherosclerosis. Early identification using ABI and GDMT interventions can delay the disease progression and prevent life-threatening cardiovascular ischemic events.

Aboyans, V., Criqui, M. H., Abraham, P., Allison, M. A., Creager, M. A., Diehm, C., . . . Treat-Jacobson, D. (2012). Measurement and interpretation of the ankle-brachial index: A scientific statement from the American Heart Association. *Circulation, 126*, 2890–2909. doi:10.1161/CIR.0b013e

Creager, M. A., White, C. J., Hiatt, W. R., Criqui, M. H., Josephs, S. C., Alberts, M. J., . . . Rocha-Singh, K. J. (2008). Atherosclerotic peripheral vascular disease symposium II: Executive summary. *Circulation, 118,* 2811–2825. doi:10.1161/CIRCULATIONAHA.108.191170

Gerhard-Herman, M. D., Gornik, H. L., Barrett, C., Barshes, N. R., Corriere, M. A., Drachman, D. E., . . . Walsh, M. E. (2016). AHA/ACC guideline on the management of patients with lower extremity peripheral artery disease: Executive summary. *Circulation.* doi:10.1161/CIR.0000000000000470

Hirsch, A. T., Haskal, J. Z., Hertzer, N. R., Bakal, C. W., Creager, M. A., Halperin, J. L., . . . Reigal, B. (2006). ACC/AHA 2005 guidelines for the management of patients with peripheral arterial disease (lower extremity, renal, mesenteric, and abdominal aortic). *Circulation, 113,* e463–e654. doi:10.1161/CIRCULATIONAHA.106.174526

Rooke, T. W., Hirsch, A. T., Mirsa, S., Sidawy, A. N., Beckman, J. A., Findeiss, L. K., . . . Zierler, R. E. (2011). ACCF/AHA focused update of the guideline for the management of patients with peripheral artery disease (updating the 2005 guidelines). *Journal of the American College of Cardiology, 58*(19), 2020–2045. doi:10.1016/j.jacc.2011.08.023

■ PERNICIOUS ANEMIA

Edwidge Cuvilly

Overview

Pernicious anemia (PA), also known as *vitamin B$_{12}$ deficiency*, is the most common vitamin deficiency in the world, affecting at least 3% of those aged 20 to 39 years, 4% of those aged 40 to 59 years, and 6% of those 60 years and older (Shipton & Thachil, 2015). PA is an insidious complex disorder, provoking a sequelae of modifications in the immunological, hematological, gastrointestinal, and neurological system over a period of time that could be fatal if left untreated. Even though PA has been found in practically every ethnic group, the highest prevalence is among individuals from Northern European countries, mainly the United Kingdom and Scandinavia (Bizzaro & Antico, 2014). Nursing care is essential in detecting the early signs and preventing the clinical manifestations of PA across the life span.

Background

PA is a macrocytic anemia caused by the inability of gastric parietal cells to produce intrinsic factor (IF). IF is a gastric protein secreted by parietal cells to allow the absorption of an adequate amount of vitamin B$_{12}$ in the diet. Vitamin B$_{12}$ is found in animal food bound to a protein that is broken down after ingestion, then further broken down in the stomach by pepsin and hydrochloric acid to release free vitamin B$_{12}$. The free vitamin B$_{12}$ is bound to IF secreted by gastric parietal cells until they bind to mucosal cell receptors in the ileum, where they gets absorbed and can be used for intracellular processes. Vitamin B$_{12}$ is an important micronutrient that aids in the formation of erythrocytes in the bone marrow. When there is a deficiency of vitamin B$_{12}$, erythrocytes are prematurely released into the systemic circulation and have a shortened life span because the premature erythrocytes are prone to early destruction, thus resulting in a reduced erythrocyte count and a state of anemia.

PA occurs as a clinical manifestation of autoimmune gastritis. Autoimmune gastritis is a disease process in which parietal cells are destroyed and a subsequent reduction in the IF results in a vitamin B$_{12}$ deficiency, or PA. Vitamin B$_{12}$ is responsible for erythropoiesis and myelin synthesis; when symptoms are present, vitamin B$_{12}$ deficiency is detected, then swift action to initiate treatment is necessary to reverse or prevent further continuation of damage.

Due to a broad spectrum of symptoms associated with severe consequences of untreated vitamin B$_{12}$ deficiency, screening is essential for high-risk patients to guarantee a quick delivery of treatment. In the elderly, the prevalence of vitamin B$_{12}$ deficiency increases with age and 20% of those 60 years or older are more prone to acquiring a vitamin B$_{12}$ deficiency (Shipton & Thachil, 2015).

There is no gold standard test to diagnose vitamin B$_{12}$ deficiency, but the World Health Organization (WHO) defined PA as having a hemoglobin concentration less than 13 g/dL for men and less than 12 g/dL for women, mean corpuscular volume (MCV) more than 100 fL, and a serum vitamin B_{12} level less than 200 pg/mL (Sun, Wang, Lin, Chia, & Chia, 2013). A low serum vitamin B_{12} that is less than 200 pg/mL is an indicator for prompt initiation of vitamin B_{12} supplementation. However, the lack of accepted value creates a vague demarcation of what is consider deficiency (Wong, 2015). In order to make a distinction between PA and other causes of low vitamin B_{12}, serum autoantibodies are imperative. Anti-IF antibody assay is the preferred test due to high specificity (more than 95%; Shipton & Thachil, 2015).

The distinction between autoimmune gastritis and other causative factors (e.g., vegetarian/vegan diet, alcoholism, poor diet) becomes important when assessing vitamin B_{12} deficiency among the elderly. The main etiology of vitamin B_{12} in the elderly can be separated into two categories: first, inadequate dietary intake (vegetarian, alcohol consumption) and impaired absorption of vitamin B_{12} (PA, atrophic gastritis, postgastrectomy). In spite of the preconception that the most common cause of vitamin B_{12} deficiency in the elderly is inadequate dietary intake, studies have shown the opposite.

Clinical Aspects

ASSESSMENT

The basic clinical features of PA are commonly associated with hypersegmented neutrophils and megaloblastic maturation of erythrocytes, sores on the tongue associated with loss of papillae, and atrophic glossitis, achlorhydria, and neurologic symptoms (paresthesia and ataxia; Bunn, 2014). A complete blood count will often confirm a low hemoglobin, hematocrit, and red blood cell count. Morphological changes of the erythrocyte are likely to occur where there is a high MCV. The megaoblastic shape of the erythrocytes contributes to clinical manifestations of anemia accompanied by pallor, fatigue, weakness, palpitations, dyspnea upon exertion, chest pain, and angina.

OUTCOMES

Evidence-based nursing care should focus on the assessment of risk factors and early identification of clinical manifestations related to PA or vitamin B_{12} deficiency. Devalia, Hamilton, and Molloy (2014) reported that the interpretation of the results should take into consideration these clinical manifestations. Clients with anemia, neuropathy, glossitis, and suspected PA should be tested for anti-IF antibodies. The specification of oral or intramuscular supplementation of vitamin B_{12} should be guided by the results of the laboratory testing, which can inform the etiology of the vitamin B_{12} deficiency.

Summary

PA or vitamin B_{12} deficiency is a treatable condition that has profound effects on the health of an individual. Nursing care for clients with PA or vitamin B_{12} deficiency should include a comprehensive physical assessment and review of pertinent laboratory tests to inform nursing management. The goal of nursing interventions for clients with PA or vitamin B_{12} deficiency is to prevent the sequelae of physiological derangements that can occur as the result of the cellular changes that occur with untreated PA or vitamin B_{12} deficiency.

Bizzaro, N., & Antico, A. (2014). Diagnosis and classification of pernicious anemia. *Autoimmunity Reviews, 13*(4–5), 565–568.

Bunn, H. F. (2014). Vitamin B_{12} and pernicious anemia—The dawn of molecular medicine. *New England Journal of Medicine, 370*(8), 773–776.

Devalia, V., Hamilton, M. S., & Molloy, A. M. (2014). Guidelines for the diagnosis and treatment of cobalamin and folate disorders. *British Journal of Haematology, 166*(4), 496–513.

Shipton, M. J., & Thachil, J. (2015). Vitamin B_{12} deficiency—A 21st century perspective. *Clinical Medicine, 15*(2), 145–150.

Sun, A., Wang, Y. P., Lin, H. P., Chia, J. S., & Chia, C. P. (2013). Do all the patients with gastric parietal cell antibodies have pernicious anemia? *Oral Diseases, 19*, 381–386.

Wong, C. W. (2015). Vitamin B_{12} deficiency in the elderly: Is it worth screening? *Hong Kong Medical Journal, 21*, 155–164.

■ POLYCYTHEMIA VERA

Sarine Beukian

Overview

Polycythemia vera (PV) is characterized by a mutation in a single amino acid that renders the Janus kinase 2 (JAK2) enzyme constitutively active. This induces cytokine-independent proliferation of cell lines that express erythropoietin (EPO) receptors and cause these cells to become hypersensitive to cytokines. Therefore, more proerythroblasts and erythrocytes are formed than are physiologically needed. PV is often discovered as an incidental finding in laboratory work or while seeking medical care in the midst of a thrombotic or hemorrhagic complication. It carries a pronounced symptom burden and can progress to myelofibrosis (9%–21% of individuals) or acute leukemia (3%–10%; Stein et al., 2015).

Background

PV is defined as elevated red blood cells (RBCs), hematocrit (Hct), and hemoglobin (Hgb) laboratory values; PV is also referred to as *erythrocytosis*. PV is further categorized as relative and absolute. Relative PV applies to patients suspected of polycythemia but are found to have a normal RBC mass and a smaller than normal plasma volume, which could be caused by dehydration. Absolute PV applies to true increase in RBC mass, which is further divided into primary and secondary PV based on etiology. The latter is more common and is caused by chronic hypoxia, EPO-producing tumors, or medications such as erythropoiesis-stimulating agents. Hypoxia stimulates EPO and increases RBC count due to bone marrow (BM) stimulation. Living in higher altitudes, smoking, carbon monoxide poisoning, chronic obstructive pulmonary disease, or heart failure can cause hypoxia. Primary polycythemia results from congenital or acquired mutations, and it includes PV and other rare familial conditions (Tefferi & Barbui, 2015). PV is one of the myeloproliferative neoplasms (MPN), alongside primary myelofibrosis and essential thrombocytopenia, among others (Tefferi & Barbui, 2017). Nearly all patients with PV hold a JAK2 mutation, involving exon 14 with JAK2V617F (96%) or exon 12 (3%; Tefferi & Barbui, 2017).

Prevalence (22 cases per 100,000 people) and yearly incidence rates are high (1.3 cases per 100,000 for women and 2.8 cases per 100,000 for men). Risk factors include old age, White race, or Ashkenazi Jewish ancestry. Male predominance with an average age of 61 years at the time of diagnosis has been reported (Scherber & Mesa, 2016; Stein et al., 2015; Tefferi & Barbui, 2015).

Patients often present with fatigue, night sweats, bone pain, fever, weight loss, splenomegaly associated with early satiety, atypical chest pain, paresthesias, and aquagenic pruritus (particularly when in contact with warm or hot water; Stein et al., 2015; Tefferi & Barbui, 2015). Patients are at risk for thrombosis at 2.5% to 4% per year. This includes cerebrovascular accidents, acute coronary syndrome, and thrombosis of the hepatic, portal, and mesenteric veins. Microvascular symptoms, such as headache, visual change, dizziness, erythromelalgia (erythema, warmth, and pain in distal extremities—most commonly palms and soles), also commonly occur and overwhelmingly perturb quality of life, with a mortality rate of 37% (Stein et al., 2015).

Persistent erythrocytosis without an obvious trigger requires workup. Presence of symptoms suggestive of a MPN should add to clinical suspicion. JAK2V617F mutation and EPO levels should be checked. Presence of the mutation makes PV a likely diagnosis. If the mutation is not present and EPO levels are normal or elevated, PV is unlikely, and other causes need to be considered. If the EPO levels are subnormal, then JAK2 (exon 12) should be checked; its presence makes the diagnosis of PV likely. However, its absence requires a BM biopsy. The World Health Organization revised its criteria for the diagnosis of PV in 2016, which includes a combination of the following: elevated Hgb/Hct levels, increased RBC mass, BM biopsy showing hypercellularity, presence of JAK2 mutation, and subnormal serum EPO level. BM biopsy is not always needed to establish the diagnosis of PV (Tefferi & Barbui, 2017).

Medical therapy has shown promising results in the prevention of thrombotic events and reducing symptom burden. However, it has failed to show a difference in disease progression or improvement in survival rates. Median survival in PV is 14 years with aggressive medical therapy, including phlebotomy. The median survival is significantly reduced to 2 years when aggressive medical therapy and the target Hct of less than 45% is not maintained (Tefferi & Barbui, 2015, 2017). Medical therapy for the prevention of thrombosis is based on risk stratification: age older than 60 years and history of thrombosis are markers of high risk. One exception is low-dose aspirin therapy: with no specific contraindication, it is prescribed to all patients regardless of risk-factor profile. It can help with managing symptoms related to microvascular complications. A twice-a-day regimen can be helpful in those who are resistant to a daily regimen or are at risk of arterial thrombus. High-risk patients who continue to be symptomatic, have extreme thrombocytosis, or are unable to tolerate phlebotomy (due to anemia) require treatment with cytoreductive therapy (Stein et al., 2015; Tefferi & Barbui, 2017).

The first line of therapy is hydroxyurea; other options are busulfan or interferon therapy, which lower the risk of thrombosis and leukemic transformation (Stein et al., 2015; Tefferi & Barbui, 2017). Busulfan shows a reduction in allele burden. Interferon therapy is prescribed to manage ongoing erythrocytosis, to reduce spleen size and control pruritus. JAK1/2 inhibitors, such as ruxolitinib, have gained a lot of interest with U.S. Food and Drug Administration approval in 2014. They have shown improvement in Hct control, splenic size reduction, and symptom burden. However, incidence of thrombosis, disease progression, and long-term safety remain questions that need to be addressed. Pipobroman is associated with a shorter survival, increased leukemic transformation, and a lower rate of fibrosis transformation. Radiophosphorus also increases the risk of leukemic transformation (Stein et al., 2015).

Clinical Aspects

ASSESSMENT

Nurses play a crucial role in identifying abnormal laboratory values and side effects of therapy, in educating and counseling patients about PV, and in appropriately intervening to reduce symptom burden and improve patients' quality of life. In the care of the patient with PV, nurses can start with assessment of the patient by reviewing the laboratory values, test results pertinent to PV, medication list, smoking history, medical and surgical history (conditions that cause chronic hypoxia), symptoms, and physical examination findings. Nursing diagnoses that apply to PV are fatigue, pain, (risk for) decreased cardiac tissue perfusion, risk for bleeding, risk for impaired skin integrity, imbalanced nutrition (patients consume less than body requirements because of early satiety), deficient knowledge regarding condition, impaired comfort related to itching, and (risk for) ineffective peripheral tissue perfusion. The following section serves as an example of a nursing care plan to discuss the last three symptoms mentioned.

Given the chronic nature of the disease, it is imperative to assess the patient's understanding of the disease process, symptoms, complications, medications, side effects, and signs and symptoms of complications such as thrombosis (Golden, 2003). Thereafter, the diagnosis of deficient knowledge can be utilized. The desired outcome would be for the patient to comprehend the disease process, medical therapy, and participate in decision making regarding therapy and interventions. Implementation can be through one-on-one discussions with the patient, providing or guiding him or her to the right resources and support groups. Evaluation should follow, in order to ensure comprehension and assessment for further needs.

All patients with PV are at risk of thrombosis. Assessment would include reviewing laboratory values, history of thrombosis, age, medications, medical history, cardiovascular risk factors, and physical examination. Nursing interventions include performing phlebotomy, medication administration, encouraging activity, and educating patients to avoid crossing legs or wearing tight-fitting clothes. Interventions specific to phlebotomy include the removal of 450 mL to 500 mL of blood every few days at first, and thereafter every 2 to 3 months in order to reach target Hct goal; encouraging hydration before and after phlebotomy; monitoring for orthostatic hypotension, headache, weakness, or chest pain postphlebotomy. Evaluation should be used as an opportunity to adjust care plans as necessary (Golden, 2003).

OUTCOMES

Aquagenic pruritus can be debilitating to PV patients. Assessment should include an observation of the patient's pattern of itching, asking the patient about the severity of the symptom, and a skin examination. Subsequently, the diagnosis can be made. One outcome is to relieve the patient or at least alleviate the symptom. Interventions include avoiding dry skin; hot temperature; encouraging tepid showers; drying the skin gently; administering antihistamines, antidepressants, or JAK inhibitors. Evaluation should follow with adjustments as necessary (Golden, 2003; Tefferi & Barbui, 2017).

Summary

PV affects about 148,000 people in the United States alone (Stein et al., 2015). JAK2 mutation remains the most important diagnostic test to identify PV. Phlebotomy and aspirin are the cornerstones of therapy. Patients' symptoms, life expectancy, and risk factors should be evaluated before selecting medical therapy for PV. One of the challenges is to identify and link elevated laboratory values to an underlying disease process; "more is not better" when it comes to RBC, Hgb, and Hct levels, as they may suggest PV.

Golden, C. (2003). Polycythemia vera: A review. *Clinical Journal of Oncology Nursing,* 7(5), 553–556.

Scherber, R. M., & Mesa, R. A. (2016). Elevated hemoglobin or hematocrit level. *Journal of the American Medical Association, 315*(20), 2225–2226.

Stein, B. L., Oh, S. T., Berenzon, D., Hobbs, G. S., Kremyanskaya, M., Rampal, R. K., . . . Hoffman, R. (2015). Polycythemia vera: An appraisal of the biology and management 10 years after the discovery of JAK2 V617F. *Journal of Clinical Oncology, 33*(33), 3953–3960.

Tefferi, A., & Barbui, T. (2015). Essential thrombocythemia and polycythemia vera: Focus on clinical practice. *Mayo Clinic Proceedings, 90*(9), 1283–1293.

Tefferi, A., & Barbui, T. (2017). Polycythemia vera and essential thrombocythemia: 2017 Update on diagnosis, risk-stratification, and management. *American Journal of Hematology, 92*(1), 94–108.

■ PROSTATE CANCER

Erin H. Discenza

Overview

Prostate cancer is the most common cancer in males following nonmelanoma skin cancer and is one of the leading causes of cancer death in males, exceeded only by lung cancer (Centers for Disease Control and Prevention [CDC], 2016). The manifestations, progressive course, and prognosis of the disease vary and are reliant on factors such as extent of the tumor, aggressiveness of the malignancy, comorbidities, and age of the patient (National Cancer Institute [NCI], 2017). The key focus of nursing care of the patient with prostate cancer should be good communication and patient education. There are numerous psychological aspects pertaining to the diagnosis and treatment of prostate cancer and these must be addressed to provide excellent patient-centered nursing care and to ensure desired outcomes.

Background

The prostate gland is located in the pelvis below the bladder and just in front of the rectum. The urethra travels through the center of the prostate. As men age, the prostate may grow benignly larger and cause urinary symptoms such as hesitancy. However, when the cells of the gland grow uncontrollably, cancer is suspected (American Cancer Society [ACS], 2017).

Although the incidence and mortality rates have decreased significantly among all races, prostate cancer remains the second most common cancer in males. According to the CDC (2016), 176,450 men were diagnosed with prostate cancer in 2013, and 27,681 men died from the disease. The NCI estimates those numbers will decrease in 2017 to 161,360 new cases and 26,730 deaths. The average age of diagnosis is 66 years (CDC, 2016).

The primary risk factors associated with prostate cancer are age, family history, and race. The older a man is, the greater his risk for developing prostate cancer. Men younger than 40 years rarely develop the disease, but the risk rises expeditiously after the age of 50 years. Approximately 60% of cases are found in men older than the age of 65 years (CDC, 2016; NCI, 2017). Family history may also affect a man's chance of developing prostate cancer. Having a first-degree relative diagnosed with prostate cancer increases an individual's risk, particularly if the relative was diagnosed at a young age; the risk increases with the number of affected relatives. African American males are at greater risk of developing the disease and are more than twice as likely to die as a result of the cancer. Geography may also play a role in the risk of developing prostate cancer. It is more common in North America and parts of Europe. The exact geographical impact is unknown, but it is posited that more extensive screening practices in developed countries or diets consisting of excessive amounts of red meat or high-fat dairy products may be a contributor to this phenomenon (ACS, 2017).

The early stages of prostate cancer rarely yield symptoms, but in advanced stages the symptoms can be detrimental to the patient's quality of life. The most common symptoms are lower urinary tract symptoms (LUTSs) and include urinary urgency, hesitancy, nocturia, dysuria, and incontinence. Other symptoms include blood in the urine or semen; intractable pain in the back, hips, or pelvis; painful ejaculation; and erectile dysfunction (ED). If the cancer spreads to the bone, there may also be spontaneous fractures (ACS, 2017; CDC, 2016).

Clinical Aspects

ASSESSMENT

Extensive history taking and a complete physical examination are the first steps in the assessment process. Because genetics may play a part in the risk of developing the disease, the nurse should be aware of any family history of prostate cancer. A digital rectal examination (DRE) is also useful in determining whether the prostate is enlarged. The clinician inserts a finger into the rectum to estimate the size of the gland and to feel for lumps or other anomalies (CDC, 2016). Prostate-specific antigen (PSA) is a protein secreted by the prostate. When higher PSA levels are found in the serum, the clinician may suspect cancer but other causes must be ruled out. PSA is specific to the prostate, but it is not specific to cancer (Paterson, Alashkham, Windsor, & Nabi, 2016). Certain medications, medical procedures, infections of the prostate, and enlargement of the prostate can all be possible origins of elevated serum PSA (CDC, 2016).

If cancer is suspected, a transrectal ultrasound guided-needle biopsy is the most common method for a definitive diagnosis (NCI, 2017). MRI produces a clearer picture and is sometimes used for biopsy and to determine whether the cancer has spread outside of the prostate gland. It is important to note that antibiotics may be prescribed prophylactically due to the increased risk of sepsis after needle biopsy (NCI, 2017).

NURSING INTERVENTIONS, MANAGEMENT, AND IMPLICATIONS

There are many factors to be considered when deciding on a treatment strategy for prostate cancer. They include the age of the patient and his life expectancy, comorbidities, stage and grade of the cancer, potential for cure, and possible side effects of the treatment modalities (Williams, Hemphill, & Knowles, 2017).

Active surveillance (AS), including a PSA test and DRE every 6 months, is rapidly becoming a preferred method of management due to the slow progression of the disease. This treatment requires active patient participation in the medical decision-making process (Jayadevappa et al., 2017). When the cancer is confined to the gland and the patient's life expectancy is at least 10 years, therapy with curative intent is most often selected. The most common procedure in this instance is radical prostatectomy (RP), in which the surgeon removes the entire gland (NCI, 2017). Urinary incontinence and ED are both major side effects of RP. If left untreated, the patient's quality of life is severely impacted, leading to depression, anxiety, and decreased feelings of well-being (Jayadevappa et al., 2017).

Radiation therapy (RT) is also a choice for low-grade cancer that is confined to the prostate gland, but may also be used in more advanced cases (ACS, 2017; Williams et al., 2017). RT is accomplished by either external beam radiation or brachytherapy, an implanted RT. Compared with RP, RT is associated with higher risk of hospitalization, need for open surgical procedures, and development of secondary malignancies (Williams et al., 2017).

A relatively new treatment method involves the development of new-generation genomic biomarkers and tissue-based gene expression tests. These biomarkers can indicate whether a prostate cancer is more aggressive than average and more likely to metastasize; however, there are no available recommendations regarding the routine use of these tests (Eapen & Meng, 2017).

Other treatment modalities include cryotherapy, hormone therapy, chemotherapy, and vaccine treatments (ACS, 2017). The choice of treatment method is an important one that should be based not only on the aforementioned factors, but also on the potential for negative impact on quality of life.

The nursing-related problems and the associated nursing interventions are directly related to the diagnosis and treatment of the disease. Many of the problems arise from the psychological impact of the side effects of treatment, such as anxiety and deficient knowledge related to the diagnosis and treatment plan, as well as sexual dysfunction related to effects of treatment. The interventions for these problems are based on open communication and patient education. A more patient-centered approach is needed to support patients and their caregivers to reduce anxiety and encourage self-management. Nurses must also better understand the role of culture, spirituality, and religion in their patients' treatment course (Allchorne & Green, 2016; Baker, Wellman, & Lavender, 2016; Paterson et al., 2016; Williams et al., 2017).

OUTCOMES

The goal of evidence-based nursing care is to ameliorate the effects of the devastating diagnosis of cancer, as well as the psychosocial ramifications of the therapies. Reduction of stress and increased ability to cope are paramount. Patient education must be a key focus as the patient moves from diagnosis to treatment to survivorship. Open lines of communication between the patient and the nurse are of utmost importance to the patient's well-being and quality of life. Along with the psychosocial needs of the patient, there are the problems of pain caused by the procedures, urinary problems such as retention, and infection risks that must be addressed by the nurse. The objective is symptom management. With good nursing care, the prospect of full recovery to prediagnosis functionality is excellent.

Summary

Although prostate cancer is one of the most common cancers in men and a leading cause of cancer death, it can be treated and cured successfully. The treatment modalities induce several undesirable side effects, but these can be mitigated with excellent nursing care. Evidence-based nursing interventions include patient education and open lines of communication, and are vital to the attainment of desired outcomes.

Allchorne, P., & Green, J. (2016). Identifying unmet care needs of patients with prostate cancer to assist with their success in coping. *Urologic Nursing, 36*(5), 224–232.

American Cancer Society. (2017). About prostate *cancer*. Retrieved from https://www .cancer.org/cancer/prostate-cancer/about.html

Baker, H., Wellman, S., & Lavender, V. (2016). Functional quality-of-life outcomes reported by men treated for localized prostate cancer: A systematic literature review. *Oncology Nursing Forum, 43*(2), 199–218.

Centers for Disease Control and Prevention and National Cancer Institute, U.S. Department of Health and Human Services. (2016). United States cancer statistics: 1999–2013 incidence and mortality web-based report [Data file]. Retrieved from https://nccd.cdc.gov/uscs

Eapen, R. S., & Meng, M. V. (2017). Role of molecular biomarkers in localized prostate cancer. *Urology Times, 45*(4), 14–16.

Jayadevappa, R., Chhatre, S., Wong, Y. N., Wittink, M. N., Cook, R., Morales, K. H., . . . Gallo, J. J. (2017). Comparative effectiveness of prostate cancer treatments for patient-centered outcomes: A systematic review and meta-analysis (PRISMA Compliant). *Medicine, 96*(18), e6790.

National Cancer Institute. (2017). *PDQ Prostate cancer treatment*. Bethesda, MD: Author. Retrieved from https://www.cancer.gov/types/prostate/hp/prostate -treatment-pdq

Paterson, C., Alashkham, A., Windsor, P., & Nabi, G. (2016). Management and treatment of men affected by metastatic prostate cancer: Evidence-based recommendations for practice. *International Journal of Urological Nursing, 10*(1), 44–55.

Williams, S., Hemphill, J. C., & Knowles, A. (2017). Confidence of nursing personnel in their understanding of the psychosocial impact of prostate cancer. *Urologic Nursing, 37*(1), 23–30.

■ RHEUMATOID ARTHRITIS

Susan V. Brindisi

Overview

There are hundreds of different types of arthritis. Rheumatoid arthritis (RA) is one specific type that is considered an autoimmune disease that occurs when antibodies in the body attack the joints. Inflammation occurs in the synovium, the joint lining, which then causes cartilage inflammation. If cartilage inflammation goes unchecked irreversible damage can occur, narrowing the joint space, which can cause loose and unstable joints, joint deformity, and pain. Complications of RA include systemic damage of the heart, lungs, and gastrointestinal tract. RA is a chronic health condition that can be a comorbidity for nurses caring for patients in every setting. Pain management and a clear understanding of current medication treatments are a priority for the nurse taking care of the RA patient. Knowledge of disease progression and its stage will determine the nursing care. It is also important to know what the patient can or cannot do in terms of activities of daily living. Knowledge of assistive devices, including mobility aids, is also essential in the care of the RA patient.

Background

RA is commonly defined as a chronic inflammatory disease of unknown etiology that attacks the articular structures and lining of the joints or synovium (Pinto & Schub, 2016). The disease can cause joint deformity, pain, swelling, tenderness, and various extra-articular manifestations. There is no cure for RA; however, it can go into remission (Schub & Uribe, 2016). According to the Arthritis Foundation (2017), 1.5 million Americans have RA and it is more common in women between 30 and 60 years of age. In men, RA is more common later in life. RA is common in families, although it can manifest in individuals without a family history. RA is also more common in Native Americans. According to Schub and Holle (2016), approximately 50% of patients with RA become disabled after 10 years of disease onset. The overall mortality rate in patients with RA is 2.5 times that of the general population and globally, RA occurs in all people and in all countries.

Clinical Aspects

ASSESSMENT

A diagnosis of RA is made based on classification criteria developed by the American College of Rheumatology/European League Against Rheumatism, 2015 version. A diagnosis of RA includes the presence of synovitis in at least one joint that is not explained by another disease; a calculated score of the number and site of joints involved allows for zero to five possible points. The smaller joints (hand, wrist, feet) score a higher number in that RA tends to effect smaller joints first. After the smaller joints, the larger weight-bearing joints may be affected. Joint symptoms are usually bilateral and symmetrical. Also included are blood tests: a positive serum rheumatoid factor and symptom duration.

Early signs and symptoms of RA can include joint pain, stiffness, fatigue, lethargy, and anorexia. Patients may present to emergency rooms with flare-ups of RA later in the disease progression. Patients with RA may participate in rehabilitation multiple times throughout the course of their lives. Working closely with physical and occupational therapists can improve quality of life and independence for the RA patient. The certified rehabilitation registered nurse (CRRN) serves as a clinical expert and important part of the rehab team in the care of the RA patient.

Serious systemic problems can arise if RA is not treated. These problems can affect the skin, eyes, muscles, blood vessels, heart, and lungs (Pinto & Schub, 2016; Schub & Uribe, 2016). Cardiovascular disease is one serious systemic problem. This is likely due to chronic inflammation that is combined with the often sedentary lifestyle of the RA patient, who might also be overweight. Complications of RA can also include temporomandibular joint disease. This could impair the patient's chewing and ability to eat. In addition, the following can also occur: infection, osteoporosis, lymphadenopathy, and peripheral neuritis. Additional potential complications of RA include pericarditis, pleuritis, pleural effusion, cervical spine instability, anemia, gastrointestinal problems, Sjögren's syndrome, Felty syndrome, lymphoma, and other cancers. Mental health issues include anxiety and depression (Schub & Holle, 2016).

NURSING INTERVENTIONS, MANAGEMENT, AND IMPLICATIONS

Pharmacologic management has progressed in the past 10 years and has made RA a more manageable condition. Drug therapy can slow the progression of RA and treat symptoms. According to Schub and Uribe (2016), drug therapy is most effective when initiated in the early stages of the disease. Disease-modifying antirheumatic drugs (DMARDs) are often the first line of therapy. These include methotrexate, hydroxychloroquine, sulfasalazine, and leflunomide. A second type of drug therapy includes tumor necrosis factor-alpha (TNF-α) antagonists. These include drugs such as etanercept, infliximab, and adalimumab. There are other biologic agents not targeting TNF-α that can reduce inflammation. This includes abatacept, which is a fusion protein that inhibits T-cell activation. Combinations of these agents can often treat RA. Side effects include infection and increased risk of cancer.

Pain management is an important part of RA management. Nonsteroidal anti-inflammatory drugs (NSAIDs) can be used for swelling and pain. They relieve symptoms but do not stop the progression of RA as do the biologic agents. Steroids, especially corticosteroids like prednisone or hydrocortisone, can also be used to decrease inflammation. Other pain management includes acetaminophen, codeine, hydrocodone, morphine, and topical capsaicin (Schub & Uribe, 2016). Nonpharmacologic approaches to treating RA-associated pain include hot and cold therapy and guided imagery.

The nurse assessing the RA patient needs to know the current stage of the disease. In unidentified RA, the nurse can refer to laboratory assessment data and a rheumatologist to make the initial diagnosis. The nurse must assess vital signs and all systems to identify risk for or actual systemic complications. During a clinical assessment, the nurse can palpate the joint for pain, swelling, warmth, erythema, lack of function, or boggy tissue (Smeltzer & Bare, 2004). RA can also cause fever, weight loss, fatigue, anemia, lymph node enlargement, lymphedema, and Raynaud's phenomena (Smeltzer & Bare, 2004). The nurse should note any decreased range of motion and assess for mobility status. Because the RA patient can also experience anorexia, the nurse must also weigh the patient and include a thorough nutrition assessment. RA nursing care includes managing pain, sleep disturbance, altered mood, and limited mobility (Smeltzer & Bare, 2004).

Nursing interventions include application of heat and cold, massage, position change, using a firm mattress, use of splints and pillows, administering antiinflammatory medications as well as other disease-modifying medication. Patient teaching about managing pain and continually monitoring joints in order to maximize lifestyle needs are paramount. The nurse should encourage verbalization about the disease, assessing the need for physical and/or occupational therapy, promoting the use of assistive devices, and encouraging rest after periods of activity. Patient teaching on pain management and medication regimen is a priority to manage activity with RA. Patient teaching should include helping the patient to identify activities that interfere with self-care activities and devising a plan to manage the difficult activities of daily living. Additional nursing interventions include teaching use of appropriate assistive devices for self-care and making a referral to a community agency for help.

OUTCOMES

Expected outcomes as a result of the nursing care of the RA patient focus on the patient living fully and managing disability associated with RA. The patient and family should be comfortable with identifying and managing pain exacerbation, proficient with the use of mobility devices, and identifying community resources that support full living with RA.

Summary

Living with RA is manageable especially with early intervention. Nursing management of RA is crucial to the patient living a fulfilling lifestyle. Teaching must focus on management of disease progression, medication management, positioning, mobility, assistive devices, and working to maintain a healthy lifestyle so that the patient will achieve a positive state of living. Future trends may reflect a larger percentage of patients going into remission as biologic medications for RA become more prevalent.

Arthritis Foundation. (2017). Rheumatoid arthritis. Retrieved from http://www.arthritis
.org/about-arthritis/types/rheumatoid-arthritis/what-is-rheumatoid-arthritis.php

Pinto, S., & Schub, T. (2016). *Arthritis, rheumatoid arthritis (evidence-based care sheet).*
Glendale: CA: CINAHL Information Systems, a division of EBSCO Information
Services.

Schub, T., & Holle, M. N. (2016). *Arthritis, rheumatoid: Complications (quick lesson).*
Glendale, CA: CINAHL Information Systems, a division of EBSCO Information
Services.

Schub, T., & Uribe, L. M. (2016). *Arthritis: Rheumatoid: Drug therapy (quick lesson).*
Glendale, CA: CINAHL Information Systems, a division of EBSCO Information
Services.

Singh, J. A., Saag, K. G., Bridges, L. S., Akl, E. A., Bannuru, R. R., Sullivan, M. C.,
. . . McAlindon, T. (2016). Arthritis and rheumatology: 2015 American College
of Rheumatology guideline for the treatment of rheumatoid arthritis. *Arthritis &
Rheumatology, 68*(1), 1–26. doi:10.1002/art.39480

■ SEPSIS

Sharon Stahl Wexler
Catherine O'Neill D'Amico

Overview

Sepsis is defined as the presence of infection in conjunction with a systemic inflammatory response. The response of the body to infection leads to life-threatening organ dysfunction. Septic shock is defined as sepsis that results in tissue hypoperfusion, hypotension requiring vasopressors, and elevated lactate levels (Howell & Davis, 2017). It is difficult to provide incidence or prevalence data for sepsis as there is no confirmatory diagnostic test for sepsis; diagnosis is based on the evidence of infection and the clinical judgment of the provider (Epstein, Dante, Magill, & Fiore 2016). Sepsis is common and is a leading cause of death, contributing to one third to one half of deaths in hospitalized patients. Patients who develop sepsis have an increased risk of complications and death and face higher health care costs and longer treatment.

Background

Older adults have increased susceptibility to sepsis. This increased susceptibility is due to the many normal age-related changes as well as increased number of comorbid conditions present in many older adults (Umberger, Callen, & Brown, 2015). It is estimated that up to 65% of patients who develop severe sepsis in the United States are older than 65 years (Umberger et al., 2015). Recent years have seen the development of sepsis "bundles" to deal with this serious issue. Major recommendations in these bundles include a focus on identifying infection, managing infection, fluid resuscitation, the use of vasopressors in patients with septic shock, and mechanical ventilation as indicated (Howell & Davis, 2017).

Clinical Aspects

Sepsis is defined as the presence of infection together with systemic manifestations of infection. Sepsis is frequently associated with other conditions such as pneumonia, intestinal obstruction, gallbladder disease, pyelonephritis, or peritonitis. Sepsis is an important complication of major trauma, burns, cancer, and major surgical procedures. Urosepsis is common in older adults. General signs and symptoms of sepsis include fever (often with shaking chills), increased respiratory rate, impaired mental status, and either warm or cold skin.

ASSESSMENT

Diagnostic criteria for sepsis include a documented or suspected infection and some of the following general manifestations, which include alterations in body temperature (fever or hypothermia), increased heart rate, increased respiratory rate, altered mental status, a positive fluid balance, or significant edema and hyperglycemia in the absence of diabetes. Inflammatory manifestations may include leukocytosis, leukopenia, elevated plasma C-reactive protein, elevated plasma procalcitonin, or a normal white blood cell count with more than 10% immature forms. Hemodynamic manifestations include arterial hypotension. Organ dysfunction variables may include arterial hypoxemia, acute oliguria, increased creatinine, coagulation abnormalities, thrombocytopenia, hyperbilirubinemia, or absent bowel sounds.

Diagnostic testing for sepsis includes a variety of laboratory studies, including a complete blood count (CBC), blood cultures, and urine cultures. The specific laboratory study recommended depends on the suspected cause of sepsis, for example, a central line infection would include a culture of the catheter tip. A CBC may show an elevated or low white blood cell count, anemia, or thrombocytopenia. Imaging studies that may be helpful in the diagnosis of sepsis also depend on the suspected cause. A chest x-ray is indicated to rule out pneumonia and other pulmonary causes. An abdominal ultrasound is useful when there is a suspected biliary tract obstruction. An abdominal CT or MRI may be useful in assessing other intra-abdominal sources of infection.

Hospitalized patients and individuals presenting in a local emergency room may or may not have the "usual signs of infection," including elevated body temperature; skin lesions; inflammatory signs and symptoms affecting the gastrointestinal, respiratory, or urinary tract. Some individuals, particularly older adults, may present with nonspecific and nonlocalized symptoms, including complaints of not feeling well, no elevation of body temperature, or family members who indicate that the individual is experiencing changes in usual behavior or complaints of inability to do usual tasks (Englert & Ross, 2015; Quan et al., 2013; Umberger et al., 2015). A thorough history followed by head-to-toe assessment of these individuals and individuals who present with the usual signs of infections and inflammation should be initiated by the nurse (Agency for Healthcare Research and Quality [AHRQ], 2013; Umberger et al., 2015).

NURSING INTERVENTIONS, MANAGEMENT, AND IMPLICATIONS

Individuals with other identified comorbidities are at greater risk for having sepsis (Englert & Ross, 2015; Novosad et al., 2016; Quan et al., 2013; Umberger et al., 2015). These comorbidities, which increase the risk for sepsis, include age greater than 75 years, immunosuppression (cancer and cancer treatments, treatment with corticosteroids), recent invasive procedure or surgery, diabetes, cardiovascular diseases, chronic kidney disease, and chronic obstructive pulmonary disease, indwelling urinary catheters, or intravenous access (Novosad et al., 2016; Quan et al., 2013; Umberger et al., 2015).

Initial management of sepsis typically includes transfer to a hospital setting if the patient is not in an acute care setting. Within the acute care setting, transfer to an intensive care setting for close monitoring and treatment is usually indicated. Swan–Ganz catheterization is frequently used to help manage fluid status.

Supportive therapy to maintain organ perfusion and respiration is initiated based on individual patient presentation. Empiric antibiotic therapy is initiated followed by antibiotic therapy that is specific to the infecting organism presumed to be the source of the sepsis. Appropriate antibiotics to treat sepsis are usually combinations of two or three antibiotics given at the same time. Surgery may be indicated to drain or remove the source of infection.

The interdisciplinary team initiates the following laboratory tests: blood gases, including glucose and lactate measurement, blood culture, CBC, C-reactive protein, blood urea nitrogen (BUN) and electrolytes, creatinine, and clotting screening. Central intravenous access is initiated in addition to any peripheral access that was initiated during the assessment. Based on the AHRQ (Quan et al., 2013) criteria, acute care facilities begin intravenous fluid bolus and broad spectrum antibiotics are initiated within 1 hour after the lactate and blood cultures are obtained. Intravenous fluids are given as a bolus of 500 mL within 15 minutes. The broad spectrum antibiotics recommended are typically those in the penicillin, sulfonamides, glycopeptide, and aminoglycoside classes. Antibiotics are to be initiated immediately after the blood cultures are obtained and within 1 hour of meeting the criteria that sepsis is likely. Usually two medications are prescribed in combination based on the assessment and the likely source of the initial infection.

The individual with sepsis or septic shock is moved to the intensive care unit (ICU) where additional measures to support hypovolemia, ventilation and oxygenation, and urinary output are initiated and level of consciousness is monitored closely. Life-support measures include the administration of fluids and vasopressors, anticoagulation, mechanical ventilation, and oxygen supplementation. Changes in the antibiotic regimen and monitoring the effectiveness of the treatment should be continuously evaluated. As the individual responds to the antibiotics and vasopressor use is diminished, the individual can be moved out of the critical care environment.

OUTCOMES

Sepsis in the adult and older adult is a medical emergency requiring quick and effective action by the interdisciplinary team. Early recognition of sepsis may be the best hope for a positive outcome (Howell & Davis, 2017). Multiple authors cite early recognition and initiation of treatment as the factor that decreases the odds that the patient will die from sepsis (DeBacker & Dorman, 2017; Howell & Davis, 2017; Stoller et al., 2016). It has been noted recently that sepsis accounts for more hospital readmissions than any of the four conditions currently tracked by the federal government for guiding reimbursement and quality care, and remains one of the leading causes of death for hospitalized patients (DeBacker & Dorman, 2017; Mayr et al., 2017). Studies identify that despite new treatments and early-recognition practices, 20% to 45% of those diagnosed do not survive (Novosad et al., 2016; Stoller et al., 2016). The recognition of this problem has led to the development of interdisciplinary best practices for the early identification and treatment of sepsis of the hospitalized adult and older adult.

The prognosis of a patient with sepsis is related to the severity of the sepsis, the underlying condition of the patient, and the stage at which the sepsis is diagnosed. Patients with sepsis and no signs of organ failure at the time of diagnosis have about a 15% to 30% chance of death. Elderly patients have the highest death rates (DeBacker & Dorman, 2017).

Because the sepsis morbidity and mortality rate is high, nurses and the interdisciplinary staff must keep families informed about the potential outcomes for the individual. The nurse and the interdisciplinary team need to be aware of the advanced directives that are in place before and during aggressive resuscitation as well as the potential for progressive organ failure. Planning for the end of life or palliative care should be considered if the individual or the family want to limit resuscitation measures (Englert & Ross, 2015; Quan et al., 2013; Umberger et al., 2015). Discharge instructions by the nurse to the individual and family should include instructions about symptoms to monitor, how to seek medical attention if these symptoms occur, including how to get urgent medical attention (Quan et al., 2013). The nurse should provide the individual and the family time to ask questions and address concerns, including whether this will happen again, how to prevent it from happening again, and details of arrangements made for the care of any residual treatments (tracheostomy care, peripherally inserted central catheter [PICC] line care; Quan et al., 2013).

Summary

Sepsis is a medical emergency with significant morbidity and mortality. It is a leading cause of hospitalization and mortality for patients of all ages. Older adults are of particular risk due to the many normal age-related changes and possible multiple comorbidities, making diagnosis a challenge. The role of the nurse in caring for patients with sepsis begins with infection prevention and progresses to recognition of the signs and symptoms of sepsis and the early initiation of fluids, vasopressors, and antibiotics for the treatment of sepsis. Current treatment of sepsis includes the use of bundles to simplify the complex processes of care of the patient with sepsis.

DeBacker, D., & Dorman, T. (2017). Surviving sepsis guidelines: A continuous move toward better care of patients with sepsis. *Journal of the American Medical Association.* Advance online publication. doi:10.1001/jama.2017.0059. Retrieved from http://jamanetwork.com/pdfaccess.ashx?url=/data/journals/jama/0

Englert, N. C., & Ross, C. (2015). The older adult experiencing sepsis. *Critical Care Nursing Quarterly, 38*(2), 175–181.

Epstein, L., Dantes, R., Magill, S., & Fiore, A. (2016). Varying estimates of sepsis mortality using death certificates and administrative codes—United States, 1999–2014. *Morbidity and Mortality Weekly Report, 65*(13), 342–345.

Howell, M. D., & Davis, A. M. (2017). Management of sepsis and septic shock. *Journal of the American Medical Association, 317*(8), 847–848.

Mayr, F. B., Talisa, V. B., Balakumar, V., Chang, C. H., Fine, M., & Yende, S. (2017). Proportion and cost of unplanned 30-day readmissions after sepsis compared with other medical conditions. *Journal of the American Medical Association, 317*(5), 530–531.

Novosad, S. A., Sapiano, M. R., Grigg, C., Lake, J., Robyn, M., Dumyati, G., . . . Epstein, L. (2016). Vital signs: Epidemiology of sepsis: Prevalence of health care factors and opportunities for prevention. *Morbidity and Mortality Weekly Report, 65*(33), 864–869.

Quan, H., Eastwood, C., Cunningham, C. T., Liu, M., Flemons, W., De Coster, C., & Ghali, W. A.; IMECCHI investigators. (2013). Validity of AHRQ patient safety indicators derived from ICD-10 hospital discharge abstract data (chart review study). *BMJ Open, 3*(10), e003716.

Stoller, J., Halpin, L., Weis, M., Aplin, B., Qu, W., Georgescu, C., & Nazzal, M. (2016). Epidemiology of severe sepsis: 2008-2012. *Journal of Critical Care, 31*, 58–62.

Umberger, R., Callen, B., & Brown, M. L. (2015). Severe sepsis in older adults. *Critical Care Nursing Quarterly, 38*(3), 259–270.

■ SICKLE CELL DISEASE

Consuela A. Albright

Overview

Sickle cell disease is a heritable, chronic disorder of the blood. Abnormalities in the composition of hemoglobin give red blood cells a sickle shape and affect the viscosity, life span, and oxygen-carrying capacity of the cell. Sickle cell disease affects multiple organs, including the brain, heart, eyes, lungs, kidneys, liver, and spleen. Acute symptoms may lead to organ damage, organ failure, and death. Care for persons with acute exacerbation of sickle cell disease should focus on reversal of symptoms through replacement of red blood cells, hydration, oxygenation, pain management, and early recognition and treatment of underlying causes to prevent secondary complications (Yawn et al., 2014).

Background

The National Heart, Lung, and Blood Institute (NHLBI) reports that sickle cell disease affects individuals of African, Hispanic, Southern European, Middle Eastern, and Asian Indian descent (NHLBI, 2016). The Centers for Disease Control and Prevention (CDC) estimate that approximately 100,000 Americans are currently affected by sickle cell disease (CDC, 2016). Sickle cell disease is caused by an autosomal recessive inheritance; a child born with sickle cell disease receives two copies of the recessive gene, one from each parent. One of every 365 African American children born in the United States has sickle cell disease, and one of every 16,300 Hispanic American children born in the United States has sickle cell disease (CDC, 2016).

All children born in the United States are tested for sickle cell disease and sickle cell trait with newborn screening. One in 13 African American babies is born with one copy of the sickle cell gene, known as sickle cell trait. Carriers of sickle cell trait do not exhibit any symptoms of sickle cell disease (CDC, 2016). Individuals with sickle cell trait have a 50% chance of passing the trait to their children, and two carriers of sickle cell trait have a 25% chance of conceiving a child with sickle cell disease (CDC, 2016).

Sickle cell disease is the result of a point mutation of the amino acids at the sixth position of the beta chain of the hemoglobin molecule. Normal adult hemoglobin (HbA) contains glutamic acid at the sixth position of the beta chain, whereas sickle hemoglobin (HbS) has valine at its sixth position. HbS makes red blood cells sickle shaped, rigid, and sticky (Yosmanovich, Rotter, Aprelev, & Ferrone, 2016). HbS is sensitive to dehydration, hypoxia, infectious processes, and temperature changes; these stressors trigger clumping of red blood cells in the vascular space, known as sickle cell crisis.

The long-term effects of sickle cell disease are the result of vaso-occlusion in sickle cell crises. Damage to the neurologic, cardiovascular, respiratory, renal, musculoskeletal, hepatic, and genitourinary systems causes complications secondary to sickle cell disease. Chronic pain is another secondary complication of sickle cell disease. The prognosis for an individual with sickle cell disease is dependent on the type and severity of sickle cell disease. Patients with HbSS and HbS/β^0 thalassemia experience marked severity of disease than do patients with HbSC, HbS, and HbS/β^+ thalassemia. Rarer forms of sickle cell disease are HbSD, HbSE, and HbSO, and each varies in severity (CDC, 2015). The mean age of mortality for sickle cell patients by disease type is HbSS (35.19 years), HbSC (44.47 years), HbS/β^0 thalassemia (41 years), and HbS/β^+ thalassemia (30.5 years; Ngo et al., 2014).

Sickle cell disease presents once levels of fetal hemoglobin (HbF) fall and HbS levels rise between 6 and 12 months (Bender & Douthitt Seibel, 2014). HbF has a high affinity for oxygen and inhibits sickling of blood cells. The life span of a sickled blood cell is 10 to 20 days, compared to healthy red blood cells' life span of 100 to 120 days, causing a decrease in the number of circulating mature red blood cells, resulting in an anemic state (NHLBI, 2014). Adult and pediatric patients may present with yellowing of the sclera (icterus), a sign of jaundice. Jaundice is caused by rapid lysis of red blood cells, buildup of excess bilirubin in tissues, and inability of the liver to process bilirubin at the same rate of cell lysis (Bender & Douthitt Seibel, 2014).

Clinical Aspects

ASSESSMENT

History and physical assessment are key to treating a patient in sickle cell crisis. A detailed medical history, including the type of sickle cell disease, should be taken. The history must also include information about the onset, duration, and location of symptoms, and baseline vital signs, paying close attention to pulse oximetry. Ongoing, thorough physical assessment and vital sign monitoring will alert a nurse in the acute care setting to changes from baseline in the patient's condition.

Sickle cell crises vary in presentation, but pain is a hallmark finding. Pain may be localized to the head, face, bones, abdomen, back, or chest with a sudden, severe onset. Vaso-occlusion in the brain is a risk for stroke in children and adults with sickle cell. Strokes in children with sickle cell are responsible for long-term cognitive deficits. The initial presentation of sickle cell crisis in a young child could present as painful swelling of the hands and feet (dactylitis). Adults may report hand and foot pain, as well as pain in the long bones of the upper and lower extremities. Male patients may experience priapism, a penile erection caused by vaso-occlusion. Abdominal pain in a patient with sickle cell crisis should be evaluated to rule out splenic sequestration, a life-threatening complication in which sickled red blood cells become trapped in the spleen, causing a drop in the volume of circulating red blood cells, leading to hypovolemic shock. Splenic sequestration may require surgical removal of the spleen (Bender & Douthitt Seibel, 2014).

Acute chest syndrome is a complication of sickle cell disease affecting adults and children alike. A vaso-occlusive crisis decreases perfusion of the lungs and leads to respiratory failure and death. Acute chest syndrome is triggered by infection, pneumonia, respiratory disease, emboli, or any other stressor that initiates hypoxemia and sickling. Clinically, acute chest syndrome is defined as new pulmonary infiltrate on chest x-ray, accompanied by fever, hypoxemia, tachypnea, wheezing, or cough (Bender & Douthitt Seibel, 2014).

A nurse should anticipate diagnostic testing and laboratory workup for appropriate treatment of symptoms. Diagnostic testing will include chest x-ray, CT scan, complete blood count with differential, electrolytes, renal function panel (blood urea nitrogen [BUN]/creatinine), urinalysis, hepatic function (alanine transaminase [ALT], bilirubin), blood culture, and arterial blood gases.

OUTCOMES

The goal of treatment for sickle cell crisis is immediate reversal of symptoms and treatment of the underlying cause (Lentz & Kautz, 2017). The amount of sickled blood cells may require exchange transfusion, in which the recipient's blood is phlebotomized and replaced in equal volumes with donor blood to reduce the amount of sickled blood in circulation. Intravenous fluid resuscitation reverses dehydration. The nurse should be prepared to administer analgesics, supplemental oxygen, and pharmacologic treatment of the underlying cause to prevent deterioration of the patient's condition. Initiation of treatment with hydroxyurea may also occur in the acute care setting. Hydroxyurea increases the levels of HbF, which increases the amount of normal red blood cells in circulation (Yawn et al., 2014).

Summary

Sickle cell disease is a lifelong condition of varying severity. Patients with sickle cell disease may have frequent admissions to the acute care setting for exacerbation of symptoms. Pain in the patient with sickle cell anemia is poorly understood in the acute care setting, as it is chronic and patient responses to pain vary significantly among individuals. Nurses in the acute care setting should be reminded that pain is a very real symptom of sickle cell crisis that should be assessed frequently and treated as needed. Aggressive treatment of sickle cell crisis and underlying causes of symptoms is necessary to prevent life-threatening complications of the disease.

Bender, M. A., & Douthitt Seibel, G. (2014). Sickle cell disease. Retrieved from https://www.ncbi.nlm.nih.gov/books/NBK1377

Centers for Disease Control and Prevention. (2015). Sickle cell trait. Retrieved from https://www.cdc.gov/ncbddd/sicklecell/traits.html

Centers for Disease Control and Prevention. (2016). Data & statistics. Retrieved from https://www.cdc.gov/ncbddd/sicklecell/data.html

Lentz, M. B., & Kautz, D. D. (2017). Acute vaso-occlusive crisis in patients with sickle cell disease. *Nursing, 47*(1), 67–68.

National Heart, Lung and Blood Institute. (2014). Sickle cell anemia. Retrieved from https://www.ncbi.nlm.nih.gov/pubmedhealth/PM

National Heart, Lung, and Blood Institute. (2016). Who is at risk for sickle cell disease? Retrieved from https://www.nhlbi.nih.gov/health/health-topics/topics/sca/atrisk

Ngo, S., Bartolucci, P., Lobo, D., Mekontso-Dessap, A., Gellen-Dautremer, J., Noizat-Pirenne, F., . . . Habibi, A. (2014). Causes of death in sickle cell disease adult patients: Old and new trends. *Blood, 124*(21), 2715. Retrieved from http://www.bloodjournal.org/content/124/21/2715

Yawn, B. P., Buchanan, G. R., Afenyi-Annan, A. N., Ballas, S. K., Hassell, K. L., James, A. H., . . . Tanabe, P. J. (2014). Management of sickle cell disease: Summary of the 2014 evidence-based report by expert panel members. *Journal of the American Medical Association, 312*(10), 1033–1048.

Yosmanovich, D., Rotter, M., Aprelev, A., & Ferrone, F. A. (2016). Calibrating sickle cell disease. *Journal of Molecular Biology, 428*(8), 1506–1514. doi:10.1016/j.jmb.2016.03.001

■ SLEEP APNEA

Deborah H. Cantero
Leslie J. Lockett
Rebecca M. Lutz

Overview

Sleep apnea (SA) results in daily functional impairment and increases the patient's risk of multisystem health disorders. SA is characterized by repetitive apneic cycles that result in disrupted sleep. Categories of SA include obstructive sleep apnea (OSA) and central sleep apnea (CSA). Management of SA requires a long-term, multidisciplinary approach aimed at decreasing apneic episodes, thereby improving long-term health outcomes.

Background

SA is a chronic condition resulting in repeated cycles of apnea or intermittent episodes of decreased inspiratory effort (hypopnea). An apneic or hypopneic episode typically lasts a minimum of 10 seconds (Kasper et al., 2016). With each apneic or hypopneic episode, the oxygen saturation level decreases. With apneic episodes, increasing the partial pressure of carbon dioxide in the circulatory system, an individual is prone to recurrent cycles of arousal, and even awakenings, while sleeping (Semelka, Wilson, & Floyd, 2016; Zinchuk & Thomas, 2017).

The most common form of SA is OSA. In OSA, there is thoracic and diaphragmatic respiratory effort; however, the airway is partially or completely obstructed. Airway obstruction in the upper airway is due to pharyngeal muscle relaxation with collapse (Chesnutt & Prendergast, 2017). In contrast, CSA is associated with decreased or ineffective respiratory drive as a result of impaired stimulation from central nervous system injury or medications (Zinchuk & Thomas, 2017).

SA occurs across the life span. OSA is diagnosed in approximately 4% of the population, although research estimates that up to 24% of the population is undiagnosed (DiNapoli, 2014). Of all the sleep-related breathing disorders, approximately 10% are CSA in origin (Zinchuk & Thomas, 2017). Risk factors include obesity, family history of SA, age 40 to 70 years, male gender, being postmenopausal, endocrine-associated conditions, certain anatomical features, central nervous system disorders, and opioid use (Kasper et al., 2016; Semelka et al., 2016). Untreated SA increases the risk of cardiac complications due to effects on the sympathetic nervous system (Kasper et al., 2016). This impacts quality of life as patients often exhibit excessive daytime sleepiness, potential changes in mood or cognition, and increased risk for occupational injury (DiNapoli, 2014).

Clinical Aspects

ASSESSMENT

Nursing assessment begins with a thorough health history to identify key aspects to guide nursing interventions. History includes investigation of regular snoring, apneic gasps, and daytime drowsiness as well as apnea reported by a sleeping partner (Avidan & Kryger, 2017). Additional assessment would include use of opiates, morning headache, excessive sleepiness, sleep duration, decreased concentration, poor memory, and motor vehicle accidents related to sleepiness. Safety considerations regarding anesthesia and postoperative recovery should also be evaluated (Avidan & Kryger, 2017). Modifiable contributing risk factors, such as obesity, smoking, and alcohol intake, should be noted. All findings should be recorded for other providers.

Objective assessment includes the observance of physical characteristics, including excessive weight, short thick neck, and any evidence of upper airway narrowing such as tonsillar hypertrophy. Secondary conditions to assess include associated hypertension (HTN), congestive heart failure (CHF), arrhythmias, myocardial infarction, and cor pulmonale (Obstructive Sleep Apnea Task Force of the American Academy of Sleep Medicine, 2009). A thorough head-to-toe assessment is necessary to inform the nurse in developing a care plan, promoting optimal health for the patient, and preventing complications.

The clinical characteristics of OSA and CSA may overlap, and definitive diagnosis is made with a polysomnography (PSG) sleep study (Obstructive Sleep Apnea Task Force of the American Academy of Sleep Medicine, 2009; Zinchuk & Thomas, 2017). The PSG study and the apnea–hypopnea index (AHI) allow the provider to distinguish between OSA and CSA (Zinchuk & Thomas, 2017). Medicare guidelines for the initiation of therapy for continuous positive airway pressure (CPAP) parameters include: (a) AHI greater than 15, eligible for CPAP and (b) AHI of 5 to 14, eligible if excessive sleepiness, HTN, or cardiovascular disease is documented (Downey, 2017).

Once treatment is initiated, nurses should continually assess and monitor for evidence of hypoxia or hypoxemia. In addition, nurses should focus on interventions regarding assessment, education, and interdisciplinary referrals. This is particularly important because compliance is a documented issue within this population. Therefore, education is critical for the patient's understanding of the increased risk for complications associated with SA (DiNapoli, 2014). Adherence, comfort, knowledge of therapy, and readiness to learn should also be assessed.

Using principles of adult learning and patient-centered care, nurses should convey the pathophysiology, risk factors, natural history, and clinical consequences of SA to both the patient and the caregiver (DiNapoli, 2014). This encourages engagement in the treatment plan. Including the caregiver is also important due to the potential for neurocognitive and physiological consequences of hypoxia, which may limit the patient's full understanding of SA and therefore limit compliance with therapy (DiNapoli, 2014; Obstructive Sleep

Apnea Task Force of the American Academy of Sleep Medicine, 2009). On initiation of therapy, and with all subsequent reevaluations, education on CPAP device usage and cleaning procedures, sleep position, and good sleep hygiene is essential (Downey, 2017; Obstructive Sleep Apnea Task Force of the American Academy of Sleep Medicine, 2009). Risk reduction education on the impact of weight loss, sleep positions, alcohol avoidance, and risks of driving while drowsy should be included to promote self-care with this chronic condition (Obstructive Sleep Apnea Task Force of the American Academy of Sleep Medicine, 2009).

OUTCOMES

Interdisciplinary referrals for care collaboration, including respiratory therapy, sleep specialists, and group behavioral therapy, have demonstrated increased compliance (DiNapoli, 2014). Prompt attention to adverse effects of CPAP (nasal stuffiness, dry eyes, skin irritation, and claustrophobia) and adjustments in the treatment plan promote compliance (DiNapoli, 2014; Downey, 2017). Finally, follow-up with the provider to evaluate effectiveness within 2 months is recommended (Downey, 2017). The major outcomes of the interventions include patient report of resolution of sleepiness, patient/spouse satisfaction, adherence to therapy, and improvement in quality of life (Freedman, 2017; Obstructive Sleep Apnea Task Force of the American Academy of Sleep Medicine, 2009).

Summary

SA, whether obstructive or central, disrupts sleep patterns and may result in increased morbidity and mortality. Causes of SA are variable, therefore medical and nursing interventions must also be customized for each patient. Nursing care begins with a thorough assessment of the physical, social, and psychological impact SA has on the patient's quality of life. Nursing interventions include an emphasis on patient and caregiver education aimed at improving understanding and compliance. The primary goal of care is to decrease the frequency of apneic episodes, improve quality of life, and ultimately decrease multiorgan impairment or death.

Avidan, E. Y., & Kryger, M. (2017). Physical examination in sleep medicine. In M. H. Kryger & T. Roth (Eds.), *Principles and practice of sleep medicine* (6th ed., pp. 587–606). Philadelphia, PA: Elsevier. Retrieved from http://www.sciencedirect.com.ezproxy.lib.usf.edu/science/article/pii/B9780323242882000593

Chesnutt, M. S., & Prendergast, T. J. (2017). Pulmonary disorders. In M. A. Papadakis, S. J. McPhee, & M. W. Rabow (Eds.), *Current medical diagnosis & treatment 2017* (56th ed). New York, NY: McGraw-Hill. Retrieved from http://accessmedicine.mhmedical.com.ezproxy.hsc.usf.edu/content.aspx?bookid=1843&sectionid=135704883

DiNapoli, C. M. (2014). Strategies to improve continuous positive airway pressure: A review. *Journal of Nursing Education and Practice, 5*(2), 110–116. doi:10.5430/jnep.v5n2p110

Downey, R. (2017). Obstructive sleep apnea. *Medscape*. Retrieved from http://emedicine .medscape.com/article/295807-overview

Freedman, N. (2017). Positive airway pressure treatment for obstructive sleep apnea. In M. H. Kryger & T. Roth (Eds.), *Principles and practice of sleep medicine* (6th ed., pp. 1125–1137). Philadelphia, PA: Elsevier. Retrieved from http://www.sciencedirect .com.ezproxy.lib.usf.edu/science/article/pii/B978032324288200115X

Kasper, D. L., Fauci, A. S., Hauser, S. L., Longo, D. L., Jameson, J., & Loscalzo, J. (2016). Sleep apnea. In D. L. Kasper, A. S. Fauci, S. L. Hauser, D. L. Longo, J. Jameson, & J. Loscalzo (Eds.), *Harrison's manual of medicine* (19th ed., pp. 745–746). New York, NY: McGraw-Hill. Retrieved from http://access medicine.mhmedical.com/Book.aspx?bookid=1820

Obstructive Sleep Apnea Task Force of the American Academy of Sleep Medicine. (2009). Clinical guideline for the evaluation, management and long-term care of obstructive sleep apnea in adults. *Journal of Clinical Sleep Medicine, 5*(3), 263–276. Retrieved https://www.ncbi.nlm.nih.gov/pmc/articles/PMC2699173

Semelka, M., Wilson, J., & Floyd, R. (2016). Diagnosis and treatment of obstructive sleep apnea in adults. *American Family Physician, 94*(5), 355–360. Retrieved from http://www.aafp.org/afp/2016/0901/p355.html

Zinchuk, A. V., & Thomas, R. J. (2017). Central sleep apnea: Diagnosis and management. In M. H. Kryger & T. Roth (Eds.), *Principles and practice of sleep medicine* (6th ed., pp. 1059–1074). Philadelphia, PA: Elsevier. Retrieved from http://www.science direct.com.ezproxy.lib.usf.edu/science/article/pii/B9780323242882001100

■ SPINAL STENOSIS AND DISC HERNIATION

Steven R. Collier

Overview

Spinal stenosis and disc herniation are common findings in the general population. Spinal stenosis has been defined in many studies as having a spinal canal dimension of 10 mm or less in the anterior–posterior plane of measurement, and the symptoms of pain, paresthesias, and dysesthesias in the legs. Although these patients may have spinal stenosis diagnosed by imaging, they are not always symptomatic (Kalichman et al., 2009). Disc herniation is defined as a focal projection of disc material into the spinal canal or neural foramina greater than 3 mm and may be situated posteriorly, cephalad, caudally, or can form a free-floating disc fragment (Fardon et al., 2014). Nursing care for these patients focuses on rehabilitation, mobilization, identification of surgical emergencies, and perioperative care for patients treated with surgical intervention.

Background

Neck pain and low-back pain are common medical conditions in the United States and around the world. The global prevalence of neck pain is 4.9% and is 6.5% in the United States (March et al., 2014). Low-back pain has a global prevalence rate of 9.4% and 7.7% in the United States (March et al., 2014). Neck pain tends to occur at a younger age with a mean age of 45 years, and is more common in females, whereas back pain peaks later in life with a mean age of 80 years and is seen more frequently in males (March et al., 2014). Spinal stenosis and disc herniation are leading causes of neck pain and low-back pain.

Lumbar spinal stenosis occurs most often in patients who are 65 years or older and occurs slightly more often in men than in women (Weinstein et al., 2008). The findings for cervical stenosis are similar, with the incidence increasing with advancing age, and occurring slightly more often in men than in women (Nagata et al., 2012). Risk factors include being overweight, having elevated body mass index (BMI), occupations involving manual labor, and for men, diabetes (Abbas et al., 2013). Smoking was not linked to an increased risk of spinal stenosis (Abbas et al., 2013). Spinal stenosis can be caused by degenerative disc disease (DDD), spondylosis, spondylolisthesis, hypertrophy of the ligamentum flavum, tumors, cysts, infection, and congenital narrowing of the spinal canal. Lumbar stenosis can occur at any level in the lumbar spine, but occurs more frequently at L4–L5, then L3–L4 centrally; neural foraminal stenosis occurs most frequently at L5–S1, followed by L4–L5 (Ishimoto et al., 2013). Cervical stenosis is noted most frequently at C5–C6, followed by C4–C5, then C6–C7 (Nagata et al., 2012).

The diagnosis of cervical spinal stenosis is made by a combination of MRI/CT findings of decreased spinal canal diameter and physical exam findings of arm and possibly leg paresthesias and dysesthesias, hyperreflexia, Hoffman's sign, up-going Babinski reflex, discoordination, and possibly gait instability (Nagata et al., 2012). Diagnosis of lumbar spinal stenosis is made by a combination of MRI/CT findings of decreased spinal canal diameter and physical exam findings of leg paresthesias and dysesthesias that can occur at rest, but are exacerbated with ambulation or standing and spinal extension, and usually improve with rest or spinal flexion (Kreiner et al., 2013).

The incidence and prevalence of cervical disc herniation is difficult to define because approximately 10% of herniations found on imaging in persons younger than 40 years and 5% in persons more than 40 years are asymptomatic (Hammer, Heller, & Kepler, 2015). Cervical disc herniation may be caused by trauma or jobs that require heavy lifting or repeated stress to the spine (Hammer et al., 2015).

The mean age for diagnosis of lumbar disc herniation is 41 years and is slightly more prevalent in males than in females (Schroeder, Guyre, & Vaccaro, 2015). Risk factors include obesity, heavy lifting with twisting and bending, and family history of herniated disc (Schroeder et al., 2015). Patients with increased stress and time-sensitive jobs also appear to be at higher risk for lumbar disc herniation (Schroeder et al., 2015). The symptoms for cervical and lumbar disc herniation are largely the same as listed previously for stenosis, but can occur more acutely when the result of trauma.

Spinal disorders are a major source of health care spending. Patients with spine problems are more likely to limit their social interactions, have decreased physical functioning, and miss school or work than persons without spine disease.

Clinical Aspects

ASSESSMENT

Nursing management of patients with spinal stenosis and disc herniation is heavily reliant on an accurate physical assessment with a focus on the neurological exam. The history should focus on the temporal aspect of the onset of the pain or the decrease in neurological function. An accurate history of the patient's current and past medical problems, along with any interventional or surgical procedures should be recorded. Medication lists should be obtained and accurately verified for any history of spinal injections or use of immunosuppressants within the last several months.

The physical exam consists of a head-to-toe assessment focusing on the neurological exam. Special attention is paid to any areas of spinal tenderness with palpation, any deformities of the spine, or abnormal posture. Strength testing of all major extremity muscle groups along with reflex testing and sensation testing are crucial to accurate diagnosis. Special reflex testing should include testing for the Hoffman and Babinski reflexes and for clonus. The gait should be observed for any alterations, inability to heel or toe walk, and inability to walk heel to toe in a straight line. Rectal tone should be assessed if the patient reports any bowel or bladder incontinence, or saddle area anesthesia.

Imaging for patients with spine pain that is consistent with stenosis or disc herniation is often appropriate for MRI, or if contraindicated, CT imaging of the spine (Kreiner et al., 2014). Plain film x-rays can be helpful in the examination of posture, or initial rapid imaging for fracture, or checking of previous spinal hardware. There are no specific laboratory tests for spinal stenosis or disc herniation, but an elevated white blood cell count and C-reactive protein (CRP) may indicate spinal infection, although these findings are nonspecific.

NURSING INTERVENTIONS, MANAGEMENT, AND IMPLICATIONS

The nursing care of patients with spinal stenosis or disc herniation focuses on promoting mobility and managing pain. Many patients need assistance with mobility, and even assistance with passive and active range of motion (PROM and AROM). If bracing is used as treatment or postoperatively, assuring proper fit and application along with checking of the skin under the brace is required.

Patients with cervical stenosis with myelopathy or cervical disc herniation with Brown–Sequard syndrome can have special needs ranging from total care to assistance with toileting, feeding, and hydration. Patients with lumbar stenosis or disc herniation may require assistance with ambulation and range of motion, as well as assistance with bladder catheterization and bowel regimens for neurogenic bowel and bladder dysfunction. Cauda equina is characterized by an acute onset of severe radicular leg pain, bowel and bladder dysfunction, and saddle area anesthesia. Cauda equina is a surgical emergency and prompt recognition of symptoms is crucial; the degree of patient recovery depends on rapid diagnosis and treatment. The opioid epidemic must be taken into account when managing patients with spinal disorders. Acute spine pain can be appropriately managed with opiate pain medication; however, there is no sufficient evidence to support the use of opiates for the chronic management of spinal pain management (Simon, Conliffe, & Kitei, 2015).

OUTCOMES

Rapid identification of neurological changes based on serial neurological examinations is critical in preserving function and limiting loss of function in the patient with a spinal disorder. Evidence-based nursing interventions are similarly focused on preservation and maximization of neurological function. Promotion of rehabilitation and therapy with the use of AROM and PROM, along with medication management, supports the achievement of optimal patient recovery, and limits permanent disabilities from occurring.

Summary

Most patients diagnosed with spinal stenosis or disc herniation can usually be managed conservatively and return to their baseline functional status. Spinal stenosis and disc herniation are prevalent in the adult population and are a leading cause of disability and decreased productivity. Early intervention and recognition of neurological decline in these patients is essential and evidence-based rehabilitation leads to optimal recovery.

Abbas, J., Hamoud, K., May, H., Peled, N., Sarig, R., Stein, D., . . . Hershkovitz, I. (2013). Socioeconomic and physical characteristics of individuals with degenerative lumbar spinal stenosis. *Spine, 38*(9), E554–E561. doi:10.1097/BRS.0b013e31828a2846

Fardon, D. F., Williams, A. L., Dohring, E. J., Murtagh, F. R., Gabriel Rothman, S. L., & Sze, G. K. (2014). Lumbar disc nomenclature: Version 2.0: Recommendations of the combined task forces of the North American Spine Society, the American Society of Spine Radiology and the American Society of Neuroradiology. *Spine Journal, 14*(11), 2525–2545. doi:10.1016/j.spinee.2014.04.022

Hammer, C., Heller, J., & Kepler, C. (2015). Epidemiology and pathophysiology of cervical disc herniation. *Seminars in Spine Surgery, 28*(2), 64–67. doi:10.1053/j.semss.2015.11.009

Ishimoto, Y., Yoshimura, N., Muraki, S., Yamada, H., Nagata, K., Hashizume, H., . . . Yoshida, M. (2013). Associations between radiographic lumbar spinal stenosis and clinical symptoms in the general population: The Wakayama Spine Study. *Osteoarthritis and Cartilage, 21*(6), 783–788. doi:10.1016/j.joca.2013.02.656

Kalichman, L., Cole, R., Kim, D. H., Li, L., Suri, P., Guermazi, A., & Hunter, D. J. (2009). Spinal stenosis prevalence and association with symptoms: The Framingham Study. *Spine Journal, 9*(7), 545–550. doi:10.1016/j.spinee.2009.03.005

Kreiner, D. S., Hwang, S. W., Easa, J. E., Resnick, D. K., Baisden, J. L., Bess, S., . . . Toton, J. F. (2014). An evidence-based clinical guideline for the diagnosis and treatment of lumbar disc herniation with radiculopathy. *Spine Journal, 14*(1), 180–191. doi:10.1016/j.spinee.2013.08.003

Kreiner, D. S., Shaffer, W. O., Baisden, J. L., Gilbert, T. J., Summers, J. T., Toton, J. F., . . . Reitman, C. A. (2013). An evidence-based clinical guideline for the diagnosis and treatment of degenerative lumbar spinal stenosis (update). *Spine Journal, 13*(7), 734–743. doi:10.1016/j.spinee.2012.11.059

March, L., Smith, E. U., Hoy, D. G., Cross, M. J., Sanchez-Riera, L., Blyth, F., . . . Woolf, A. D. (2014). Burden of disability due to musculoskeletal (MSK) disorders. *Best Practice & Research: Clinical Rheumatology, 28*(3), 353–366. doi:10.1016/j.berh.2014.08.002

Nagata, K., Yoshimura, N., Muraki, S., Hashizume, H., Ishimoto, Y., Yamada, H., . . . Yoshida, M. (2012). Prevalence of cervical cord compression and its association with physical performance in a population-based cohort in Japan: The Wakayama Spine Study. *Spine, 37*(22), 1892–1898. doi:10.1097/BRS.0b013e31825a2619

Schroeder, G. D., Guyre, C. A., & Vaccaro, A. R. The epidemiology and pathophysiology of lumbar disc herniations. *Seminars in Spine Surgery, 28*(1), 2–7. doi:10.1053/j.semss.2015.08.003

Simon, J., Conliffe, T., & Kitei, P. Non-operative management: An evidence-based approach. *Seminars in Spine Surgery, 28*(1), 8–13. doi:10.1053/j.semss.2015.08.004

Weinstein, J. N., Lurie, J. D., Tosteson, T. D., Tosteson, A. N., Blood, E. A., Abdu, W. A., . . . Fischgrund, J. (2008). Surgical versus nonoperative treatment for lumbar disc herniation: Four-year results for the Spine Patient Outcomes Research Trial (SPORT). *Spine, 33*(25), 2789–2800. doi:10.1097/BRS.0b013e31818ed8f4

■ SYNDROME OF INAPPROPRIATE ANTIDIURETIC HORMONE SECRETION

Carrie Foster

Overview

Syndrome of inappropriate antidiuretic hormone secretion (SIADH) was first discussed in 1957 in relation to patients with bronchogenic lung carcinoma (Schwartz, Bennett, Curelop, & Bartter, 1957). The classic description still holds true today. Characteristics of SIADH include hypotonic hyponatremia and inappropriate release of antidiuretic hormone (ADH) causing excessive renal water reabsorption, resulting in inadequately diluted urine (Grant et al., 2015). The causes of SIADH are multiple and varied, but generally fit into three categories: malignant disease; pulmonary, central nervous system (CNS) and genetic disorders; or medication induced (Spasovski et al., 2014).

Background

SIADH is a biochemical syndrome of euvolemic hyponatremia resulting from inappropriate secretion of ADH independent of plasma osmolality (Cuesta & Thompson, 2016). SIADH has been reported in association with many disease processes and as a complication from medications. Increased incidence is noted with conditions such as intracranial processes, lung carcinoma, and other pulmonary illness (Spasovski et al., 2014). An estimated 15% of patients with small cell lung cancer experience SIADH (Cuesta & Thompson, 2016). Generally, it is likely that about 5% to 10% of hospital admissions may have a component of SIADH, with highest rates in neurosurgical units (Cuesta & Thompson, 2016). SIADH is the most common cause of hyponatremia in specific patient populations, including nursing home residents and oncology patients (Shepshelovich et al., 2015). Recent data indicate the most frequent causes of SIADH include malignancy and as a result of administered medication (Shepshelovich et al., 2015). Morbidity and mortality are typically driven by the causative factor, with worse outcomes in malignancy-induced versus idiopathic or medication-induced SIADH, as the pathophysiology between the two processes is different.

The pathophysiology behind SIADH can vary by cause. In general, the sodium concentration in the plasma is the primary osmotic determinant of arginine vasopressin (AVP) secretion. AVP is the naturally occurring form of ADH found in humans, and is stored in the posterior pituitary gland. Baroreceptors and osmoreceptors detect changes in circulating volume depletion and hyperosmolality, and, as plasma osmolality rises, AVP secretion is stimulated. AVP is released from the posterior pituitary and binds to cell membranes of target tissues, causing an increase in water reabsorption and an increase in urine osmolality. Typically, AVP secretion stops when the plasma osmolality drops below 275 mOsm/kg. This decrease in AVP causes increased water excretion, creating dilute urine. Malignancy-associated SIADH is usually the result of an ectopic secretion of AVP (Cuesta & Thompson, 2016). Tumors may cause SIADH by creating physical interference with the osmoregulatory pathways. The mechanism of action behind medication-induced SIADH is incredibly variable, but is commonly seen with cytotoxic agents (Cuesta & Thompson, 2016).

The most serious complications from SIADH primarily arise from too rapid correction of hyponatremia or rapid initial development. When osmolality changes faster than 10 mOsm/kg per hour, patients are at increased risk for cerebral herniation, central pontine myelinolysis, and severe neurological impairment (Grant et al., 2015). Risk factors for increased morbidity and mortality rates include being hospitalized, rapid onset of hyponatremia, and severity of hyponatremia (Mocan, Terhes, & Blaga, 2016). Hyponatremia can result in gait instability and neurological impairment, placing elderly patients at higher risk for falls (Mocan et al., 2016). Multifactorial SIADH is associated with increased mortality, with the etiology as the key prognostic indicator.

Clinical Aspects

ASSESSMENT

The primary presentation of a patient experiencing SIADH is usually related to hyponatremia, with two factors influencing presentation: degree of hyponatremia and rate of development (Mocan et al., 2016). Serum sodium less than 135 mmol/L is considered hyponatremia (Spasovski et al., 2014). Patients will have plasma serum osmolality less than 275 mOsm/kg as well as urine sodium concentration greater than 30 mmol/L with normal dietary salt and water intake (Grant et al., 2015). Depending on the rate of development and biochemical degree of hyponatremia, patients may be asymptomatic. Patients may have symptoms that correlate to increased ADH secretion, including increased thirst, chronic pain, symptoms associated with CNS or pulmonary tumors, head injury, or drug use. Rapid-onset hyponatremia can manifest with confusion, disorientation or change in mental status, muscle weakness, and decreased reaction times. Because the patient is often euvolemic, signs of fluid overload are typically absent (Mocan et al., 2016).

TREATMENT

SIADH is a diagnosis of exclusion, and can be made if a patient meets the established six essential criteria originally proposed by Schwartz, Bennett, Curelop, and Bartter in 1957 (Spasovski et al., 2014). The diagnostic criteria are effective serum osmolality less than 275 mOsm/kg; urine osmolality greater than 100 mOsm/kg at some level of decreased effective osmolality; clinical euvolemia; urine sodium concentration greater than 30 mmol/L with normal dietary salt and water intake; absence of adrenal, thyroid, pituitary, or renal insufficiency; and no recent use of diuretics. After a diagnosis has been made, the mainstay of treatment for SIADH is fluid restriction, the degree of which is driven by the patient's ability to excrete electrolyte-free urine (Grant et al., 2015). Fluid restriction allows for a more gradual correction of hyponatremia. Rapid correction of sodium imbalances can have catastrophic outcomes, including central pontine myelinolysis and permanent neurological deficits (Spasovski et al., 2014). Second-line treatments include increasing solute intake with 0.25 to 0.50 g/kg per day of urea or using a combination of low-dose loop diuretics and oral sodium chloride to correct electrolyte imbalance (Spasovski et al., 2014). If possible, it is important to treat and diagnose the underlying cause of SIADH, as this may correct symptoms.

NURSING INTERVENTIONS, MANAGEMENT, AND IMPLICATIONS

Patients with SIADH are typically euvolemic and normotensive, but clinical changes can be seen in severe or rapid-onset scenarios (Mocan et al., 2016). Nevertheless, nursing staff must be vigilant in monitoring fluid balance for patients with SIADH. Careful attention should be paid to fluid intake and urine output. Nurses should monitor skin turgor, condition of mucous membranes, and changes in weight, noting that rapid changes of 0.5 to 1 kg/day can be related to fluid status. Mental status assessments are critical in hyponatremic patients. Nurses must monitor level of consciousness, orientation, and presence of muscle weakness and alert providers to changes. Serious consequences of hyponatremia include seizure and coma, although this is unlikely in a patient with SIADH (Grant et al., 2015). Patients are at risk for neurological changes as sodium levels are being corrected and careful monitoring is critical during this period.

OUTCOMES

Best practice recommends correcting hyponatremia gradually, with the best patient outcomes occurring when correction occurs over 24 to 48 hours (Grant et al., 2015). Hyponatremia is the most clinically significant problem with SIADH and is associated with multiple diseases. Hyponatremia may be a poor prognostic marker, but is not a disease state in itself. The prognosis for SIADH greatly correlates to the underlying cause. A complete recovery is commonly seen with drug or anesthesia-induced SIADH once the causative agent is removed. Effective treatment of a CNS or pulmonary infection also often results in correction of SIADH (Cuesta & Thompson 2016).

Summary

SIADH is a complex phenomenon with multiple etiologies. ADH is secreted independently of osmolality, placing the patient in a hyponatremic, hypoosmolar state. The excessive ADH secretion leads to renal water reabsorption and subsequent diuresis. The severity of symptoms is correlated to the degree of hyponatremia; patients most at risk are those with rapid onset of symptoms, or severe levels of hyponatremia. The current best practice for treatment is fluid restriction with gradual correction of sodium levels.

Nursing interventions revolve around careful monitoring of intake and output for patients with SIADH. Frequent and careful neurological assessment may be indicated for patients with severe hyponatremia, or during the process for corrections. Elderly patients are at an increased risk for falls due to gait instability and changes in mental status associated with hyponatremia, and should be assisted with ambulation. It is imperative that nursing staff notify providers to any acute changes in level of consciousness or orientation, as rapid correction of hyponatremia can have profoundly adverse side effects on neurological status. As the frontline caregivers, nursing staff should feel empowered to notice changes in their patient's assessment, intake and output, as well as abnormal lab values when caring for patients at risk or currently experiencing SIADH.

Cuesta, M., & Thompson, C. J. (2016). The syndrome of inappropriate antidiuresis (SIAD). *Best Practice & Research Clinical Endocrinology & Metabolism, 30*(2), 175–187.

Grant, P., Ayuk, J., Bouloux, P. M., Cohen, M., Cranston, I., Murray, R. D., . . . Grossman, A. (2015). The diagnosis and management of inpatient hyponatraemia and SIADH. *European Journal of Clinical Investigation, 45*(8), 888–894.

Mocan, M., Terhes, L. M., & Blaga, S. N. (2016). Difficulties in the diagnosis and management of hyponatremia. *Clujul Medical, 89*(4), 464–469.

Schwartz, W. B., Bennett, W., Curelop, S., & Bartter, F. C. (1957). A syndrome of renal sodium loss and hyponatremia probably resulting from inappropriate secretion of antidiuretic hormone. *American Journal of Medicine, 23*(4), 529–542.

Shepshelovich, D., Leibovitch, C., Klein, A., Zoldan, S., Milo, G., Shochat, T., . . . Lahav, M. (2015). The syndrome of inappropriate antidiuretic hormone secretion: Distribution and characterization according to etiologies. *European Journal of Internal Medicine, 26*(10), 819–824.

Spasovski, G., Vanholder, R., Allolio, B., Annane, D., Ball, S., Bichet, D., . . . Nagler, E.; Hyponatraemia Guideline Development Group. (2014). Clinical practice guideline on diagnosis and treatment of hyponatraemia. *Nephrology, Dialysis, Transplantation, 29*(Suppl. 2), i1–i39.

■ SYSTEMIC LUPUS ERYTHEMATOSUS

Merlyn A. Dorsainvil

Overview

The word *lupus* originates from the Latin word for wolf. Wolf, a legendary predator, is a fitting name for a disease that is referred to as *the cruel mystery* (Lupus Foundation of America, 2017). Lupus is a mystery because it has remained elusive for much of its long history. To date, its cause remains unknown and there is no known cure for it. Lupus is cruel for the various degrees of debilitation that it causes. Systemic lupus erythematosus (SLE) is an autoimmune disease that causes widespread inflammation throughout various body tissues, including the kidneys, heart, lungs, brain, and blood vessels. There are different types of lupus: (a) cutaneous lupus, (b) drug-induced lupus, and (c) neonatal lupus. However, SLE is the most common and serious type. SLE is a chronic disease marked by periods of flares and remissions. Symptoms can range from mild to life-threatening, but with effective management the prognosis can be good. It is estimated that 1.5 million Americans have SLE, with more than 16,000 new cases detected annually. Women of color and of childbearing age are two to three times more likely to develop SLE than Caucasians (Lupus Foundation of America, 2017).

Background

SLE is a chronic, autoimmune disease that causes widespread inflammation throughout the body. Individuals with SLE often present with generalized symptoms such as fatigue, fever, and weight loss. Diagnosis is made by a clinical assessment, ideally by an experienced rheumatologist. The American College of Rheumatology (ACR) has developed criteria for diagnosing SLE. Individuals are diagnosed with SLE if they report at least four of these symptoms, with no other cause:

- ■ Rashes:
  - ● Butterfly-shaped rash over the cheeks—referred to as *malar rash*
  - ● Red rash with raised round or oval patches—known as *discoid rash*
  - ● Rash on skin exposed to the sun
- ■ Mouth sores: sores in the mouth or nose lasting from a few days to more than a month
- ■ Arthritis: tenderness and swelling lasting for a few weeks in two or more joints
- ■ Lung or heart inflammation: swelling of the tissue lining the lungs (referred to as *pleurisy* or *pleuritis*) or the heart (pericarditis), which can cause chest pain when breathing deeply
- ■ Kidney problem: blood or protein in the urine, or tests that suggest poor kidney function
- ■ Neurologic problem: seizures, strokes, or psychosis
- ■ Abnormal blood tests such as:
  - ● Low blood cell counts: anemia, low white blood cells, or low platelets
  - ● Positive antinuclear antibodies (ANA) test result
  - ● Certain antibodies that show an immune system problem (ACR, 2015).

Based on the ACR criteria for SLE, the estimated prevalence of SLE in the United States is 72.8 to 74.4 per 100,000 and the incidence is 5.5 to 5.6 per 100,000 of population. Prevalence of SLE is more than 2 times higher among African Americans than among Caucasians and the incidence is three times higher. The burden of the disease is on women, with nine to 10 times higher prevalence among women than men (Lim et al., 2014; Somers et al., 2014). The average age of diagnosis is 39 to 41 years (Lim et al., 2014; Somers et al., 2014).

The cause of SLE is unknown but, based on the disproportionate burden on women and people of color, it is believed to be linked to genetic and hormonal factors. Exogenous and endogenous environmental exposures, such as infections, ultraviolet light, and stress, are linked to SLE (Sakkas & Bogdanos, 2016). The most common clinical manifestations of SLE among new cases include (a) arthritis, (b) hematologic disorders, (c) and serologic disorders. African Americans have a higher proportion of renal disease and end-stage renal disease compared to Caucasians (Somers et al., 2014).

There is no cure for SLE and treatment is based on the severity of symptoms. Nonsteroidal anti-inflammatory drugs (NSAIDs) are commonly used to treat inflammation and pain. Antimalarial drugs are used to treat symptoms such as fatigue and rashes. The biologic belimumab was approved in 2011 by the U.S. Food and Drug Administration for the treatment of active, nonsevere SLE. And for severe symptoms of SLE, corticosteroids and immunosuppressants are prescribed (ACR, 2015).

SLE has among the highest 30-day hospital readmission rates among chronic conditions. Following hospitalization for SLE, about one in six patients return within 30 days. Patients who are more likely to be initially hospitalized and readmitted within 30 days with SLE are those who (a) are young, (b) are African American or Hispanic, and (c) have Medicare or Medicaid as the primary payer. Renal disease, thrombocytopenia, serositis, and seizures are the SLE manifestations that are associated with readmissions (Yazdany et al., 2014). Pregnant women with SLE are at increased risk for stillbirths and early-onset preeclampsia (Simard et al., 2017; Vinet et al., 2016). Hospital admissions can pose financial burdens to patients and result in high health care costs. The average cost of a hospitalized patient with SLE is $51,808.41 per year (Anandarajah, Luc, & Ritchlin, 2016). Further financial burden comes from loss of productivity and loss of work days. SLE also significantly impacts quality of life. Most of the symptoms of SLE are not visible to others; common symptoms, such as fatigue and joint pain, are experienced by the individual but are not apparent to others. Subsequently this limits the amount of social support, validation, and medical care that individuals suffering with SLE receive (Brennan & Creaven, 2016).

Clinical Aspects

ASSESSMENT

The invisibility of SLE (Brennan & Creaven, 2016) can lead to feelings of powerlessness among those suffering with the condition. A thorough nursing assessment can be the first step in putting a face to this invisible condition. The nursing assessment should begin qualitatively with a history, examining onset of symptoms as well as exacerbating and relieving factors. Psychosocial aspects should be examined also: How has the disease impacted the client's life? What types of support does the client currently have? The history should be followed with a comprehensive physical examination, with focused assessments to the following systems: dermatologic, cardiovascular, renal, musculoskeletal, neurological, and pain. Nurses should anticipate laboratory tests, including an ANA test, complete blood count, erythrocyte sedimentation rate, C-reactive protein, and urinalysis. Although no two people with SLE will present with identical symptoms, some symptoms are commonly seen. Rashes are a classical symptom and, at some stage in the disease process, individuals with SLE will present with a rash. Fatigue is often a common and initial complaint. Many clients will also have joint pain.

The goals of nursing care for the client with SLE are to control flare-ups, prevent damage to organs, and promote overall health. Nursing-related problems clients can experience include (a) fatigue related to SLE disease process, (b) disturbed body image related to rashes, and (c) social isolation due to overall lack of public awareness of SLE. Clients should be encouraged to see a rheumatologist for the medical management of SLE. In addition, clients should also have routine primary health care for overall health promotion. For women of childbearing age, primary care from a women's health provider is ideal. Clients with SLE should be encouraged to maintain healthy, balanced diets and exercise. Frequent rest periods and energy conservation techniques should be discussed with clients. Nurses can assist clients in identifying essential versus nonessential activities so that their energy can be put to the most productive use. Clients with rashes should avoid direct sunlight and use sunscreen whenever outdoors. Nurses can use advocacy skills to educate and raise awareness of SLE to family, friends, and the public.

OUTCOMES

The outcome of nursing care for the client with SLE should be the client's confidence in managing the disease and improved quality of life. This outcome is achieved when nurses utilize the Quality and Safety Education for Nurses (QSEN) competency of patient-centered care. Nurses assist clients in the process of self-discovery of how SLE impacts their body and lives and ways to mitigate any potential or actual damages.

Summary

SLE has been deemed a "cruel mystery" because little is known about this debilitating, chronic disease. There is no known cause, no known cure, and minimal epidemiological data. Therefore, it remains a mystery to the health care community and the public; those with SLE often suffer in silence. However, the Centers for Disease Control and Prevention has recently funded research throughout the United States to obtain more accurate estimates of the disease. With better estimates of SLE prevalence and incidence, more resources can be allocated for research. Organizations, such as the Lupus Foundation of America, promote advocacy, research, and support for the disease so that SLE will no longer be a mystery. Until a cause and cure are found, clients with SLE can live long, productive lives with effective medical management and self-management. Nurses can support clients with SLE in their self-management and help to increase public awareness of this chronic condition.

American College of Rheumatology. (2015). Lupus. Retrieved from http://www .rheumatology.org/i-am-a/patient-caregiver/diseases-conditions/lupus

Anandarajah, A., Luc, M., & Ritchlin, C. (2016). Hospitalization of patients with systemic lupus erythematosus is a major cause of direct and indirect healthcare costs. *Lupus, 26*(7), 1–6. doi:10.1177/0961203316676641

Brennan, K. A., & Creaven, A. M. (2016). Living with invisible illness: Social support experiences of individuals with systemic lupus erythematosus. *Quality of Life Research, 25*(5), 1227–1235.

Lim, S. S., Bayakly, A. R., Helmick, C. G., Gordon, C., Easley, K. A., & Drenkard, C. (2014). The incidence and prevalence of systemic lupus erythematosus, 2002–2004: The Georgia Lupus Registry. *Arthritis & Rheumatology, 66*(2), 357–368.

Lupus Foundation of America. (2017). What is lupus? Retrieved from http://www.lupus .org/answers/entry/what-is-lupus

Sakkas, L. I., & Bogdanos, D. P. (2016). Infections as a cause of autoimmune rheumatic diseases. *Auto-Immunity Highlights, 7*(1), 13.

Simard, J. F., Arkema, E. V., Nguyen, C., Svenungsson, E., Wikström, A. K., Palmsten, K., & Salmon, J. E. (2017). Early-onset preeclampsia in lupus pregnancy. *Paediatric and Perinatal Epidemiology, 31*(1), 29–36.

Somers, E. C., Marder, W., Cagnoli, P., Lewis, E. E., DeGuire, P., Gordon, C., . . . McCune, W. J. (2014). Population-based incidence and prevalence of systemic lupus erythematosus: The Michigan Lupus Epidemiology and Surveillance program. *Arthritis & Rheumatology, 66*(2), 369–378.

Vinet, É., Genest, G., Scott, S., Pineau, C. A., Clarke, A. E., Platt, R. W., & Bernatsky, S. (2016). Brief report: Causes of stillbirths in women with systemic lupus erythematosus. *Arthritis & Rheumatology, 68*(10), 2487–2491.

Yazdany, J., Marafino, B., Dean, M., Bardach, N., Duseja, R., Ward, M., & Dudley, R. (2014). Thirty-day hospital readmissions in systemic lupus erythematosus: Predictors and hospital and state-level variation. *Arthritis& Rheumatology, 66*(10), 2828–2836. doi:10.1002/art.38768

■ THROMBOCYTOPENIA

Maria A. Mendoza

Overview

Thrombocytopenia is a blood disorder characterized by low platelet (thrombocyte) count caused by deficient marrow production, increased destruction, and splenic sequestration. Normal platelet count is between 150,000 and 400,000/μL and thrombocytopenia in adults is defined as a platelet count below 150,000/μL (Krisnegowda & Rajashekaraiah, 2015).

Thrombocytopenia may be associated with many diseases and syndromes and in some cases is drug induced, making it the most common blood disorder (Izak & Bussel, 2014). It is common among hospitalized and critically ill adults. It is believed to be present in as much as 67.6% of adult patients on admission to the intensive care unit (ICU) and acquired by up to 44% of patients while in the ICU (Hui, Cook, Lim, Fraser, & Arnold, 2011). It may sometimes be the first sign of hematologic cancers. In many situations, the patient suffering from thrombocytopenia is clinically asymptomatic. Low platelet count is often found during a routine complete blood count (CBC) test. Patients with count less than 30,000/μL have potential for bleeding but it is generally a count below 10,000/μL that clinically presents with spontaneous bleeding from skin, wounds, or body cavities (Izak & Bussel, 2014).

Background

Platelets are tiny (1–3 μm) anucleated cells produced in the large bone marrow cells called *megakaryocytes*. The fragmentation of megakaryocytes in the presence of a hormone called *thrombopoietin* results in the release of platelets (1,000 platelets per megakaryocyte). The main functions of platelets are hemostasis and wound healing. Their sticky consistency plus ability to change shape make them efficient in sealing off the bleeding site.

Identifying the etiology of thrombocytopenia is part of the diagnostic process. The major laboratory tests are CBC, blood smear (to analyze blood cell morphology), and coagulation tests (prothrombin time and activated partial thromboplastin time). Other tests ordered to help with the differential diagnosis include direct Coombs, fibrinogen, D-Dimer, lactate dehydrogenase (LDH), alkaline phosphatase, liver and renal function tests, vitamin B_{12}, folic acid level, and serological tests. In some cases, a bone marrow biopsy may be performed.

Treatment of thrombocytopenia is directed at eliminating the etiology. However, in the majority of cases, the etiology is not very clear. First-line pharmacotherapy includes corticosteroids, intravenous immunoglobulin G (IV IgG), and intravenous anti-D (Krisnegowda & Rajashekaraiah, 2015). When first-line drugs have failed, immunosuppressants, such as azathioprine, cyclophosphamide, and cyclosporine, may be tried (Krisnegowda & Rajashekaraiah, 2015).

The American Association of Blood Banks (AABB) recommends platelet transfusion in hospitalized adult patients with a platelet count of 10,000/μL or less to reduce spontaneous bleeding (Kaufman et al., 2015). Packed cell transfusion is administered to replace blood loss. In case of increased destruction of platelets by the spleen, a splenectomy (laparoscopic, if possible) may be done.

Clinical Aspects

ASSESSMENT

A comprehensive history helps to identify the etiology of the disease. The nurse is part of the health care team who may collect this information, which includes presence of family history of thrombocytopenia, recent infection (viral and bacterial), vaccinations, history of cancer, treatment with chemotherapy, pregnancy, recent travels (for possible exposure to malaria, dengue fever, rickettsiosis), recent transfusions, alcohol intake, dietary habits, risk factors for or history of HIV, and hepatitis C. A review of all medications with focus on medications started in the past 2 weeks should also be done. Verify symptoms such as muscle/joint pain, dizziness, persistent headache, blurred or double vision, and abdominal pain.

Physical assessment should include thorough examination of the skin to identify signs of bleeding such as ecchymosis (bruising), petechiae, purpura, and frank hemorrhage. Bleeding from body cavities is also checked, including the oral cavity (gums), eyes, nose (epistaxis), lungs (hemoptysis), gastrointestinal tract (hematemesis, melena, and occult bleeding), urinary tract (hematuria), and vaginal tract (vaginal bleeding or increased menstrual flow). A neurological assessment should be done, especially in patients at risk for and/or with suspicion of cerebral bleeding. Careful palpation for lymphadenopathy (enlarged lymph nodes) and for organomegaly of the liver and spleen should be performed. Skeletal malformations of the thumbs and forearm, and short stature present in certain forms of thrombocytopenia should be noted (Izak & Bussel, 2014).

NURSING INTERVENTIONS, MANAGEMENT, AND IMPLICATIONS

Patient education is needed to prevent bleeding and injury. The nurse reviews with the patient/family the disease condition, etiology (if known), complications, treatment, and how to prevent and manage bleeding. A review of all medications (prescribed and over-the-counter) should be done (Winkeljohn, 2013). General instructions should include medications to avoid such as aspirin and drugs containing aspirin. The patient is informed to check with health care provider before using over-the-counter medication. Promote activities to prevent bleeding such as using soft-bristle toothbrush, electric shaver when shaving, and emery board to trim nails. Patient should avoid using household tools, such as scissors, knives, and sharp objects, to prevent injuries. Counsel the patient not to drink alcohol. Patient has to check with his or her health care provider before undergoing dental work or other procedures that can cause bleeding. Patient should avoid heavy lifting, contact sports, and strenuous activities that can lead to a fall or injury.

The patient/family should know what to report to the health care provider, such as observation of any kind of bleeding, as listed earlier. Teach the patient/family how to control bleeding such as applying pressure over a cut with a clean cloth or gauze until bleeding is controlled. Hemostatic agents, such as Gelfoam, may be used to cause vasoconstriction (Winkeljohn, 2013). The health care provider and emergency medical service phone numbers should be handy in case of emergency.

Teaching directed toward medication(s) prescribed to treat thrombocytopenia should be provided to patient/family. The nurse should teach proper administration and side/adverse effects of medications such as corticosteroids and other immunosuppressants.

For severe states of thrombocytopenia, a platelet transfusion may be included in the patient's plan of care. The nurse assists in the administration of a platelet transfusion and performs the following nursing interventions to ensure the patient's safety:

1. Obtain an informed consent after explaining the procedure, purpose, possible complications, and necessary monitoring during and after the procedure. Use the laboratory results to explain the need for transfusion and target levels posttransfusion (Winkeljohn, 2013). Proper identification of the patient before transfusion is imperative. The platelet bags and tubing should be checked for integrity. The procedure should be done under strict aseptic technique.
2. Establish baseline vital signs and lab values before transfusion. Allergic and hemolytic reactions, such as fever, isolated pruritus and urticaria, bronchoconstriction, hypotension, and shock, may occur. Febrile nonhemolytic transfusion reaction (FNHTR) with or without chills may occur within the first 4 hours of transfusion followed by normalization of the temperature within 48 hours. FNHTR is confirmed once bacterial infection and hemolytic causes are ruled out. Bacterial sepsis, caused by contaminated platelets, is manifested by high fever, chills, vomiting, tachycardia, hypotension, and shock.
3. Monitor patient's vital signs during and after transfusion. Check platelet count 15 minutes to 1-hour posttransfusion. As indicated, CBC, coagulation, and renal function tests are done. Continue to monitor for bleeding.
4. Maintain good oral hygiene using soft swabs, normal saline rinse, and mouthwash as appropriate to prevent dry mucous membranes and minimize bleeding.

OUTCOMES

The major role of the nurse in managing thrombocytopenia is to work and collaborate with the health care team to collect data and provide safe patient care. Nursing assessment includes a thorough history to identify etiology and a physical examination to check for bleeding. Patient education is very important to promote safety and prevent injuries that may lead to bleeding.

Summary

Thrombocytopenia is a common blood disorder defined as platelet count less than 150,000/μL. Etiology can be due to deficient marrow production, increased destruction, and splenic sequestration. Diagnosis is primarily established by laboratory studies. In few cases, bone marrow biopsy may be done to identify deficient marrow production. Treatment is focused on removing the causative factor. First-line drug therapy includes corticosteroids, IV IgG, and intravenous anti-D. Platelet transfusion may be necessary when platelet count falls below 10,000/μL and there is high risk of spontaneous bleeding.

Hui, P., Cook, D. J., Lim, W., Fraser, G. A., & Arnold, D. M. (2011). The frequency and clinical significance of thrombocytopenia complicating critical illness: A systematic review. *Chest, 139*(2), 271–278.

Izak, M., & Bussel, J. B. (2014). Management of thrombocytopenia. *F1000Prime Reports, 6*, 45.

Kaufman, R. M., Djulbegovic, B., Gernsheimer, T., Kleinman, S., Tinmouth, A. T., Capocelli, K. E., . . . Tobian, A. A. (2015). Platelet transfusion: A clinical practice guideline from the AABB. *Annals of Internal Medicine, 162*(3), 205–213.

Krisnegowda, M., & Rajashekaraiah, V. (2015). Platelet disorders: An overview. *Blood Coagulation and Fibrinolysis, 26*(5), 479–491. doi:10.1097/01.mbc .0000469521.23628.2d

Winkeljohn, D. (2013). Diagnosis, treatment and management of immune thrombocytopenia. *Clinical Journal of Oncology Nursing, 17*(6), 664–666. doi:10.1188/ 13.CJON.664-666

■ TUBERCULOSIS

Christina M. Canfield

Overview

A disease of historical significance, tuberculosis (TB) has caused more deaths worldwide than any other infectious disease, including plague, smallpox, and malaria (Heemskerk, Caws, Marais, & Farrar, 2015). One third of the world's population is infected with TB and there is one new case of TB diagnosed every 4 seconds (Centers for Disease Control and Prevention [CDC], 2016). Nurses must be aware of the risk factors associated with transmission, symptoms, and treatment of a TB infection.

Background

The global incidence of TB varies widely. In 2015 an estimated 10.4 million new cases of TB were identified worldwide. Incidence of TB is higher in underdeveloped countries. The World Health Organization (Global Tuberculosis Report, 2016) reports that 60% of new cases were identified in just six countries: India, Indonesia, China, Nigeria, Pakistan, and South Africa. The CDC (2016) noted a rate of 3.0 cases per 100,000 persons in the United States in 2015. HIV-infected adults, persons born in foreign countries, and those of lower socioeconomic status make up the majority of active TB cases in the United States (Raviglione, 2015). TB is a treatable disease that may be cured; however, drug-resistant strains of *Mycobacterium tuberculosis* are becoming more prevalent. Untreated TB is often fatal and carries a 1-year mortality of 30%.

TB has been known by many names, including consumption, Pott's disease, shaky oncay, and the white plague (Heemskerk et al., 2015). It is a disease caused by the bacterium *M. tuberculosis*. Mycobacteria have a unique lipid-rich cell wall, which makes them resistant to many disinfectants and antibiotics. *M. tuberculosis* is an acid-fast bacilli (AFB) usually transmitted when an infectious person coughs, sneezes, or speaks. Droplets may remain suspended in the air for hours and then be inhaled into the airways. An infected individual may expel up to 3,000 infectious nuclei per cough. It is estimated that up to 20 contacts may be infected by each positive case. This is due to delays in pursuing care and in making a diagnosis (Raviglione, 2015).

TB transmission occurs in high population density locations such as hospitals, nursing facilities, prisons, and hostels (Heemskerk et al., 2015).

Clinical Aspects

Exposure to *M. tuberculosis* activates the immune system. In most cases, the body will contain the infection and form a granuloma around it. Cases in which the infection is controlled but not fully eliminated are referred to as *latent TB*.

Latent TB may become an active infection if the infected individual suffers from an impaired immune system. In 5% to 10% of exposed individuals, the bacteria cannot be contained and TB occurs soon after the initial exposure. The lungs are affected in two thirds of TB cases and the middle and lower lungs are most commonly involved. Pulmonary TB may be asymptomatic or the infected individual may present with fever and pleuritic chest pain. In young children or immuno-compromised individuals, TB may progress rapidly. All HIV-positive patients should be screened for TB (Heemskerk et al., 2015).

ASSESSMENT

Symptoms may mimic the flu and therefore patients may not immediately seek treatment. Diagnosis is commonly made based on finding evidence of AFB testing on a sputum sample.

Symptoms include:

■ Fever
■ Night sweats
■ Weight loss
■ Loss of appetite
■ Malaise
■ Weakness
■ Cough
■ Sputum (purulent or bloody)

NURSING INTERVENTIONS, MANAGEMENT, AND IMPLICATIONS

The nurse should suspect TB in the patient who presents with persistent cough and unexplained weight loss. A heightened suspicion should be given to patients who are infected with HIV, who are homeless, or who have emigrated from a county of high incidence of TB. Abnormal findings on a chest x-ray may lead to further testing. Follow the facility's procedure for use of personal protective equipment and establishing isolation. Anticipate placing the patient in a negative pressure airflow room.

The nurse should expect to collect or facilitate the collection of two to three samples gathered first thing in the morning on consecutive days (Raviglione, 2015).

There are four medications that are considered to be first-line agents for the treatment of active TB: isoniazid, rifampin, pyrazinamide, and ethambutol.

Patients will receive a 2-month initial course of all four medications followed by up to 4 months of rifampin and isoniazid. Up to 90% of patients will be cured following 6 months of active treatment (Raviglione, 2015). The long course of therapy and multiple medications required present a challenge for medication adherence. The multidisciplinary team may engage the assistance of a TB control program to help with medication management. Administration of medications using directly observed therapy (DOT) improves adherence to the medication regimen and is strongly recommended for individuals who require treatment for TB in the community setting. Medications provided during DOT are given directly to the patient by a health care provider or trained worker. The patient is monitored during administration to ensure that medications have been taken. Use of DOT is essential for patients with drug-resistant TB and those with HIV infection. The effectiveness of treatment is monitored by repeating sputum cultures.

Patients with known latent TB infections may also receive treatment with isoniazid. This treatment may last 9 months. Presence of HIV infection is the strongest risk factor associated with conversion of a latent TB infection to an active TB infection (Heemskerk et al., 2015).

There is only one vaccine available for prevention of TB. The bacillus Calmette-Guérin (BCG) vaccine has been administered around the world since 1921. The effectiveness of the vaccine varies from 0% to 80% and it has been found to be most effective in preventing meningitis associated with TB (Heemskerk et al., 2015).

The nurse should consider including the following problems and interventions when creating the patient-specific plan of care (Garvey, 2014): ineffective airway clearance, risk for impaired gas exchange, impaired nutrition, and knowledge deficit.

OUTCOMES

Expected nursing outcomes are focused on maintaining and improving oxygenation and nutrition while assuring adherence to prescribed therapies. The nurse should perform ongoing assessments of the patient's and significant other(s)' understanding of the medication regimen and actions necessary to prevent the spread of infection. Those who will be in close contact with the patient during the anticipated course of treatment must be able to verbalize an understanding of the signs and symptoms of TB and must know when to seek medical treatment.

Summary

The worldwide burden of TB remains significant. TB is a curable disease but commitment to completion of the long course of treatment requires significant personal effort, social support, and access to resources. Wide-scale elimination efforts hinge on the identification of an effective vaccine. The nurse must become familiar with the signs and symptoms of active TB infection to prevent the spread of disease and protect vulnerable individuals. Nursing care of the patient with active TB infection involves medication delivery, monitoring for adverse effects, and frequent education of the patient and his or her support systems.

Centers for Disease Control and Prevention. (2016). TB data and statistics. Retrieved from https://www.cdc.gov/tb/statistics/default.htm

Garvey, C. (2014). Respiratory disorders. In S. M. Nettina (Ed.), *Lippincott manual of nursing practice* (10th ed., 277–323). Philadelphia, PA: Lippincott Williams & Wilkins.

Global Tuberculosis Report. (2016). (1st ed., pp. 5–82). Retrieved from http://apps.who .int/iris/bitstream/10665/250441/1/9789241565394-eng.pdf?ua=1

Heemskerk, D., Caws, M., Marais, B., & Farrar, J. (2015). *Tuberculosis in adults and children* (1st ed., pp. 1–55). Springer International.

Raviglione, M. (2015). Tuberculosis. In D. Kasper, A. Fauci, S. Hauser, D. Longo, J. Jameson, & J. Loscalzo (Eds.), *Harrison's principles of internal medicine* (19th ed.). New York, NY: McGraw-Hill. Retrieved from http://accessmedicine.mhmedical .com/content.aspx?bookid=1130&Sectionid=79737003

■ VALVULAR HEART DISEASE

Rebecca Witten Grizzle

Overview

Valvular heart disease (VHD) encompasses health conditions affecting the four heart valves: aortic, pulmonic, mitral, and tricuspid. Common disorders include valvular stenosis and regurgitation; the aortic and mitral valves are most commonly affected. In the United States, the prevalence of VHD is 2.5% in the general population and 13% in persons over the age of 75 years (Iung & Vahanian, 2014). VHD results in significant morbidity and mortality and burden to the health care system (Moore, Chen, Mallow, & Rizzo, 2016). Therefore, patient management and quality of life are important concerns to nurses, especially those who care for special populations such as pediatric, athletic, obstetric, perioperative, and geriatric patients.

Background

The most common types of VHD among European populations are aortic stenosis (43%) and mitral regurgitation (32%), followed by aortic regurgitation (13%) and mitral stenosis (12%; Iung & Vahanian, 2014). In the United States, mitral valve disease is more prevalent than aortic valve disease and rates of both increase with age (Moore et al., 2016). The etiology of VHD is predominantly degenerative in nature, although rheumatic heart disease still accounts for many cases worldwide (Moore et al., 2016). The remaining causes are infective endocarditis, congenital heart disease, inflammatory processes, mediastinal radiation, or cardiotoxic drug exposure. Degeneration is the result of progressive calcification of the valve cusps in a process similar to atherosclerosis, although there are no known evidence-based strategies to slow its progression (Iung & Vahanian, 2014). The risk factors for progression of aortic valve calcification include age, hypertension, diabetes mellitus, hypercholesterolemia, hypercalcemia, and smoking (Carità et al., 2016). Rates of aortic valve calcification vary from person to person and may be influenced by genetic factors that result in higher plasma lipoprotein(a) levels (Rahimtoola, 2014).

Approximately one third of VHD patients are symptomatic, reporting significant chest pain, palpitations, shortness of breath, dizziness, and syncope (Moore et al., 2016). Medical management of symptomatic patients appears largely ineffective, and the only definitive treatment is repair or replacement of the affected valve. Thus, the risks and benefits of surgery must be considered given the patient's comorbidities, expected outcome, quality of life, and personal wishes. There were approximately 133,000 heart valve surgeries in 2013 in the United States partly due to the increasing incidence of transcatheter aortic valve implantation (TAVI) procedures (Miller & Flynn, 2015). The health care expenditure for all types of mitral and aortic valve diseases is estimated at

$23.4 billion annually. Successful surgery decreases the patient's symptom burden and is seen as cost-effective compared to medical management in the long term (Moore et al., 2016).

Individuals with VHD are at higher risk of thromboembolic events due to changes in blood flow from valve pathology. However, the population also has higher bleeding risks such as age, hypertension, medication usage, liver dysfunction, alcohol use, and renal disease. Careful consideration must be given to patient selection for anticoagulation management. For example, the annual risk of thromboembolism among patients with mitral stenosis is 1% to 6% (Iung & Vahanian, 2014). However, patients with mitral valve disease were considerably undertreated with oral anticoagulants when compared to patients with aortic valve disease, even though their risk for stroke is much higher (Başaran et al., 2017).

Other comorbidities, such as atrial fibrillation, carry an elevated risk for stroke, based on the risk stratification score. In patients with nonvalvular atrial fibrillation, at least one third have significant valvular disease. Patients with significant valvular disease are at greater risk of stroke and simultaneously have higher risks for bleeding (Başaran et al., 2017). These caveats make patient management challenging and complex.

Living with VHD significantly impacts an individual's quality of life due to physical, psychological, and social factors (dos Anjos, Rodrigues, Padilha, Pedrose, & Gallani, 2016). Patients with VHD worry about exacerbations and decompensating, thus affecting their health self-perception. Fatigue, dyspnea, palpitations, chest pain, syncope, and edema affect their daily lives. Patients are prescribed an average of four medications. Diuretic use can have a significant impact on the individual's physical, social, and emotional well-being due to the drug's effects on activities of daily living. A high percentage of these patients are unemployed or on disability, and many have lower educational and income levels (dos Anjos et al., 2016). In addition, symptomatic aortic valve disease patients are more likely to have higher rates of depression and anxiety (Moore et al., 2016).

Clinical Aspects

ASSESSMENT

Special populations with different VHD management concerns include infants and children, adolescent and young adult athletes, pregnant women, and older adults. Nurses must continue to maintain physical assessment skills across the life span, particularly in auscultating cardiovascular sounds and documenting findings pertaining to rhythm, pitch, tone, timing, and radiation to carotid arteries and thorax. Nurses must also be able to anticipate patients' cardiac complaints and pose appropriate assessment questions to elicit signs and symptoms. In short, patients with VHD must be properly assessed in order to be efficiently diagnosed, evaluated, and treated. Diagnostic tests, such as electrocardiogram, chest radiography, and echocardiography, are used to evaluate cardiac function to determine the extent of valve pathology. Cardiac stress testing is discouraged in symptomatic VHD patients.

Symptomatic or undiagnosed heart murmur in surgical patients may present a dilemma to the perioperative team. Given the high prevalence of untreated aortic stenosis among older adults, the perioperative team may consider obtaining an echocardiogram to evaluate cardiac function and valvular anatomy. A higher degree of suspicion is supported by the presence of signs and symptoms of heart failure, history of heart failure and worsening dyspnea, or dyspnea of unknown origin (Fleisher et al., 2014). Research findings suggest that patients with severe aortic stenosis can undergo noncardiac surgery if consideration is given to enhanced anesthetic management. Careful monitoring with an arterial line to monitor and prevent hypotension on induction and during anesthesia will help prevent intraoperative events, by maintaining the pressure gradient to overcome the stenotic aortic valve (Rahimtoola, 2014).

The American Heart Association and American College of Cardiology updated management guidelines for patients with VHD, including recommendations regarding dental prophylaxis, diagnostic imaging, surgical intervention, prosthetic valve selection, and anticoagulation (Nishimura et al., 2017). These recommendations highlight the need for a comprehensive team approach for care of patients with VHD. Although nurses may not be central in the medical decision making, they are essential in supporting, teaching, and advocating for these patients. Nurses' integral involvement on a dedicated heart team provides clinical leadership for promoting excellent outcomes among VHD patients (Lauck, McGladrey, Lawlor, & Webb, 2016).

Perioperative nursing interventions include monitoring for hemodynamic instability, such as hypotension, bleeding, tamponade, and arrhythmias. Patients are at risk for paravalvular leak, ventricular dysfunction, atrioventricular conduction abnormalities, atrial fibrillation, and pulmonary hypertension. All are conditions that can lead to decompensation. In general, patients undergoing aortic and mitral procedures have higher risk than those undergoing pulmonic and tricuspid procedures. Postoperative patients need frequent neurological assessments to evaluate for stroke or transient ischemic attacks (Miller & Flynn, 2015). Anticoagulation therapy is often indicated, requiring careful lifelong follow-up care.

OUTCOMES

Nurses play an important role in teaching and supporting patients in the management of VHD. Patient education for this population focuses on smoking cessation, health-promotion strategies, medication therapies, anticoagulation monitoring, thromboembolic risk reduction, and endocarditis prophylaxis. Nurses have a unique perspective in that they can promote lifestyle changes while addressing diverse social, cultural, emotional, and financial concerns (McLachlan, Sutton, Ding, & Kerr, 2015). By understanding the influence of socioeconomic factors on the clinical management of VHD patients, nurses can plan more effective interventions that are tailored to the individual patient's needs (dos Anjos et al., 2016).

Summary

VHD is a worldwide concern affecting newborns to older adults, although prevalence increases with age. Patients should be evaluated thoroughly if they exhibit signs and symptoms of VHD. Given the tremendous implications for morbidity and quality of life, a team approach is needed to determine the best plan of care. Often surgical valve repair or replacement is the only definitive treatment in symptomatic severe VHD. Patients will require lifelong monitoring and continuous support. Nurses play a key role in planning patient management strategies that are tailored to the individual's needs. Trends indicate more catheter-based procedures will increase the demand for highly trained nurses who can care for the growing population of VHD patients.

Başaran, Ö., Dogan, V., Beton, O., Tekinalp, M., Aykan, A. Ç., Kalaycioglu, E., . . . Biteker, M. (2017). Impact of valvular heart disease on oral anticoagulant therapy in non-valvular atrial fibrillation: Results from the RAMSES study. *Journal of Thrombosis and Thrombolysis, 43*(2), 157–165.

Carità, P., Coppola, G., Novo, G., Caccamo, G., Guglielmo, M., Balasus, F., . . . Corrado, E. (2016). Aortic stenosis: Insights on pathogenesis and clinical implications. *Journal of Geriatric Cardiology, 13*(6), 489–498.

dos Anjos, D. B., Rodrigues, R. C., Padilha, K. M., Pedrosa, R. B., & Gallani, M. C. (2016). Influence of sociodemographic and clinical characteristics at the impact of valvular heart disease. *Revista Brasileira De Enfermagem, 69*(1), 33–39.

Fleisher, L. A., Fleischmann, K. E., Auerbach, A. D., Barnason, S. A., Beckman, J. A., Bozkurt, B., . . . Wijeysundera, D. N. (2014). 2014 ACC/AHA guideline on perioperative cardiovascular evaluation and management of patients undergoing noncardiac surgery: Executive summary: A report of the American College of Cardiology/ American Heart Association Task Force on Practice Guidelines. *Circulation, 130*(24), 2215–2245.

Iung, B., & Vahanian, A. (2014). Epidemiology of acquired valvular heart disease. *Canadian Journal of Cardiology, 30*(9), 962–970.

Lauck, S. B., McGladrey, J., Lawlor, C., & Webb, J. G. (2016). Nursing leadership of the transcatheter aortic valve implantation Heart Team: Supporting innovation, excellence, and sustainability. *Healthcare Management Forum, 29*(3), 126–130.

McLachlan, A., Sutton, T., Ding, P., & Kerr, A. (2015). A nurse practitioner clinic: A novel approach to supporting patients following heart valve surgery. *Heart, Lung & Circulation, 24*(11), 1126–1133.

Miller, S., & Flynn, B. C. (2015). Valvular heart disease and postoperative considerations. *Seminars in Cardiothoracic and Vascular Anesthesia, 19*(2), 130–142.

Moore, M., Chen, J., Mallow, P. J., & Rizzo, J. A. (2016). The direct health-care burden of valvular heart disease: Evidence from US national survey data. *ClinicoEconomics and Outcomes Research, 8*, 613–627.

Nishimura, R. A., Otto, C. M., Bonow, R. O., Carabello, B. A., Erwin, J. P., Fleisher, L. A., . . . Thompson, A. (2017). 2017 AHA/ACC focused update of the 2014 AHA/ACC guideline for the management of patients with valvular heart disease: A report of the American College of Cardiology/American Heart Association Task Force on Clinical Practice Guidelines. *Journal of the American College of Cardiology, 70*(2), 252–289.

Rahimtoola, S. H. (2014). The year in valvular heart disease. *Journal of the American College of Cardiology, 63*(19), 1948–1958.

Index